Cardiac Surgery and Concomitant Disease

J. Ennker
Editor

Cardiac Surgery and Concomitant Disease

Incidence, Preoperative Preparation, and Prognostic Relevance

STEINKOPFF
DARMSTADT

Springer

J. Ennker M.D.
Heart Institute Lahr/Baden
P.O.B. 1340
D-77933 Lahr
Germany

ISBN 978-3-642-48845-0 ISBN 978-3-642-48843-6 (eBook)
DOI 10.1007/978-3-642-48843-6

Die Deutsche Bibliothek – CIP-Einheitsaufnahme

Cardiac surgery and concomitant disease : incidence, preoperative preparation and prognostic relevance / J. Ennker, ed. – Darmstadt : Steinkopff ; New York : Springer, 1999

Softcover reprint of the hardcover 1st edition 1999
Medical Editor: Beate Rühlemann, English Editor: Mary K. Gossen, Production: Heinz J. Schäfer
Cover Design: Erich Kirchner, Heidelberg

Typesetting and Printing: VEBU Druck GmbH, Bad Schussenried
Printed on acid-free paper

Preface

The contributions to this volume were originally presented on October 24th and 25th, 1997 at the symposium on "Cardiac surgery and concomitant disease-Incidence, preoperative preparation, perioperative importance and prognostic relevance" in Baden-Baden, Germany.

In 1960 the development of coronary artery cinearteriography by Sones and Shirey at the Cleveland Clinic realized the direct identification of stenotic and obstructive artheriosclerotic lesions in coronary arteries during life possible and laid the basis for coronary artery surgery. From time to time attempts had been performed to restore impaired coronary artery perfusion by various surgeons, however these efforts suffered due to the deficit of precise anatomic diagnostics. Thirteen years after Vineberg had reported the direct implantation of an internal mammary artery into the myocardium in Montreal, Kolesov in St. Petersburg employed the internal thoracic artery for anastomosis to the left anterior descending artery for the first time. In May 1967 Favaloro and Effler at the Cleveland Clinic initiated the technique of using reversed saphenous vein bypass grafting to a stenosed right coronary artery. Their description of the benefits of the saphenous vein for bypass grafting demonstrated it's later wide spread applicability. Quickly afterwards Johnson in Milwaukee extended the procedure to the left coronary artery which was a major step ahead at that time. In 1968 Green in New York reported the anastomosis of the internal mammary artery to the left internal descending artery using the dissecting microscope. The first bilateral internal mammary artery bypass was performed in 1969 by Kay in Cleveland. In 1971 the technique and the advantages of sequential grafting with only one vein used for several distal anastomoses was described by Flemma. These first steps evolved towards a tremendous success story which led to the nowadays recognised principles of coronary artery revascularisation. This became the surgical operation performed with the highest frequency today.

Coronary artery disease in industrialized countries is still the number one cause of death. In Germany the number of coronary artery bypass operations increased from 4268 operations in 1980 to 69 888 operations in 1997. Early mortality decreased from 4.0% in 1980 to 3.3% in 1996. The average age of patients scheduled for cardiac surgery rose 10 years within the last decade, thus substantially increasing the incidence of cardiac operations which previously would not have been performed on as the risks of operation were estimated as being too high.

The proceedings of the symposium concentrated on the problems of concomitant diseases demonstrated by patients refered for cardiac surgery especially coronary artery surgery. Prominent authorities and experts from the field of internal medicine, cardiac surgery, and related subjects shared with us their experience in handling severely ill and "difficult" patients.

In particular the problems of patients with endocrine disorders, liver disease, pulmonary dysfunction, obesity, connective tissues disease, and hematologic diseases were analyzed in addition to skeletal and renal disorders, the problems of cardiac surgery and pregnancy, hyperlipidemia or dental problems. Another point of interest commented in the book is the following: As the use of the extracorporeal circulation (ECC) aggravates many of the above mentioned problems in our patients, cardiac operations without ECC, thus, reducing neurological and other ECC related problems are increasingly frequent in many surgical centers.

We would like to thank the authors for their support and contributions. We are also indebted to Ms. Ibkendanz and Ms. Rühlemann and others from the Steinkopff Verlag for assembling and publishing this book. Our special gratitude belongs to our coworker Stefan Bauer for his support in organizing the symposium and his share in the collection and revision of the presented articles.

We hope that this book will serve as a useful synopsis of current knowledge of How to handle patients with concomitant diseases and complex clinical disorders.

Lahr, November 1998 J. Ennker

Contents

List of Contributors

Alexander Albert, M. D.
Heart Institute Lahr/Baden
Department of Thoracic
and Cardiovascular Surgery
77933 Lahr, Germany

Matthias Angrés, M. D.
Department of Anesthesiology
and Intensive Care
Cottbus Heart Center
Thiemstr. 111
03048 Cottbus, Germany

Knut Ansorge, M. D.
Department of Thoracic
and Cardiovascular Surgery
Klinikum Karlsburg
Greifswalder Straße 11A
17495 Karlsburg, Germany

Prof. M. Barthels, M. D.
Division of Hematology and Oncology
Hannover Medical School
Carl-Neuberg-Straße 1
30625 Hannover, Germany

Sven Beholz, M. D.
Department of Cardiovascular Surgery
Klinikum Karlsburg
Greifswalder Str. 11A
17495 Karlsburg, Germany

Andreas Böning, M. D.
Department of Thoracic
and Cardiovascular Surgery
Hannover Medical School
30623 Hannover, Germany

Mathias M. Borst, M. D.
Department of Internal Medicine III
University Hospital
Ruprecht-Karls-University Heidelberg,
Bergheimer Str. 58
69115 Heidelberg, Germany

Antonio Maria Calafiore, M. D.
Department of Cardiac Surgery
"G. D'Annunzio" University
Camillo de' Lellis Hospital
Via C. Forlanini 50
66100 Chieti, Italy

Joseph S. Coselli, M. D.
6560 Fannin, #1100
Houston, TX 77030, USA

Jochen Cremer, M. D.
Department of Thoracic
and Cardiovascular Surgery
Hannover Medical School
30623 Hannover, Germany

Ingo Dähnert, M. D.
German Heart Institute Berlin
Department of Paediatric Cardiology
Augustenburger Platz 1
13353 Berlin, Germany

Gabriele Di Giammarco, M. D.
Clinica Cardiochirurgica
Ospedale San Camillo de' Lellis
Via Forlanini, 50
66100 Chieti, Italy

Prof. Curt Diehm, M. D.
Department of Internal Medicine/
Vascular Medicine
Karlsbad Clinic
Academic Hospital University
of Heidelberg
76307 Karlsbad, Germany

Ina Carolin Ennker, M. D.
Heart Institute Lahr/Baden
Department of Thoracic
and Cardiovascular Surgery
77933 Lahr, Germany

J. Ennker, M. D.
Heart Institute Lahr/Baden
Department of Thoracic
and Cardiovascular Surgery
77933 Lahr, Germany

Charlotte Fischer, M. D.
Department of Thoracic
and Cardiovascular Surgery
University Hospital
Josef-Schneider-Str. 6
97080 Würzburg, Germany

M. K. H. Fritz, M. D.
Department of Cardiac
and Thoracic Surgery
Berufsgenossenschaftliche Kliniken
Bergmannsheil
Bürkle-De-La-Camp-Platz 1
44789 Bochum, Germany

Herko Grubitzsch, M. D.
Department of Thoracic
and Cardiovascular Surgery
Klinikum Karlsburg
Greifswalder Str. 11A
17495 Karlsburg, Germany

C. Hanefeld, M. D.
Department of Cardiology
St. Josef- Hospital
Ruhr-University Bochum
Gudrunstr. 56
44791 Bochum, Germany

Eberhard von Hodenberg, M. D.
Heart Institute Lahr/Baden
Department of Internal Medicine
and Cardiology
77933 Lahr, Germany

Andreas Hoffmeier, M. D.
Department of Cardiothoracic Surgery
Westphalian Willhelms-University
Albert-Schweitzer-Str. 33
48149 Münster, Germany

Rolf Kaiser, M. D.
Department of Thoracic
and Cardiovascular Surgery
Klinikum Karlsburg
Greifswalder Straße 11A
17495 Karlsburg, Germany

W. Kallweit, M. D.
Clinic for Thoracic
and Cardiovascular Surgery
Klinikum Karlsburg
Greifswalder Str. 11A
17495 Karlsburg, Germany

Prof. W. Konertz, M. D.
Department of Cardiac Surgery
Charité
Schumannstraße 20/21
10098 Berlin, Germany

M. Loebe, M. D.
German Heart Institute Berlin
Augustenburger Platz 1
13353 Berlin, Germany

Prof. F. W. Mohr, M. D.
Department of Cardiac Surgery
Heart Institute Leipzig, University
Russenstraße 19
04289 Leipzig, Germany

Karl J. Oldhafer
Abdominal and Transplantation Surgery
Hannover Medical School
Carl-Neuberg-Straße 1
30625 Hannover, Germany

Andrew Parry, Assistant Professor, M. D.
Box 0118
University of California, San Francisco
505 Parnassus Ave.
San Francisco, CA 94143-0118, USA

Si M. Pham, M. D.
Assistant Professor of Surgery
Division of Cardiothoracic Surgery
University of Pittsburgh
School of Medicine
Suite C-700 PUH
200 Lothrop Street
Pittsburgh, PA 15213, USA

Friedrich-Christian Riess, M. D.
Department of Cardiac Surgery
Albertinen-Krankenhaus
Suentelstraße 11A
22457 Hamburg, Germany

Ø. Risum, Ph. D., M. D.
Surgical Department A
University of Oslo
Pilestredet 32
N-0027 Oslo, Norway

Francis Robicsek, M. D., Ph. D.
Carolinas Heart Institute
1000 Blythe Boulevard
Charlotte, North Carolina 23203, USA

U. P. Rosendahl, M. D.
Heart Institute Lahr/Baden
Department of Thoracic
and Cardiovascular Surgery
77933 Lahr, Germany

Jürgen Rötker, M. D.
Thoracic and Cardiovascular Surgery
Westphalian Willhelms-University
Albert-Schweitzer-Str. 33
48129 Münster, Germany

Luay Salaymeh, M. D.
Department of Cardiac Surgery
University Hospital
Auenbruggerplatz 29
8036 Graz, Austria

Arnulf Schiessler, M. D.
Leibnizstr. 44
10629 Berlin, Germany

Ulrike Schindel, M. D.
Cardio Clinic Frankfurt
Fachkrankenhaus für Herzchirurgie
Usinger Str. 5
60389 Frankfurt/Main, Germany

A. Schmidt-Westhausen, M. D.
Department for Oral Surgery
and Dental Radiology
Center for Dental Medicine, Charité
Campus Virchow-Klinikum
Humboldt University Berlin
Föhrer Str. 15
13353 Berlin, Germany

Prof. Volker Schuchardt, M. D.
Department of Neurology
Klinikum Lahr
Klostenstraße 19
77933 Lahr, Germany

Prof. V. Schusdziarra, M. D.
Department of Medicine II
Klinikum rechts der Isar
Ismaninger Straße 20
81675 München, Germany

Paul Stelzer, M. D.
Division of Cardiac Surgery
Beth Israel Medical Center
317 East 17th Street 11th Floor
New York, NY 10003, USA

Professor Tom Treasure, M. D.
Cardiothoracic Unit
St. George's Hospital
Blackshaw Road, Tooting
London Sw17 0QT, England

Prof. Alexander Tschirkov, M. D.
University Hospital 'St. Ekaterina'
2, P. Slaveikov blvd.
1431 Sofia, Bulgaria

Prof. K.-H. Usadel, M. D.
Department of Internal Medicine I
University Hospital
Johann Wolfgang Goethe-University
Theodor-Stern-Kai 7
60590 Frankfurt am Main, Germany

H.-G. Wollert, M. D.
Department of Thoracic
and Cardiovascular Surgery
Klinikum Karlsburg
Greifswalder Str. 11A
17495 Karlsburg, Germany

Coexisting peripheral arterial obliterative disease (PAOD) in patients with coronary artery (CAD) and cerebral vascular disease (CVD)

C. Diehm

Department of Internal Medicine/Vascular Medicine, Academic Hospital University of Heidelberg, Karlsbad, Germany

Epidemiology and prognosis of PAOD

Epidemiological research into vascular disease has largely concentrated on ischemic heart disease and stroke, because of their high mortality and morbidity. However interest in vascular disease of the lower extremities has increased in recent years, particularly with the advent of new techniques for diagnosis and treatment.

Peripheral arterial disease is a significant cause of morbidity in the community, especially in the elderly. The prevalence increases with age and is higher in males than females, although the sex difference narrows with increasing age. The Framingham Study has reported age – and sex – specific population data on the incidence of intermittent claudication that show a sharp increase in incidence already in late middle age and somewhat higher rates in men than in women.
Population surveys have reported a prevalence of intermittent claudication between 1% and 7% for men aged 50–75 years (14). The incidence of symptoms increases

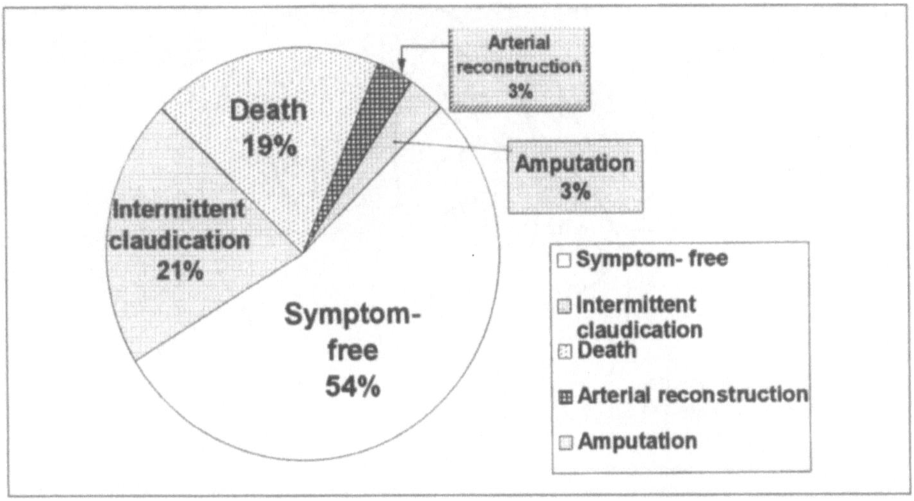

Fig. 1. Outcome of patients with claudication at 5 years in Edinburgh Artery Study (adapted from 15)

with age, from around 0.2 % per year for men aged 35–45 years to more than 1 % per year for men older than 65 years.

Atherothrombosis is a generalized disease, and most patients with peripheral vascular disease have occlusive arterial disease elsewhere in the body. As a result of the generalized nature of the arterial disease, patients with intermittent claudication have a mortality rate two to three times higher than age-matched, sex-matched controls (14). Men with intermittent claudication (IC) have 5-year cumulative mortality rates of around 15%. About half of the deaths are secondary to coronary artery disease (CAD), a quarter from stroke or abdominal vascular disease and a quarter from noncardiovascular causes (15; Fig. 1).

Coexisting Vascular Diseases in Patients with PAOD

There is very little reliable information on the overlap between significant arterial disease in the three areas: leg, heart, and brain. Most studies have concentrated on one area only and recorded only superficially, if at all, the coexistence of significant arterial disease elsewhere. The large CAPRIE study is an example of this, where for instance the presence or absence of claudication in the patients entered following myocardial infarction was based on a single question (7). However, the evidence available from all the relevant studies suggests that approximately 30% of patients with coronary disease or significant cerebral circulatory disease will also have PAOD.

Aronow and Ahn evaluated the prevalence of CAD, PAOD, and CVD (diagnosed by clinical history/ECG), and their coexistence in a prospective study of 1,886 patients aged ≥ 62 years (2). CAD, PAOD, and CVD were all more prevalent among men than women (Table 1 and Fig. 2). Only 37% of these patients had none of these coexisting diseases.

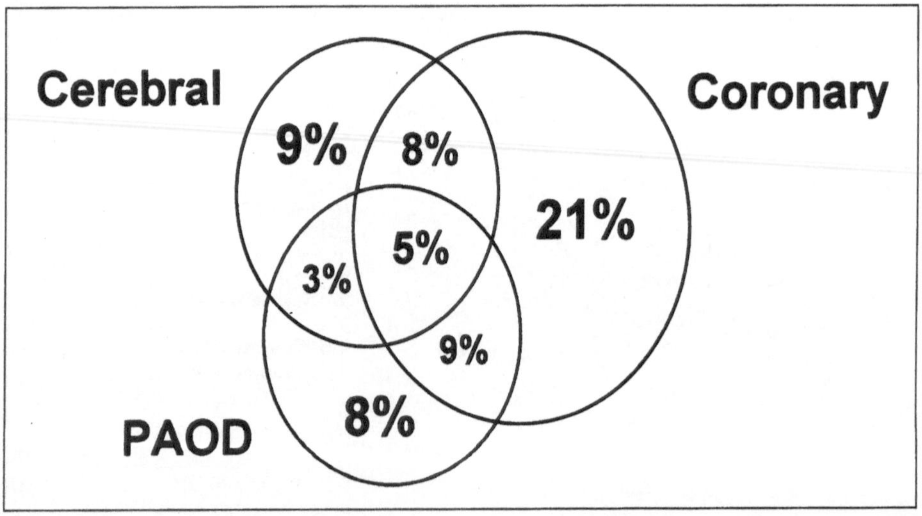

Fig. 2. Overlap between PAOD, CHD, and CVD in 1886 patients aged > 62; 37% of whom had no CHD, CVD or PAOD (adapted from 2)

Table 1. Prevalence of CAD, PAOD and CVD in elderly men and women ≥ 62 years (2)

Disease	Men (n = 580 (%)	Women (n = 11306) (%)
CAD	274 (47)	536 (41)
PAOD	167 (29)	301 (23)
CVD	169 (29)	316 (24)

Table 2. Prevalence of CHD in patients presenting with Intermittent Claudication (adapted from Dormandy et al. 12 and 13)

Reference	No of patients	Screening method	CAD (%)
History			
Taylor & Calo 1962 (33)	412	History	17
Murabito et al. 1997 (26)	5209	Questionnaire/examination	34
History/ECG			
Begg & Richards 1962 (4)	198	History/ECG	19
De Weese & Richards 1962 (11)	103	History/ECG	34
Mallone et al. 1977 (24)	180	History/ECG	58
Hughson et al. 1978 (20)	160	History/ECG	36
Szilagyi et al. 1979 (31, 32)	531	History/ECG	38.5
Crawford et al. 1981 (8)	949	History/ECG	38
Hertzer 1981 (18)	256	History/ECG	47
Szilagyi et al. 1986 (31, 32)	1748	–	47
Dormandy & Murray 1991 (13)	1969	History/ECG	47
Aronow & Ahn 1994 (2)	1886	History/ECG	58
von Kemp et al. 1997 (22)	200	History/ECG	46
Other diagnostic tests			
Vecht et al. 1982 (35)	100	Stress ECG	62
Hertzer et al. 1984 (19)	381	Angiography	90
Brewster et al. 1985 (6)	54	Thallium scan	63

Studies consistently show that individuals with PAOD are more likely to have coronary heart disease and cerebrovascular disease than those without PAOD. The degree of overlap between PAOD and other clinical manifestations of atherosclerotic disease increases with both the severity of atherosclerotic disease and the sensitivity of the diagnostic work-up for atherosclerotic disease.

In the study by Criqui et al. patients with PAOD also had an assessment of other cardiovascular disease (CAD and CVD), based on a history of myocardial infarction, coronary bypass surgery, stroke, or stroke related surgery. This study found that cardiovascular disease was 2–3 times more frequent among people with PAOD than those without PAOD (9).

Peripheral arterial occlusive disease and coronary artery disease

Table 2 summarizes some of the published studies on the prevalence of coronary artery disease (CAD) in patients with intermittent claudication and shows that history, clinical examination, and electrocardiography consistently reveal the presence of CAD in typically 40-60% of such patients, althought it may be asymptomatic if exercise is severely limited by claudication. In one study in which coronary angiograms were performed, the prevalence was as high as 90% (17). Among individuals with IC identified in the general population, the prevalence of CHD varied between 20 and 52% and was between two and four times higher than that in non-PAOD individuals (5, 20, 28).

All patients presenting to the Cleveland Clinic from 1978–1981 for elective peripheral vascular surgery had cardiac catheterization to determine whether prophylactic treatment of severe CAD could improve long-term survival. Only 10% of the patients (n = 381) presenting with IC had normal coronary arteries on angiography, while 28% had severe three vessel disease that merited revascularization or which was already inoperable (17–19).

The prevalence of CAD seems to be proportional to the severity of the PAOD. In the Basle study, 27% of a study group with asymptomatic PAOD, detected by oscillometry, had "symptoms of coronary insufficiency" compared with 10% in an age-matched control group. Fowkes studied a group who probably had more severe asymptomatic disease (ABPI<0.7) and found CAD in 54%, which is similar to the

Table 3. Prevalence of CVD at presentation of IC to a clinician-selected studies (adapted from Dormandy et al., 12, 13)

Reference	No of patients	Screening method	CAD (%)
Begg & Richards 1962 (4)	198	Clinical history	0.5
De Weese & Richards 1962 (11)	103	Clinical history	4
Mallone et al. 1977 (24)	180	Questionnaire/examinati on (incl. cervical bruit)	45
Hughson et al. 1978 (20)	54	Clinical history	6
Szilagyi et al. 1979 (32)	531	Clinical history ± angiography	13
Szilagyi et al. 1986 (32)	1748	–	18.5
Turnipseed 1980 (34)	160	Cervical bruit + non-invasive tests (Doppler)	44 52
von Kemp et al. 1997 (22)	200	Clinical history/ECG	32

rate found in claudicants (9). Hertzer found that angiographically documented severe CAD occurred in 17% of patients who had an ABPBI>0.75 (17, 18).

The converse is also true; among individuals with CAD, the prevalence of PAOD is higher than in non-CAD individuals (29,30). The relative risk of IC among Finnish men and women with angina pectoris compared with controls was 7.2 and 4, respectively. Aronow found that 33% of CAD patients also had PAOD (2). In the Framingham study the relative risk of IC in patients with angina pectoris was 2.8 in men and 5.2 in women (21, 36). Probably the risks are even higher, because the development of IC is often masked by the exercise-limiting effects of angina. As with CAD in patients with IC, the prevalence of PAOD tends to increase with more severe CAD. In a study of 58 CAD patients examined with coronary angiography, using digital volume pulse plethysmography and ankle and toe blood pressure measurements, the overall prevalence of PAOD was found to be 22% which is in agreement with the results from other studies (3). However, the prevalence of PAOD was 14% in patients with no or minimal coronary atheromatous lesions, 18% in patients with moderate coronary atheromatous lesions, and 32% in patients with marked coronary atheromatous disease.

Peripheral arterial occlusive disease and cerebrovascular disease

Table 3 lists some selected studies of patients with PAOD who have assessed the prevalence of concomitant cerebrovascular disease (CVP). Here, even more than with coronary artery disease, prevalence varies depending on the type of population and the screening method.

The link between PAOD and CVD seems to be weaker than that with CAD, while about half of all patients with IC have CAD detectable by simple clinical techniques, a much lower proportion have demonstrable CVD Hughson found that 6% of individuals gave a history of a previous stroke compared with non in age and sex-matched controls (20). In the Basle-Study 12% of male survivors with PAOD developed a stroke during 11 years of follow-up compared with 4% of controls (10). Also, more cases had evidence of carotid stenosis. However, Aronow et al. found that 34% of PAOD patients aged ≥ 62 years also had CVD (2). Ögren et al. found that men with PAOD were twice as likely to have a cerebrovascular event then those without PAOD (Relative risk 2.1 (95% CI 1.1–8.7) (27) using duplex examination, carotid disease has been found in 26–50% of claudicants (1, 16, 23, 34). Most of these patients will have a history of cerebral events or a carotid bruit and seem to be at increased risk of further events (25). Aronow et al. found that 33% of patients with CVD also had PAOD (2).

References

1. Alexandrova NA, Gibson WC, Norris JW, Maggisano R (1996) Carotid artery stenosis in peripheral vascular disease. J Vasc Surg 23:645–649
2. Aronow WS, Ahn C (1994) Prevalence of coexistence of coronary artery disease, peripheral arterial disease, and atherothrombotic brain infarction in men and women 62 years of age. Am J Cardiol 74:64–65.
3. Atmer B, Jogestrand T, Laska J, Lund F (1995) Peripheral artery disease in patients with coronary artery disease. Int Angiol 4:89–93.

4. Begg TB, Richards RL (1962) The prognosis of intermittent claudication. Scott Med J 7:342–352
5. Böthig S. Metelitsa VI, Barth W et al. (1976) Prevalence of ischemic heart disease, arterial hypertension and intermittent claudication, and distribution of risk factors among middle-aged men in Moscow and Berlin. Cor Vasa 8:104–118
6. Brewster DC, Okada RD, Strauss HW et al. (1985) Selection of patients for preoperative coronary angiography: Use of dipyridamole stress-thallium myocardial imaging. J Vasc Surg 2:504
7. CAPRIE Steering Comittee (1996) A randomised, blinded, trial of clopidogrel versus aspirin in patients at risk of ischemic events (CAPRIE). Lancet 348:1329–1339
8. Crawford ES, Bomberger RA, Glaeser DH et al. (1981) Aortoiliac occlusive disease: factors influencing survival and function following reconstructive operation over twenty-five year period. Surgery 90:1055–1067
9. Criqui MH, Denenberg JO, Langer RD, Fronek A (1997) The epidemiology of peripheral arterial disease: importance of identifying the population at risk. Vasc Med 81:551–555
10. Da Silva A, Widmer LK, Muller HR. Cardiovascular disease and occlusive peripheral artery disease (OPAD). In: Proceedings of the 13th International Congress of Angiology. Athens, Greece, 9-14 June 1985
11. De Weese JA, Rob CG (1962) Autogenous vein grafts ten years later. Surgery 6:775–784
12. Dormandy J, Mahir M, Ascady G et al. (1989) Fate of the patient with chronic leg ischaemia. J Cardiovasc Surg 30:50–57
13. Dormandy JA, Murray GD (1991) The fate of the claudicant – a prospective study of 1969 claudicants. Eur J Vasc Surg 5:131–133
14. Fowkes FGR, Housley E, Cawood EHH et al. (1991) Edinburgh Artery Study: prevalence of asymptomatic and symptomatic peripheral arterial disease in the general population. Int J Epidemiol 20:384–392
15. Golledge J (1997) Lower – limb arterial disease. Lancet 350:1459–65
16. Hennerici M, Aulich A, Sandeman W, Freund H-J (1981) Incidence of asymptomatic extracranial arterial disease. Stroke 12:750–758
17. Hertzer NR, Beven EG, Young JR et al. (1984) Coronary artery disease in peripheral vascular patients – a classification of 1000 coronary angiograms and results of surgical management. Ann Surg 199:223–233
18. Hertzer NR (1981) Fatal myocardial infarction following lower extremity revascularization: two hundred and seventy-three patients followed six to eleven postoperative years. Ann Surg 193:492–436
19. Hertzer NR (1991) The natural history of peripheral vascular diseas 3. Implications for its management. Circulation 83(Suppl. 1):12–19
20. Hughson WG, Mann JI, Garrod A (1978) Intermittent claudication: Prevalence and risk factors. Br Med J 1:1379–1381
21. Kannel WB, Skinner JJ Jr, Schwartz MJ, Shurtleff D (1970) Intermittent claudication: Incidence in the Framingham Study. Circulation 41:875–883
22. von Kemp K, van den Brande P, Peterson T, Waegeneers S, Scheerlinck T, Danau W, van Tussenbroek F, Debing E, Staelens I (1997) Screening for concomitant diseases in peripheral vascular patients. Int Angiol 16:114–122
23. Klop RBJ, Eikelboom BC, Taks ACJM (1991) Screening of the internal carotid arteries in patients with peripheral vascular disease by colour-flow Duplex scanning. Eur J Vasc Surg 5:41–45
24. Mallone JM, Moore WS, Goldstone J (1977) Life expectancy following aortofemoral arterial grafting. Surgery 81:551–555
25. Mc Daniel MD, Cronenwett JL (1989) Basic data related to the natural history of intermittent Claudication. Ann Gasc Surg 3:271–377
26. Murabito JM, D'Agostino RB, Silbershatz H, Wilson PWF (1997) Intermittent claudication. A risk profile from the Framingham Heart Study. Circulation 96:44–49
27. Örgen M, Hedblad B, Isacsson SO, Janzon L, et al. (1995) Ten year cerebrovascular morbidity and mortality in 68-year-old men with asymptomatic carotid stenosis. Br Med J 310:1294–1298
28. Reid DD, Holland WW, Hummerfelt S, Rose G (1966) A cardiovascular survey of British postal workers. Lancet 1:614–61
29. Reunanen A, Takkunen H, Aromaa A (1982) Prevalence of intermittent claudication and its effect on mortality. Acta Med Scand 211:249–256

30. Schroll M, Munck O (1981) Estimation of peripheral arteriosclerotic disease by ankle blood pressure measurements in a population study of 60-year-old men and women. J Chron Dis 34:261–269
31. Szilagyi DE, Elliott JP, Smith RF, Reddy DJ, McPharlin M (1986) A thirty-year survey of the reconstructive surgical treatment of aortoiliac occlusive disease. J Vasc Surg 3:421–436
32. Szilagyi DE, Hageman JH, Smith RF et al. (1979) Autogenous vein grafting in femoropopliteal atherosclerosis: the limits of its effectiveness. Surgery 86:836–851
33. Taylor MS, Calo MR (1962) Atherosclerosis of arteries of lower limbs. Br Med J 24:507–519
34. Turnipseed WD, Berkoff HA, Belzer FO (1980) Postoperative stroke in cardiac and peripheral vascular disease. Ann Surg 192:365–368
35. Vecht RJ, Nicolaides AN, Brandao E et al. (1982) Resting and treadmill electrocardiographic findings in patients with intermittent claudication. Inter Angio 1:119–121
36. Widmer LK, Greensher A, Kannel WB (1964) Occlusion of peripheral arteries. A study of 6400 working subjects. Circulation 30:836–842

Author's address:
Prof. Dr. med. Curt Diehm
Department of Internal Medicine/Vascular Medicine
Karlsbad Clinic
Academic Hospital University of Heidelberg
76307 Karlsbad

Cardiac surgery and simultaneous repair of abdominal aortic aneurysm

F.W. Mohr, V. Falk

Department of Cardiac Surgery University of Leipzig, Germany

Introduction

The overall mortality for elective repair of abdominal aortic aneurysms has constantly declined in recent decades (8, 29). Besides the use of better diagnostic tools, refinements in both surgical and anesthesiological techniques, and the use of shielded vascular grafts, it was recognized that concomitant diseases play a major role in patients undergoing abdominal aortic aneurysm repair. Half of the patients scheduled for abdominal aortic aneurysm repair present with coronary artery disease to some degree (4, 31) which puts them at risk for perioperative morbidity and mortality and decreased long-term survival (25). Most hospital and late deaths in patients undergoing AAA repair are due to cardiac causes (16, 26, 32). In patients with uncorrected coronary artery disease there is a two- to three-fold higher incidence of myocardial infarction, congestive heart failure, and cardiac related death after aneurysmectomy (9, 30, 33, 52). Impaired left ventricular function is an independent risk factor. In patients with an ejection fraction below 35% high rates of myocardial infarction (up to 80%) and mortality (up to 20%) as well as a poor long-term survival have been reported after major vascular surgery (37, 49, 50).

The use of preoperative screening programs to identify patients at cardiac risk can effectively lower cardiac related morbidity and mortality following AAA repair (24, 29, 55). Patients with correctable coronary artery disease (almost 10% in larger series) and a stable aortic aneurysm will have myocardial revascularization procedures (coronary artery bypass graft surgery (CABG) or PTCA) prior to AAA repair (5, 22). Nevertheless, optimal timing for aortic surgery is crucial. Perioperative stress and hemodynamic instability following cardiac surgery increase the risk of rupture of an abdominal aneurysm during the time the patient is recovering from CABG surgery (8). In addition the systemic inflammatory response to cardiopulmonary bypass may contribute to the risk of rupturing an AAA soon after cardiac surgery. From numerous studies it is known that the inflammatory response to cardiopulmonary bypass is associated with an up to ten-fold and persistent increase in plasma elastase levels probably by an adhesion-triggered degranulation of neutrophils (14, 43). Although still speculative, elevated elastase levels may increase the risk for rupture of an abdominal aortic aneurysm in patients recovering from coronary bypass surgery by an increased digestion of abdominal aortic wall proteins (39).

Eventually, some patients with extensive CAD or severely reduced left ventricular function will be denied surgery. For this high risk group of patients, a simultaneous approach has been suggested (18, 23, 46, 56).

Methods

In order to achieve an optimum of cardiac protection during aortic clamping, AAA repair is performed during cardiopulmonary bypass. While being supported by cardiopulmonary bypass (CPB) the deleterious effects of infrarenal aortic clamping and declamping on myocardial function can be effectively avoided. At the same time CABG surgery will optimize coronary blood flow. After a median sternotomy the ITA is harvested and the patient is cannulated for CPB. After completion of the distal coronary anastomoses the aortic cross-clamp is released and the proximal anastomoses are performed on the arrested heart. While the patient is still on cardiopulmonary bypass and kept moderately hypothermic, the incision is extended to the pubic bone and the aneurysm is exposed. The infrarenal aorta and iliac arteries are clamped and the aneurysm is opened. Blood that is lost during the abdominal procedure is retransfused using the cardiotomy suction. Transperitoneal abdominal aortic aneurysm repair is then performed. As soon as the proximal aortic anastomosis is performed rewarming is begun. The patient is weaned from CPB after the distal aortic, iliac or femoral anastomoses are completed. The routine use of Collagen-shielded vascular grafts allows for adequate hemostasis despite full heparinization required for CPB.

Results

35 patients (31 male) underwent combined cardiac and abdominal aortic aneurysm repair since 1992. The results have been already reported in part elsewhere (2, 20, 45). 26 patients had three vessel disease and presented either with symptoms of unstable angina and/or poor left ventricular function. At the same time all these patients had large aneurysms with a diameter exceeding 5 cm that were either acutely leaking, recently expanding, or acutely symptomatic. The mean diameter of the aneurysms was 62 mm (range 50–86 mm). Mean age was 68 ± 12 years (range 55–80) with most patients having several cardiovascular risk factors (diabetes, hypertension) and suffering from comorbid conditions (renal insufficiency, cerebrovascular disease, peripheral vascular disease). Due to high operative risk some of these patients had been denied AAA repair in other centers. All patients were operated simultaneously receiving a mean of 3.2 coronary artery bypass grafts and bifurcation (n=19) or tube grafts (n = 16) in the aortic position. In addition, in two patients with aortic stenosis had additional aortic valve replacement. Three renal and two carotid arteries were revascularized during the same procedure. ICU treatment and hospital stay averaged 4.3 days and 19.6 days, respectively.

There was considerable associated morbidity with almost half of the patients experiencing one or more complications requiring therapeutic intervention. 15 patients required inotropic support for more than two days. Pulmonary complications with prolonged ventilatory support (> 48 h) were frequent (31.4%) and most likely associated with the negative effects of the thoracoabdominal exposure on respiratory mechanics. Postoperative renal insufficiency was observed in 8 patients. Three patients required temporary hemodialysis. Neurological complications were encountered in 3 and vascular complications in 2 patients. Three patients underwent relaparotomy for bleeding (n = 2) or ileus (n = 1). Most of these complications were resolved with appropriate treatment. Besides one fatal intraoperative cardiac

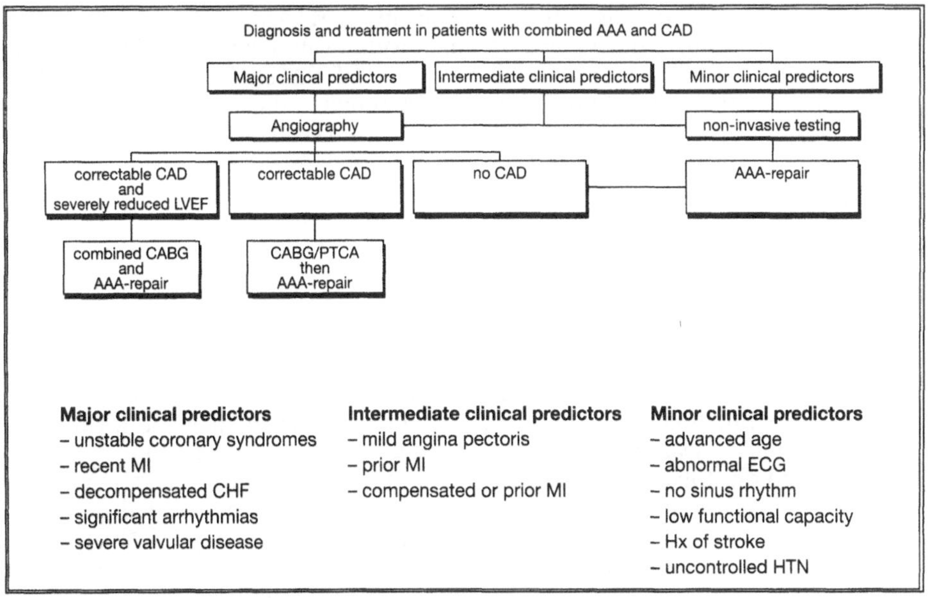

Fig. 1. Assessment of individual risk for abdominal aortic surgery in patients with concommittant cardiac disease and decision tree to perform either a staged or combined procedure. (Modified from the Guidelines for perioperative cardiovascular evaluation for noncardiac surgery, ACC / AHA Task Force Report (1996) Circulation 93:1278–1317)

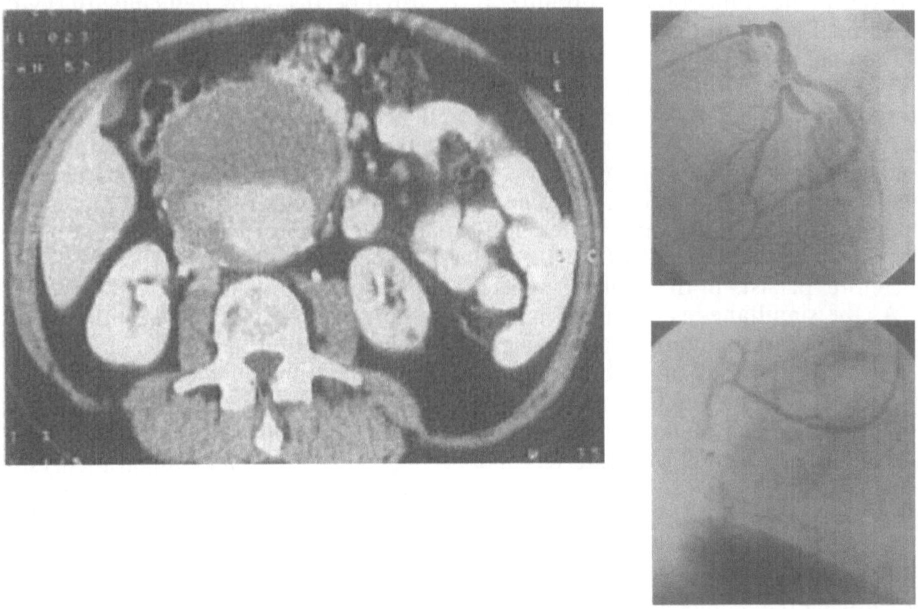

Fig. 2. Case study: 78 year old male patient with typical abdominal pain from an expanding abdominal aortic aneurysm (CT-scan). Coronary angiography revealed severe three vessel coronary artery disease with an left ventricular ejection fraction of 15%. The patient was operated simultaneously and discharged on postop. day 14

failure, there were no serious cardiac complications related to the procedure. We observed 3 perioperative deaths two of which were of non cardiac origin resulting in an hospital mortality of 8.5%. All but three of the survivors regained their preoperative health status, improved in NYHA functional class. All but 3 patients were free from angina at their last visit. Actuarial survival at four years is 73.4%.

Discussion

Infrarenal aortic crossclamping results in an acute rise of ventricular afterload due to sudden increase of systemic vascular resistance (17, 54). The otherwise healthy individual tolerates these hemodynamic changes, but in patients with decreased left ventricular function and coronary artery disease, arrhythmias and myocardial ischemia with a consecutive reduction in stroke volume and cardiac index and an increase in end diastolic volume occur (11, 13, 21, 27, 41, 42). Especially in patients with CAD the resulting increase in wall stress impairs subendocardial perfusion and can cause myocardial ischemia (1, 28). In contrast, declamping of the aorta leads to a sudden fall in SVR and large volume shifts resulting in hypotension that may also cause critical coronary perfusion (6, 41). In addition, washout acidosis with increased lactate concentration and oxygen consumption adversely affects myocardial performance (19).

When first performed CPB was terminated before aortic surgery was begun in combined CABG and AAA surgery (53, 59). This approach has certainly no advantage when compared to the two-stage procedure but carries potential risks. Since one of the major therapeutic goals following CABG in patients with poor left ventricular function is to optimize myocardial perfusion by reducing afterload, it seems illogical to discontinue cardiopulmonary bypass and then crossclamp the abdominal aorta (58).

The combined operation is currently performed with continuing CPB support during aortic surgery (7, 15, 46, 53, 58). It is well documented that a recovery period is necessary for the heart to overcome the effects of cardioplegic arrest following myocardial revascularization. In patients with poor ventricular function and severe CAD myocardial dysfunction due to incomplete myocardial protection and reperfusion injury immediately following CABG surgery is a common finding despite patent bypass grafts (10, 40). The risk associated with aortic cross clamping, therefore, persists in the short term after revascularization (44, 45, 51, 58)

As the simultaneous operation is major surgery, careful patient selection is crucial in order to maintain a reasonable risk to benefit ratio (3).

Given the high risk of perioperative myocardial infarction in patients with unstable coronary syndromes and chronic left ventricular failure undergoing abdominal aortic surgery (12, 20), a simultaneous approach is justified in patients with tender aneurysms suspicious for impending rupture, recent dissecting or expanding abdominal aneurysm. Patients with asymptomatic aneurysms and correctable CAD with normal or only moderately impaired LVF should be treated by a revascularization procedure either PTCA or CABG surgery first, followed by AAA resection at a two week interval. Both PTCA and CABG surgery have been shown to be effective in reducing the incidence of cardiac events immediately after AAA repair (18). It is debatable if patients with asymptomatic but large (> 6 cm) aneurysms who have 2–3 vessel disease and poor ventricular function should undergo a staged or a combined approach. These patients are unlikely to improve their cardiac function to an extent that would make them tolerate the rapid changes in afterload associated with AAA repair even after successful myocardial revascularization procedures.

The combined procedure is indicated for a selected high-risk subset of patients. As for patients with symptomatic or rapidly expanding AAA, there are only few relative contraindications, such as preterminal condition, incurable malignancies, and overwhelming medical problems (29). Both severe pulmonary disease and chronic renal failure will increase the risk of a combined approach and worsen the prognosis for these patients.

There is controversy whether to expand the indication of the combined operation to patients with end-stage aortic occlusive disease and impending loss of limb. Our limited experience in 6 patients with end-stage aortic occlusive disease (rest pain and ischemic ulcerations) who underwent simultaneous surgery is not encouraging as we lost two of these patients in the first two months after operation.

Obviously, these patients represent a rather morbid group with multiple vascular lesions. Furthermore, the hemodynamic benefit of having the aorta clamped during CPB will not be as great as in patients with an AAA because the aorta is already occluded (36, 47). In addition, depending on CPB flow rates, limb perfusion may further deteriorate during the cardiac procedure. As such, only patients requiring intermediate cardiac intervention are candidates for a combined operation.

An interesting alternative approach to the selected patient group with concomitant coronary and leg ischemia was recently reported by Jebara and coworkers. They performed combined coronary and and aorto-iliac revascularization in ten male patients using an ascending aorta to bifemoral bypass, thus, avoiding an intraperitoneal procedure (35).

If a combined approach is chosen, one has to consider that in patients with severe AOD, the ITA serves as an important collateral pathway to circumvent the occluded aorta. Acute lower extremity ischemia secondary to coronary artery bypass grafting has been reported in patients with severe obstruction of the aortoiliac artery system (38, 48). Especially in older patients, alternative conduits should, therefore, be used for coronary grafting (57) despite proven superior long-term patency rates of the ITA.

In conclusion, the simultaneous operation is an alternative option for selected patients with multiple cardiac and vascular disorders who are often denied surgical intervention. Continuous cardiac support by CPB during infrarenal aortic surgery offers a maximum of cardiac protection at least in patients with abdominal aortic aneurysms. The potential benefit is less evident for patients with aortic occlusive disease.

Summary

Although effective screening programs and myocardial revascularization procedures (PTCA and CABG surgery) have helped to decrease the risk of cardiac related adverse events, coronary artery disease remains the most important risk factor for morbidity and mortality in patients undergoing abdominal aortic aneurysm repair. Especially in patients with impaired left ventricular function, myocardial infarction rates up to 80% and mortality rates up to 20% due to cardiac causes have been reported after major vascular surgery. As a result almost 5% of all patients scheduled for elective AAA repair are denied surgery for their increased cardiac risk that is mainly due to extensive coronary artery disease and severely impaired ventricular function. During recent years we have focused on this multimorbid subset of patients and used a combined approach of simultaneous CABG surgery and AAA resection. The rationale for a combined operation is to optimize cardiac protection during abdominal aortic aortic surgery. After completion of the revascularization procedure and under continuous cardiac support by cardiopulmonary bypass, the deleterious effects of infrarenal aortic clamping and declamping on myocardial function can be effectively avoided. At the same time CABG surgery will optimize coronary blood flow and minimize the risk of perioperative ischemic complications. AAA repair can, therefore, be performed with maximum safety and carries low risk of adverse cardiac events. The combined operation is an attractive therapeutical option for the patient with multivascular and severe cardiac disease and should be considered in selected patients

References

1. Anguissola GB, Mangiarotti R, Pierini A, Lubatti L, Conti E, Arpesani A, Burdick L, Trazzi R (1994) Wall stress in the assessment of left ventricular function in surgery of abdominal aortic aneurysm. Validity and importance of transesophageal echocardiography (TEE) in intraoperative monitoring. Minerva Anestesiol (english abstract) 60:237–244
2. Autschbach R, Falk V, Walther T, Vettelschoß M, Diegeler A, Dalichau H, Mohr FW (1995) Simultaneous coronary bypass and abdominal aortic surgery in patients with severe coronary disease – Indications and results. Eur J Cardiothorac Surg. 9:678–784
3. Azuma K, Hirose H, Matsumoto K, Fuwa S, Mori Y, Murakawa S, Arakawa H, Ishikawa M (1995) Screening of patients with ischemic heart disease by transesophageal atrial pacing and the selection of surgical therapy in patients with arteriosclerosis obliterans and aortic aneurysm. J Cardiovasc Surg (Torino) 36:61–69
4. Bayazit M, Ǵol MK, Battaloglu B, Tokmakoglu H, Tasdemir O, Bayazit K (1995) Routine coronary arteriography before abdominal aortic aneurysm repair. Am J Surg 170:246–50
5. Bayazit M, Gol MK, Battaloglu B, Tokmakoglu H, Tasdemir O, Bayazit K (1995) Routine coronary arteriography before abdominal aortic aneurysm repair. Am J Surg 170:246–250
6. Becker H, Brinkmann H, Allenberg JR (1985) Die Bedeutung der hämodynamischen Folgen der Aortenabklemmung beim infrarenalen Bauchaortenaneurysma. Chirurg 56:522–527
7. Black JJ, Desai JB (1995) Combined coronary artery bypass surgery and abdominal aortic aneurysm repair. J R Soc Med 88:350–52
8. Blackbourne LH, Tribble CG, Langenburg SE, Mauney MC, Buchanan SA, Sinclair KN, Kron IL, Dean RH, Davidson JT (1994) Optimal timing of abdominal aortic aneurysm repair after coronary artery revascularization. Ann Surg 219:693–698
9. Blombery PA, Ferguson IA, Rosengarten DS, Stuchbery KE, Miles CR, Black AJ, Pitt A, Anderson ST, Harper RW, Federman J (1987) The role of coronary artery disease in complications of abdominal aortic aneurysm surgery. Surgery 101:150–55
10. Breisblatt WM, Stein KL, Wolfe Follansbee WP, Capozzi J, Armitage JM, Hardesty RL (1990) Acute myocardial dysfunction and recovery: a common occurence after coronary bypass surgery. J Am Coll Cardiol 15:1261–69
11. Carrel T, Niederhauser U, Laske A, Pasic M, Turina M (1993) Effect of aortic clamping on heart function in elective operation of the abdominal aorta – immediate effects of coronary revascularization. Helv Chir Acta 59:849–854
12. Carrell T, Niederhäuser U, Pasic M, von Segesser L, Turina M (1991) Simultaneous revascularization for critical coronary and peripheral vascular ischemia. Ann thorac Surg 52:805–9
13. Carrol RM, Laravuso RB, Schauble JF (1976) Left ventricular function during aortic surgery. arch Surg 111:740–743
14. Curello S, Ceconi C, de Giuli F, Panzali AF, Milanesi B, Calarco M, Pardini A, Marzallo P, Alfieri O, Messineo F (1995) Oxidative stress during reperfusion of human hearts: potential sources of oxygen free radicals. Cardiovasc Res 29:118–125
15. David TE (1984) Combined cardiac and abdominal aortic surgery. Circulation 72 (Suppl II):II-18–21
16. Diehl JT, Cali RF, Hertzer NR (1983) Complications of Abdominal Aortic reconstruction. An Analysis of perioperative risk factors in 557 patients. Ann Surg 197:49–56
17. Dunn E, Prager RL, Fry W, Kirsh M (1976) The effect of abdominal aortic cross-clamping on myocardial function. J Surg Res 22:463–468
18. Elmore JR, Hallett JW, Gibbons RJ, Naessens JM, Bower TC, Cherry KJ, Gloviczki P, Pairolero PC (1993) Myocardial revascularization before abdominal aortic aneurysmorrhaphy: Effect of coronary angioplasty. Mayo Clin Proc 68:637–641

19. Falk JL, Rackow EC, Blumenberg R, Gelfand M, Fein IA (1981) Hemodynamic and metabolic effects of abdominal aortic crossclamping. Am J Surg 142:174–177
20. Falk V, Walther T, Mohr FW (1997) Abdominal aortic aneurysm repair during cardiopulmonary bypass – Rationale for a combined approach. Cardiovasc Surg 5:271–277
21. Fiser WP, Thompson BW, Thompson AR, Eason C, Read RC (1983) Nuclear cardiac ejection fraction and cardiac index in abdominal aortic surgery. Surgery 94:736–39
22. Fleisher LA, Skolnick ED, Holroyd KJ, Lehmann HP(1994) Coronary artery revascularization before abdominal aortic aneurysm surgery: a decision analytic approach. Anesth Analg 79:661–669
23. Foster ED, Davis KB, Carpenter JA, Abele S, Fray D (1986) Risk of noncardiac operation in patients with defined coronary disease: the coronary artery surgery study (CASS) registry experience. Ann Thorac Surg 41:42–50
24. Fraedrich G, Wollschläger H, Schönbach B, Schlosser V (1991) Reduction of the risk of surgery for abdominal aortic aneurysms by extended coronary diagnostics and therapy. Thorac Cardiovasc Surg 39:255–257
25. Gajraaj H, Jamieson CW (1994) Coronary artery disease in patients with peripheral vascular disease. Br. J. Surg 81:333–342
26. Gersh BJ, Charanijt SR, Rooke TW, Ballard DJ (1991) Evaluation and management of patients with both peripheral vascular and coronary artery disease. J Am Coll Cardiol 18:203–14
27. Gooding JM, Archie JP, Mc Dowell H (1980) Hemodynamic response to infrarenal cross clamping in patients with and without coronary artery disease. Crit Care Med 8:382–385
28. Harpole DH, Clements FM, Quill T, Wolfe WG, Jones RH, McCann RL (1989) Right and left ventricular performance during and after abdominal aortic aneurysm repair. Ann Surg 209:356–62
29. Hollier LH, Taylor LM, Ochsner J (1992) Recommended indications for operative treatment of abdominal aortic aneurysms. J Vasc Surg 15:1046–1056
30. Henderson A, Effeney D (1995) Morbidity and mortality after abdominal aortic surgery in a population of patients with high cardiovascular risk. Aust N Z J Surg 65:417–20
31. Hertzer NR (1987) Basic data concerning associated coronary disease in peripheral vascular patients. Ann Vasc Surg 1:616–20
32. Hertzer NR, Beven EG, Young JR (1984) Coronary artery disease in peripheral vascular patients – a classification of 1000 coronary angiograms and results of surgical management. Ann Surg 199:223–33
33. Hertzer NR (1990) Fatal myocardial infarction following abdominal aortic aneurysm resection.Two hundred seventy-three patients followed 6 to 11 postoperative years. Ann Surg 192:667–73
34. Hollier LH (1992) Cardiac evaluation in patients with vascular disease – Overview: A practical approach. J Vasc Surg 15:726–729
35. Jebara VA, Fabiani JN, Acar C, Chardigny C, Julia P, Carpentier A (1994) Combined coronary and femoral revascularization using an ascending aorta to bifemoral bypass. Arch Surg 129:275–279
36. Johnston WE, Balestrieri FJ, Plonk G, D'Souza V, Howard G (1987) The influence of periaortic collateral vessels on the intraoperative hemodynamic effects of acute aortic occlusion in patients with aorto-occlusive disease or abdominal aortic aneurysms. Anesthesiology 66:386–389
37. Kazmers A, Cerqueira MD, Zierler RE (1988) Perioperative and late outcome in patients with left ventricular ejection fraction of 35% or less who require major vascular surgery. J Vasc Surg 8:307–15
38. Kitamura S, Inoue K, Kawachi K, Morita R, Seki T, Taniguchi S, Kawata T (1993) Lower extremity ischemia secondary to internal-thoracic-coronary bypass graft. Ann Thorac Surg 56:57–59
39. Lalak N, Englund R, Hanel KC (1995) Incidence of rupture of aortic aneurysms after coincidental operation. Cardiovasc Surg 3:30–4
40. Mangano DT (1985) Biventricular function after myocardial revascularization in humans: deterioation and recovery patterns during the first 24 hours. Anesthesiology 62:571–7
41. McCoy D, Hargaden K, Kilfeather S, Bouchier-Hayes D, Cunningham AJ (1993) Neuroendocrine and hemodynamic responses to abdominal aortic cross clamp and release during high-dose opiate-oxygen-isoflurane anesthesia. Eur J Vasc Surg 7:648–653

42. Meloche R, Pottecher T, Audet J, Dufresne O, Lepage C (1977) Heamodynamic changes due to clamping of the abdominal aorta. Can Anaesth Soc J 24:20–34
43. Menasche P, Peynet J, Haeffner-Cavaillon N, Carreno MP, de Chaumaray T, Dillisse V, Faris B, Piwnica A, Bloch G, Tedgui A (1995) influence of temperature on neutrophil trafficking during clinical cardiopulmonary bypass. Circulation 92:pII 334–340
44. Minale C, Reifschneider HJ, Schmitz E (1995) Synchronous surgical treatment of abdominal aortic aneurysms and coronary heart disease. Advantages of extracorporeal circulation. Thorac cardiovasc Surg 43 (Suppl):61
45. Mohr FW, Falk V, Autschbach R, Diegeler A, Schorn B, Weyland A, Vettelschoß M, Frank B, Gummert J, Dalichau H (1995) One stage surgery of coronary arteries and abdominal aortic aorta in patients with impaired left ventricular function. Circulation 91:379–385
46. O'Connor MS, Licina MG, Kraenzler EJ, Savage RM, Padua-Shannon N, Starr NJ (1994) Perioperative management and outcome of patients having cardiac surgery combined with abdominal aortic aneurysm resection. J Cardiothorac Vasc Anesth 8:519–526
47. O'Toole DP, Broe P, Bouchier Hayes D, Cunningham AJ (1988) Perioperative hemodynamic changes during aortic vascular surgery: comparison between occlusive and aneurysm disease states. Br J Anaesth 60:322
48. Parashara DK, Kotler MN, Ledley GS, Yazdanfar S Internal mammary artery collateral to the external iliac artery: an angiographic consideration prior to coronary bypass surgery.
49. Pasternack PF, Imparato AM, Bear G, Bauman FG, Benjamin D, Sanger J, Kramer E, Wood RP (1984) The role of radionuclide angiography as a predictor of perioperative myocardial infarction in patients undergoing abdominal aortic aneurysm resection. J Vasc Surg 1:320–5
50. Pasternack PF, Imparato AM, Riles TS, Bauman FG, Bear G, Lamarello PJ, Benjamin D, Sanger J, Kramer E (1985) The value of the radionuclide angiogram in the prediction of perioperative myocardial infarction in patients undergoing lower extremity revascularization procedures, Circulation 72 (Suppl II):II-13-II-17
51. Reul GJ, Cooley DA, Duncan JM, Frazier OH, Ott DA, Livesay JJ, Walker WE (1986) The effect of coronary bypass on the outcome of peripheral vascular operations in 1093 patients. J Vasc Surg 3:788–98
52. Roger VL, Ballard DJ, Hallett JW, Osmundson PJ, Puetz PA, Gersh BJ (1989) Influence of coronary artery disease on morbidity and mortality after abdominal aortic aneurysmectomy: a population based study. 1971–1987. J Am Coll Cardiol 14:1245–52
53. Ruby ST, Whittemore AD, Couch NP, Collins JJ, Cohn L, Shemin R, Mannick JA (1985) Coronary artery disease in patients requiring abdominal aortic aneurysm repair – selective use of a combined approach. Ann Surg 201:758–64
54. Stokland O, Miller MM, Ilebekk A, Kiil F (1980) Mechanism of hemodynamic responses to occlusion of the descending thoracic aorta. Am J Physiol 238:423–429
55. Suggs WD, Smith RB III, Weintraub WS, Dodson TF, Salam AA, Motta JC (1993) Selective screening for coronary artery disease in patients undergoing elective repair of abdominal aortic aneurysms. J Vasc Surg 18:349–57
56. Taylor SM, Fujitani RM, Myers JC, Mills JL (1993) Combined coronary artery bypass and abdominal aortic aneurysmectomy: appropriate management in selected cases. South Med J 86:974–976
57. Tsui SS, Parry AJ, Large SR (1995) Leg ischemia following bilateral internal thoracic artery and inferior epigastric artery harvesting. Eur J Cardiothorac Surg 9:218–220
58. Westaby S, Parry A, Grebenik CR, Pillai R, Lamont P (1992) Combined cardiac and abdominal aortic aneurysm operations – The dual operation on cardiopulmonary bypass. J Thorac Cardiovasc Surg 104:900–5
59. Whittemore AD, Clowes AW, Hechtman HB, Mannick JA (1980) Aortic aneurysm repair. Reduced operative mortality with maintenance of optimal cardiac performance. Ann Surg 192:414–21

Author's address:
Prof. F. W. Mohr
Universität Leipzig Herzzentrum
Klinik für Herzchirurgie
Russenstraße 19
04289 Leipzig, FRG

Surgical strategy for major aortoiliac reconstructions in patients with associated coronary artery disease

T. Zakhariev, M. Stankev, B. Baev, B. Mintchev, A. Tschirkov

Univesity Hospital 'Saint Ekaterina', Sofia, Bulgaria

Summary

The objective of this study was to evaluate the perioperative risk of simultaneous compared to staged surgery in patients with abdominal aortic aneurysm (AAA) or aortoiliac occlusive disease (AIOD) associated with coronary artery disease (CAD). The hospital data of 50 patients with coexistent severe symptomatic AAA or AIOD and significant CAD who underwent surgery of the abdominal aorta and the coronary arteries were retrospectively analyzed. Simultaneous surgical correction of both lesions was accomplished in 32 patients (group I) and two-stage procedure was performed in 18 patients (group II), coronary artery bypass grafting (CABG) as first procedure and aortoiliac reconstruction (AIR) 4–12 months later. In group I, AAA was present in 15 patients (suprarenal extension in 4, infrarenal in 11 cases) and AIOD in 17, while all patients with coexisting CAD had three vessels disease and significant impairment of left ventricular function. In group II, CAD was associated with AAA in 11 patients and with AIOD in 7. The aortoiliac reconstruction in patients undergoing the one stage procedure was performed on cardiopulmonary bypass (CPB) and moderate hypothermia. There were 3 early postoperative deaths (9.4%) and 5 major nonfatal postoperative complications (15.6%) in group I and II early postoperative deaths (11.1%) in group II. Another 2 patients (11.1%) from group II developed severe respiratory failure which necessitated prolonged ventilatory support, but were successfully weaned from the ventilator. In the two-stage group 14 patients underwent aortoiliac reconstruction 4–9 months after CABG, whereas 2 died of ruptured AAA before receiving the second procedure. Our experience with simultaneous and staged surgery of coexistent AAA/AIOD and demonstrates that a) combined procedures can be performed safely in patients with significant AAA/AIOD and CAD, b) the overall early operative morbidity and mortality after combined surgery compare favorably with the results after CABG in staged surgery as well as with the results after routine CABG in patients with impaired left ventricular function, c) simultaneous operations seem to be beneficial to patients with coexisting AAA and CAD regarding the high risk of aneurysmal rupture, and are saving them the potential morbidity linked to the second procedure, and d) even the management of suprarenal and huge infrarenal AAA can be easier and associated with fewer complications under the protection of CPB

Aims

The objectives of our retrospective non-randomized study were
A) to review our experience with combined surgery in patients with coexisting coronary artery disease (CAD) and major aorto-iliac lesions – abdominal aortic aneurysm (AAA) or severe aorto-iliac occlusive disease (AIOD) and
B) to assess the influence of combined surgery on the early postoperative mortality and complications and to compare the results with those of the two-stage approach in the same sub-group of patients

Patients and methods

In the time period between January 1984 and March 1993 fifty patients with severe CAD and marked symptomatic AI lesions (mean age of 56.6 years) underwent one stage (group I–32 patients) or two stage operation (group II–18 patients). In group II CABG was performed first, followed by the aortoiliac reconstruction 4–9 months later. The preoperative conditions of the patients are presented in Table 1.

Table 1. Preoperative patient data: there is no significant difference between the two groups, as seen by the p-value > 0.05

	group I	group II
Number of patients	32	18
Age	mean 58.7	mean 53.7
Sex male female	29 3	15 3
Stenocardia class*	25-IV 7-III	14-IV 4-III
Coronary artery lesions*	3 VD-32 11-LM	3 VD-18 5-LM
Ejection fraction* < 30% > 30 < 50% > 50%	8 12 12	1 7 p = 0.3372 10 p = 0.1921
Aortoiliac lesions	AAA-15 (4 suprarenal) AID-17	AAA-11 AID-7
Respiratory status	6 COPD	3 COPD
Diabetes	11	7
Hypertension	18	9

VD – vessels disease; LM – left main; COPD – chronic obstructive; pulmonary disease; * – p-value > 0.05

There was no significant difference between the two groups regarding their major clinical and hemodynamic characteristics.

The aortoiliac reconstruction in patients undergoing the one stage procedure was performed on cardiopulmonary bypass (CPB) and moderate hypothermia. We used Yates corrected Chi-square test for significance, 1 d f. 2×2 contengency table for statiscal analysis and comparison of important perioperative variables (stenocardia class, ejection fraction, early mortality, ventilatory support, blood loss).

We applied the following surgical strategy for one stage CABG and AIR:

- Standard preoperative assessment, premedication (Fentanyl-Droperidol), induction of anesthesia (Dromicum-Lysthenon-Pancuronium), ventilation with 100% oxygen and Isoflurane for maintenance.
- Preparation and draping of operative field as for CABG and AIR.
- Median laparotomy with inspection and evaluation of AAA or AIOD, meanwhile obtaining the saphenous vein and preparing distal iliac or femoral arteries (in cases of extended AAA or AIOD).
- Median sternotomy and harvesting of left internal mammary artery (LIMA).
- CPB and core cooling down to 26 °C
- Cross-clamping of ascending aorta and heart arrest with cold crystalloid or blood cardioplegia solution (when EF < 25 %).
- Distal anastomoses (3–5) were performed first:
  - mean clamping time 44 min (32–68)
  - mean duration of CPB 142 min (110–170)
- Following completion of proximal vein graft anastomoses under CPB and moderate hypothermia, the abdominal aorta is cross-clamped above the aneurysm (or proximal Al lesion) without clamping of iliac vessels!
- Resection of AAA and restoration of aorto-iliac continuity with Dacron prosthesis.
- Rewarming, CPB discontinued, and heparin reversal with protamine.
- Careful hemosthasis and insertion of chest and abdominal drains.
- Wound closure of the sternotomy and abdominal incisions.

Results and discussion

The operative and postoperative courses are presented in Table 2. Patients undergoing aortoiliac reconstruction for AAA or AIOD with coexisting severe CAD continue to be a therapeutic and surgical challenge (1–5). Myocardial infarction (MI) following peripheral reconstructive surgery is the leading cause for both early and late mortality.

In our practice between 1979–1984 we registered a high mortality rate (42 %) due to myocardial infarction in a group of vascular patients without clinical evidence of angina.

Consequently the meticulous evaluation of the cardiac function and angiologic status stands out as one of the most important components of the work-up before surgery for AIOD.

Most surgeons still prefer the two-stage approach (CABG first and peripheral vascular reconstruction in the second stage) despite the two ICU stays, repeated blood transfusions, sophisticated monitoring, and longer hospitalisation.

The limited number of one-stage operations may be the reason why recent publications report satisfactory results after simultaneous operative correction of coexistant coronary and vascular lesions.

Table 2. Operative and postoperative patient data. No significant difference is seen between the two groups, as reflected by the statistics (for operative mortality p = 0.7683, for postoperative complications p = 0.9865 etc.)

	group I	group II
Number of patients	32	18
CABG	28 LIMA	1 BIMA; 13 LIMA
Number of coronary grafts per patient	4.6	3.9
AIR	32, 15 resections of AAA (4 suprarenal)	4–9 months later 14 AIR 9 resections of AAA
Total bypass time	142 min (110–170)	102 min (64–140)
Aortic clamping time	44 min (32–68)	43 min (35–65)
Operative mortality*	3 9.3%	2 11.1%
Ventilatory support*	19.1 h (4–14)	36.3 h (2–26)
Postoperative blood loss*	1.58 L (0.6–4.7)	1.84 L (0.6–7.5)
Postop complications*	5 15.6%	2 11.1%
Hospitalisation*	14.8 days (7–32)	12.6 days (7–29)

LIMA – left internal mammary artery; BIMA – bilateral mammary artery; * – p-value > 0.05

Advocates of the one-stage approach point out the high risk of performing one procedure first on the ground of severe concomitant disease (severe CAD with LV disfunction or ruptured AAA) and the potential benefit of performing both at one time. Recent reviews focus predominantly on the concomitant CABG and AAA resection and reconstruction omitting the risks and benefits of the one-stage operation in the large group of patients with coexisting CAD and severe AOID.

We started our retrospective study after the observation that patients were dying of ruptured AAA or were undergoing emergency AIR for severe complicated AIOD after CABG.

The distribution of AAA and AIOD is almost uniform in group I and group II because we believe that the detrimental effect of abdominal aortic cross-clamping and declamping on LV function, the periods of hypertension (risk of AAA rupture) or hypotension (risk of leg ischemia in AIOD) necessitate the same surgical tactic.

There is some controversy between authors about the way to perform the one-stage operation. Rubi and Vicaretti recommend aneurysm repair after discontinuation of CPB. Emery supports the revised technique of Rubi with continued aortic cannulation and full heparinization during the AAA repair. Grebenic, Westaby, and Blackbourne prefer to realize the combined procedure on CPB.

There is no substantial benefit (reduction in MI or mortality) immediately after CABG and a global myocardial injury occurs during the cold cardioplegic arrest with a transient ventricular dysfunction after CPB. During aortic cross-clamping, there is an increase in after load, a rise in left ventricular wall stress, and ensuring subendocardial ischemia.

Combined procedures on CPB spare the detrimental effect of abdominal aortic cross-clamping and declamping on LV function, internal organs are protected by hypothermia, aortoiliac reconstruction is easy to perform because of the lax, non-pulsatile state of the aorta, and the otherwise significant intraoperative heat loss is avoided by rewarming before coming out of CPB.

We strongly believe that the concomitant performance of both procedures in well evaluated cases is the better strategy which saves the patient the potential morbidity and the expense of a second operation.

Future randomized studies are needed to assess the influence of one-stage surgery to coronary patients with coexistent AAA or AIOD and to compare the benefits of this approach to the results of the routine two-stage surgery.

Conclusions

Our experience with simultaneous and staged surgery of coexistant AAA/AIOD and CAD demonstrates that

- Combined procedures can be performed safely in patients with significant AAA/AIOD and CAD;
- The overall early operative morbidity and mortality after combined surgery compare favorably with the results after CABG in staged surgery as well as with the results after routine CABG in patients with impaired left ventricular function;
- Simultaneous operations seem to be beneficial to patients with coexisting AAA and CAD regarding the high risk of aneurysmal rupture and are saving them the potential morbidity and eventually fatal complications linked to the second procedure; and
- Even the management of suprarenal and huge infrarenal AAA's can be easier and associated with fewer complications under the protection of CPB

References

References are available from the author

Author's address:
Prof. Alexander Tschirkov
University Hospital 'St. Ekaterina'
2, P. Slaveikov blvd.
1431 Sofia, Bulgaria

Concomitant carotid and coronary artery disease: Is combined approach warranted?

F. Robicsek, and T. L. Pansegrau

Department of Thoracic and Cardiovascular Surgery, Carolinas Medical Center, Charlotte, North Carolina, USA

Introduction

The common occurrence of carotid artery disease in patients in need of coronary artery bypass surgery is well established with an incidence of 11 to 20% (17). The management of patients with atherosclerosis of the coronary and cerebral circulations is controversial and varies among different institutions. While some reports suggest that the staged procedure with the CEA performed first decreases the risk of cerebral vascular infarct with cardiopulmonary bypass, other investigators, however, have demonstrated that simultaneous CEA and CABG can be performed with no increase inmorbidity or mortality (1–43, 45, 46). To explain this controversy is difficult because of the lack of any controlled randomized study which demonstrates the safety of combined versus staged procedures. There are also numerous additional variables which can effect outcome. In some institutions, the CEA and CABG are performed by two different surgeons, which adds yet another variable. Although there is no hard data to support either stance, it appears each surgeon has a strong personal bias towards one method or the other, thus, making a randomized study difficult.

At our institution, our bias had been to perform a combined CEA/CABG by the same surgeon in patients with critical carotid stenosis who require coronary revascularization. This report summarizes our experience over a six year period presented in the mirror of carotid endarterectomies performed on non coronary patients by the same surgical group during the same period. In addition, we have included the results of our isolated coronary artery bypass grafting patients during this same time period.

Materials and methods

From January 1, 1991 through February 1, 1997, 146 patients underwent combined CEA/CABG. The average age was 67.6 years (range 48–84). During the same time period, there was a second group of 31 patients with average age 68.3 (range 58–84) who underwent isolated CEA followed in 1–4 days by CABG (to be referred to as "staged" CEA/CABG). During this same time period, 923 patients CEA and 5504 patients underwent isolated CABG. Patients who underwent CEA/CABG and other open cadiac procedures simultaneously, such as valve repair/replacement or ventricular aneurysm repair, were excluded from this study. This study is based upon our institutional experience of a surgeon engaged in the practice of both cardiac and vascular surgery.

All patients in either the combined or the staged CEA/CABG group were selected based on their need for coronary revascularization and the presence of severe carotid artery bifurcation stenosis. All these patients were found to have by history and/or physical exam to have significant cerebral vascular disease warranting further investigation by carotid doppler examination and arch and four vessel arteriogram. We defined those with significant carotid artery disease as: 1) a unilateral stenosis of 70% or greater with or without symptoms, 2) 50% or greater stenosis and symptoms, 3) 50% or greater stenosis and contralateral occlusion with or without symptoms. There was no randomization of patients to either group.

As far as surgical technique for combined CEA/CABG is concerned, the chest is opened first and prepared for cannulation in the event that the patient becomes unstable or ischemic based on the electrocardiogram and hemodynamic monitoring. The use of a shunt and patching of carotid arteries was done on a selective basis. Electroencephalography was not used. Perioperative events were defined as those occurring within 30 days of surgery or during the same hospitalization.

Results

The incidence of risk factors for atherosclerotic occlusive coronary and cerebral vascular disease for the combined and staged CEA/CABG group as well as those who sustained a stroke are compared in Fig. 1, 2 and 3. The incidence of a prior CEA was significantly higher in the combined group. Also of note is the fact that the presence of severe bilateral carotid artery disease was significantly higher in the staged group. This may have played a role in their selection to this method since this was a non-randomized retrospective study. A significant risk factor for sustaining a stroke when a combined CEA/CABG was performed was presence of symptomatic carotid artery disease or a contralateral occlusion. In the "staged" group there were no perioperative cardiac complications during the CEA or in the interval prior to

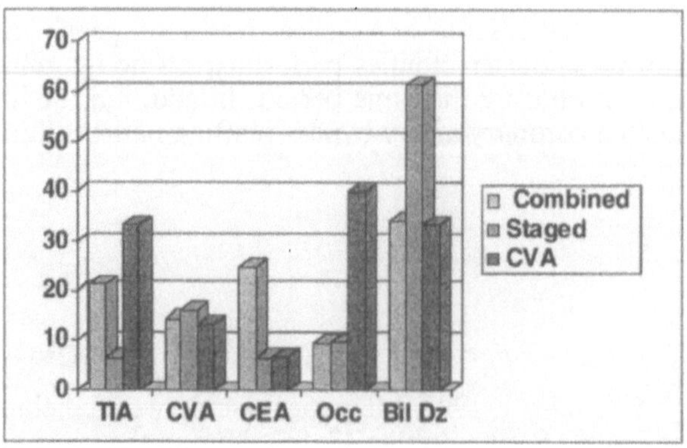

Fig. 1. TIA-Transient ischemic attack, CVA-Prior cerebrovascular accident, CEA-Prior carotid endartectomy, Occ-Contralateral carotid occlusion, Bil Dz-Bilateral carotid artery stenosis > 70%

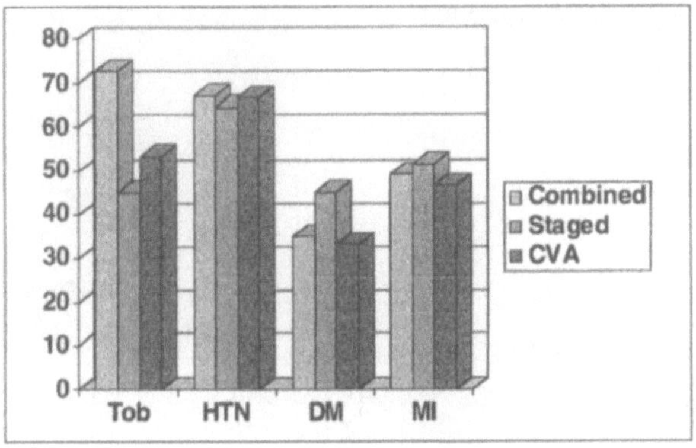

Fig. 2. Tob-History of tobacco abuse, HTN-Hypertension, DM-Diabets Mellitus, MI-prior myocardial infarction

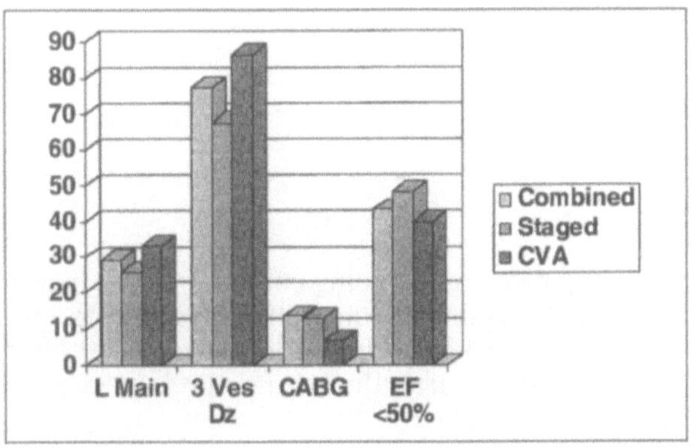

Fig. 3. L Main-Presence of Left main coronary artery disease, 3 Ves Dz-Three vessel coronary artery disease, CABG-prior coronary artery bypass grafting, EF < 50% – left ventricular function < 50%

undergoing CABG. In addition, there were no strokes within this group. The number of coronary artery bypass grafts for the combined staged and stroke group were roughly equivalent for all three groups being 2.8, 3.1, and 2.8 grafts per patients, respectively.

The morbidity and mortality for the simultaneous CEA/CABG group is listed in Table 1. The incidence of a cerebrovascular infarct is 10.3% with 6.8% of the patients sustaining a permanent deficit. Five of the fifteen CVAs (3.4%) occurred more than 48 hours postoperatively but less than two weeks and were embolic in nature and attributed to atrial fibrillation. In addition, there was one vagus nerve injury resulting in vocal cord paralysis and one hypoglossal nerve injury. The causes of death were as follows: one from adult respiratory distress syndrome, two from gastrointestinal bleeding, one from cerebral vascular infarct, respiratory arrest, and one from sepsis.

We compared the results of our combined and staged CEA/CABG to our isolated CEA and our isolated CABG. The results are shown in Table 2.

Table 1. Morbidity and mortality in combined CEA/CABG

Complication	Incidence	%
Cerebrovascular accident (CVA)	15/146	10.3%
Permanent deficit	10/146	6.8%
No deficit post CVA	5/146	3.4%
Other complications	2/146	1.4%
Death	6/146	4.1%

Table 2. Comparison of procedures performed at CMC

Procedure	# of patients	Stroke	%
Asymptomatic CEA	333	3	0.9%
All CEA	923	26	2.8%
CABG	5504	60	1.1%
Combined CEA/CABG	146	15	10.3
Staged CEA/CABG	31	0	0.0%

Discussion

The principal mechanisms of stroke in patients undergoing coronary artery bypass grafting consists of hypoperfusion, athero-embolization from aorta during cannulation, air or clot embolus in the extracorporeal circuit, left side of the heart or ascending aorta. In addition, postoperative arrhythmias, i.e., prolonged atrial fibrillation, may also be a factor as was shown in 5 of these 15 cases.

In Brener's series the rate of neurological complications was higher than anticipated in the combined CEA/CABG group, especially in the presence of a contralateral internal carotid artery occlusion. In patients undergoing only coronary revascularization with severe carotid artery stenosis, he found a 6% incidence of stroke post CABG and 15% if the contralateral carotid was also occluded. As his study progressed, he began to omit the CEA in those patients who were asymptomatic as far as their carotid disease was concerned and found that there was no increase in the incidence of neurologic events. He also favored CEA prior to CABG in those patients with symptomatic carotid artery disease in need of CABG (41). Results with simultaneous CEA/CABG vary when one reviews the literature, where perioperative stroke rates ranging from 0 to 25% (Table 3). According to Berens, the most important predictors of stroke are previous myocardial infarction, left main coronary artery stenosis, and greater than 80% stenosis of the internal carotid artery (3). It has also been shown that myocardial infarction after CEA in patients with severe symptomatic coronary artery disease can be as high as 18% (16).

Several authors have also addressed the issue of staged CEA/CABG with results showing a risk of stroke from 0 to 6.7% and a risk of death from 0 to 33% (Table 4). The "reversed" staged CEA/CABG (i.e., the CABG performed first followed in several days by CEA) has shown very poor results with an incidence of stroke of 11–14% (17, 19). Cambria concluded that optimally carotid bifurcation disease which warranted surgery should be corrected first if the coronary artery disease is clinically stable and appropriate expert anesthesia is available (7). Coyle reviewed their experience at Emory University over a ten year period with simultaneous

Table 3. Combined CEA/CABG

Author	Year	No. patients	Death	Stroke
Bernard (5)	1972	16	0.0% (0)	0.0% (1)
Urschel (46)	1976	8	0.0% (0)	0.0% (0)
Okies (39)	1977	16	6.3% (1)	12.6% (2)
Mehigan (29)	1977	29	13.8% (4)	3.4% (1)
Dalton (13)	1978	25	4.0% (1)	0.0% (0)
Morris (31)	1978	44	4.5% (2)	2.3% (1)
Hertzer (20)	1978	115	4.3% (5)	11.3% (13)
Ennix (16)	1979	51	5.9% (3)	0.0% (0)
Rice (40)	1980	54	0.0% (0)	3.7% (2)
Reichart (38)	1982	15	0.0% (0)	0.0% (0)
Craver (11)	1982	68	0.0% (0)	7.5% (5)
Korompoi (24)	1982	13	7.7% (1)	0.0% (0)
Schwartz (43)	1982	73	9.6% (7)	1.4% (1)
Curling (12)	1982	62	0.0% (0)	0.0% (0)
O'Donell (33)	1983	22	4.5% (1)	4.5% (1)
Hertzer (21)	1983	331	5.7% (19)	9.0% (30)
Emery (15)	1983	42	5.0% (2)	7.1% (3)
Jones (23)	1984	132	3.0% (4)	1.6% (2)
Berkoff (4)	1984	16	6.3% (1)	6.3% (1)
Rosenthal (42)	1984	24	0.0% (0)	0.0% (0)
Furlan (18)	1985	115	NR	7.9% (8)
Perler (35)	1985	61	11.4% (7)	4.9% (3)
Babu (1)	1985	62	4.8% (3)	4.8% (3)
Cosgrove (9)	1986	74	4.1% (3)	12.3% (6)
Lord (25)	1986	78	6.4% (5)	6.4% (5)
Ivey (22)	1986	4	25.0% (1)	25.0% (1)
Reul (39)	1986	143	4.2% (6)	2.8% (4)
Dunn (14)	1986	130	4.6% (6)	10.0% (13)
Brener (6)	1987	57	10.5% (6)	8.8% (5)
Newman (32)	1987	10	0.0% (0)	10.0% (1)
Lubicz (26)	1987	40	5.0% (2)	10.0% (4)
Perler (36)	1988	30	13.3 (4)	6.7% (2)
Minami (30)	1988	47	2.1% (1)	2.1% (1)
Cambria (7)	1989	71	2.8% (2)	4.2% (3)
Hertzer (19)	1989	131	5.3% (7)	5.3% (7)
Faggioli (17)	1990	19	0.0% (0)	0.0% (0)
Pome (37)	1991	52	0.0% (0)	5.7% (3)
Bass (2)	1992	99	12.1% (12)	17.2% (17)
Rizzo (41)	1992	127	5.5% (7)	5.5% (7)
Vermulen (45)	1992	230	3.5% (8)	6.1% (14)
Berens (3)	1992	45	11.1% (5)	11.1% (5)
Chang (8)	1994	189	2.1% (4)	3.7% (7)
Coyle (10)	1994	65	10.8% (7)	15.4% (10)
Mackey (27)	1996	100	8.0% (8)	9.0% (9)
Takach (44)	1997	255	3.9% (10)	3.9% (10)
CMC series	1997	146	4.1% (6)	10.3% (15)
Total		3315	5.0% (171)	6.8% (226)

Table 4. Staged CEA/CABG

Author	Year	No. patients	Death	Stroke
Bernhard (5)	1972	15	33.3% (5)	6.7% (1)
Urschel (46)	1976	8	0.0% (0)	0.0% (0)
Mehigan (29)	1977	23	4.3% (1)	4.3% (1)
Morris (31)	1978	35	20-0% (0)	0.0% (0)
Hertzer (20)	1978	59	1.7% (1)	3.1% (2)
Cosgrove (9)	1986	24	0.0% (0)	0.0% (0)
Ivey (22)	1986	5	0.0% (0)	0.0% (0)
Reul (39)	1986	164	4.9% (8)	2.4% (4)
Hertzer (19)	1989	24	4.2% (1)	4.2% (1)
Coyle (10)	1994	45	2.2% (1)	4.4% (2)
Takach (44)	1997	257	1.6% (4)	1.9% (5)
CMC Series	1997	29	0.0% (0)	0.0% (0)
Total		688	4.1% (28)	2.3% (16)

CEA/CABG and came to a similar conclusion that only very high risk patients with both symptomatic carotid and coronary disease should undergo a simultaneous procedure (10). Their experience, like ours, suggested that delaying CABG by several days will reduce the overall stroke morbidity and mortality.

Conclusion

Before reviewing this data, it was our impression that the management of patients with severe carotid bifurcation disease and in need of coronary revascularization was a simultaneous CEA/CABG. Our reasoning behind this was based on the beliefs that on one hand if the carotid artery were not repaired the rate of CVA would be increased because of presumed decreased perfusion pressure during cardiopulmonary bypass. On the other hand the combined operation could be done with one anesthetic, saving the patient a second operation, thus, resulting in lower risk. We also felt that the only risk would be a slightly longer operation and possible surgeon fatigue. In reviewing our data, although only retrospective and non randomized, our hypothesis was not confirmed. Based on these results, we feel that carotid endartectomy places an ischemic insult on the brain as does cardiopulmonary bypass. When both are combined in the same setting, the effect may be not merely additive but compounded, thus, increasing the observed stroke rate in the simultaneous CEA/CABG group. We also feel that a randomized study to address this issue of simultaneous versus staged CEA/CABG is greatly needed.

Summary

Purpose: The purpose of this study is to examine the ongoing controversy regarding the strategy of management of patients with severe carotid stenosis who are also in need of coronary revascularization. Methods: A retrospective review of

146 patients with simultaneous carotid endarterectomy (CEA) and coronary artery bypass grafting (CABG) between January 1, 1991 and February 1, 1997 was conducted. During this same time period 31 patients underwent "staged" CEA followed in 1–3 days by CABG. The occurrence of cerebrovascular complications in these two groups was compared to two control groups: 1) CABG only and 2 CEA only. Results: During the study period, 15 patients (10.2%) in the combined CEA/CABG group sustained a cerebral vascular accident in the post operative period with 10 patients (6.8%) having a permanent deficit as a result. This was compared to the rate of stroke which was 1.1% for CABG only, 0.9% for unilateral asymptomatic CEA and 2.8% for all CEA. There were neither cardiac nor cerebral complications in the 31 patients who had "staged" CEA followed by CABG. Conclusions: We conclude that a CEA even if uneventful is an ischemic insult to the brain to which CABG may add a second ischemic insult. Furthermore, these two events are not merely additive but compounded, which explains the higher stroke rate observed in the combined group. In reviewing this data, we conclude that the strategy of staging should be applied with the CEA first followed by CABG on a subsequent day during the same hospitalization. With the excellent quality of anesthesia today, the risk of myocardial infarction should be acceptably low.

References

1. Babu SC, Shah PM, Semel L et al. (1985) Coexisting carotid stenosis in patients undergoing cardiac surgery. Indication and guidelines for simultaneous operations. Am J Surg 150: 207–211
2. Bass A, Krupsk WC, Dilley RB, et al. (1992) Combined carotid endartectomy and coronary artery revascularization: A sobering review. Isr J Med Sci 28: 27–32
3. Behrens ES, Kouchoukos NT, Murphy SF, et al. (1992) Preoperative carotid artery screening in elderly patients undergoing cardiac surgery. J Vasc Surg 15: 313–323
4. Berkoff HA, Turnipseed W (1984) Patient selection and results of simultaneous coronary and carotid artery procedures. Ann Thorac Surg 2: 172–175
5. Bernhard VM, Johnson WD, Peterson JJ (1972) Carotid artery stenosis: Association with surgery for coronary artery disease. Arch Surg 105: 837–840
6. Brener BJ, Brief DK, Alpert J et al. (1987) The risk of stroke in patients with asymptomatic carotid stenosis undergoing cardiac surgery: a follow-up study. J Vasc Surg 5: 269–279
7. Cambria RP, Ivarson BL, Akins CW et al (1989) Simultaneous carotid and coronary disease: Safety of the combined approach. J Vasc Surg 9: 56–64
8. Chang BB, Darling C, Shah DM, et al. (1994) Carotid endartectomy can be safely performed with acceptable mortality and morbidity in patients requiring coronary artery bypass grafts. Am J. Surg 168: 94–96
9. Cosgrove DM, Hertzer NR, Loop FD (1986) Surgical management of synchronous carotid and coronary artery disease. J Vasc Surg 4: 690–692
10. Coyle KA, Gray BC, Smith RB, et al. (1995) Morbidity and mortality associated with carotid endartectomy: effect of adjunctive coronary revascularization. Ann Vasc Surg 10: 921–927
11. Craver JM, Murphy DA, Jones EL, et al. (1982) Concomitant carotid and coronary artery reconstruction. Am Surg 195: 712–720
12. Curling PE, Murphy DA, Kaplan JA, et al. (1982) Concomitant carotid and coronary artery surgery: Anaesthetic, Management, Morbidity and Mortality. Anesthesiol 57: A74
13. Dalton ML, Parker TM, Mistrot JJ, et al. (1978) Concomitant coronary artery bypass and major noncardiac surgery. J Thorac Cardiovasc Surg 75: 621–624
14. Dunn EJ (1986) Concomitant cerebral and myocardial revascularization. Surg Clin North Am 66: 385–395
15. Emery RW, Cohn LH, Wittemore AD, et al. (1983) Coexistent carotid and coronary artery disease. Surgical management. Arch Surg 118: 1035–1038

16. Ennix CL, Lawrie GM, Morris GC, et al. (1979) Improved results of carotid endartectomy in patients with symptomatic coronary disease: an analysis of 1546 consecutive carotid operations. Stroke 10: 122–125
17. Faggioli GL, Curl GR, Ricotta JJ (1990) The role of carotid screening before coronary artery bypss. J Vasc Surg 12: 724–731
18. Furlan AJ, Cracium AR (1985) Risk of stroke during coronary artery bypass graft surgery in patients with internal carotid arteryt disease documented by angiography. Stroke 16: 797–799
19. Hertzer NR, Loop FD, Beven EG, et al. (1989) Surgical staging for simultaneous coronary and carotid disease: a study including prospective randomization. J Vasc Surg 9: 455–463
20. Hertzer NR, Loop FD, Taylor PC, et al. (1978) Staged and combinedsurgical approach to simultaneous carotid and coronary vascular disease. Surgery 84: 803–811
21. Hertzer NR, Loop FD, Taylor PC, et al. (1983) Combined myocardial revascularization and carotid endartectomy. Thorac Cardiovasc Surg 85: 577–589
22. Ivey TD (1986) Combined carotid and coronary disease – A conservative strategy. J Vasc Surg 3: 687–689
23. Jones EL, Craver JM, Michalik RA, et al. (1984) Combined carotid and coronary operations: When are they necessary? J Thorac Cardivasc Surg 87: 7–16
24. Korompoi FL, Hayward RH, Knight WL (1982) Non-cardiac operations combined with coronary artery bypass. Surg Clin North Am 62: 215–224
25. Lord RSA, Graham AR, Shanahan MX, et al. (1986) Rationale for simultaneous carotid endartectomy and aortocoronary bypass. Ann Vasc Surg 1: 201–207
26. Lubicz S, Kelly A, Field PL, et al. (1987) Combined carotid and coronary surgery. Aust NZ J Surg 57: 593–597
27. Mackey WC, Khabbaz K, Bojar R, et al. (1996) Simultaneous carotid endartectomy and coronary bypass: Perioperative risk and long-term survival. J Vasc Surg 24: 58–64
28. McKhann GM, Goldsborough MA, Borowicz LM, et al. (1997) Predictors of stroke risk in coronar artery bypass patients. Ann Thorac Surg 63: 516–521
29. Mehigan JT, Buch WS, Pipkin RD, et al. (1976) A planned approach to coexistent cerebrovascular disease in coronary arteries. J Thorac Cardiovasc Surg 72: 829–834
30. Minami K, Sago KS, Breymann T, et al. (1988) Operative strategy in combined coronary and carotid artery disease. J Thorac Cardiovasc Surg 95: 303–309
31. Morris GC, Ennix CL, Lawrie GM, et al. (1978) Management of coexistent carotid and coronary artery occlusive atherosclerosis. Clev Clin Q 45: 125–127
32. Newman DC, Hicks RG, Horton DA (1987) Coexistent carotid and coronary arterial disease. J Cardiovasc Surg 28: 599–606
33. O'Donnell TF, Callow AD, Willet C, et al. (1983) The impact of coronary artery disease on carotid endartectomy. Ann Surg 198: 705–712
34. Okies JE, McManus Q, Starr A (1977) Myocardial revascularization and carotid endartectomy. A combined approach. Ann Thorac Surg 23: 560–563
35. Perler BA, Burdick JF, Williams GM (1985) The safety of carotid endartectomy at the time of coronary artery bypass surgery. Analysis of results in a high risk patient population. J Vasc Surg 2: 558–562
36. Perler BA, Burdick JF, Minken SL, et al. (1988) Should we perform carotid endarterectomy synchronously with cardiac surgical procedures? J Vasc Surg 8: 402–409
37. Pome G, Passini L, Colucci V, et al. (1991) Combined surgical approach to coexistent carotid and coronary artery disease. J Cardiovasc Surg 32: 787–793
38. Reichart B, Becker HM, Autenrieth G, et al. (1982) Stenosis of the supraaortic branches combined with coronary artery disease: One-staged surgical treatment. Thorac Cardiovasc Surgeon 30: 269–372
39. Reul GJ, Cooley DA, Duncan M, et al. (1986) The effect of coronary bypass on the outcome of peripheral vascular operations in 1093 patients. J Vasc Surg 3: 788–798
40. Rice PL, Pifarre R, Sullivan HJ et al. (1980) Experience with simultaneous myocardial revascularization and carotid endartectomy. J Thorac Cardiovasc Surg 79: 922–925
41. Rizzo RJ, Whittemore AD, Couper GS, et al. (1992) Combined carotid and coronary revascularization: the preferred approach to the severe vasculopath. Ann Thorac Surg 54: 1099–1109
42. Rosenthal D, Caudill DR, Lamis PA, et al. (1984) Carotid and coronary arterial disease: a ratinal approach. Am Surg 50: 233–235
43. Schwartz RL, Garrett JR, Karp RB, et al. (1982) Simultaneous myocardial revascularization and carotid endartectomy. Circulation 66: I, 97–101

44. Takach TJ, Reul GJ, Cooley DA, et al. (1997) Is an integrated approach warranted for severe concomitant coronary artery and carotid artery occlusive disease? Ann Thor Surg 64: 16–22
45. Vermulen FEE, Ruben PH, Hamerlijnck M, et al. (1992) Synchronous operation for ischemic cardiac and cerebrovascular disease: early results and long-term follow-up. Ann Thorac Surg 53: 381–390
46. Urschel HC, Razzuk MA, Gardner MA (1976) Management of concomitant occlusive disease of the carotid and coronary arteries. J Thor Cardiovasc Surg 72: 829–834

Author's address:
Francis Robicsek, M.D., Ph.D.
Carolinas Heart Institute
1000 Blythe Boulevard
Charlotte, North Carolina 28203, USA

Indication and results of combined CABG and carotid endarterectomy

L. Salaymeh, W. Amann, H. E. Mächler, G. Gutschi, D. Dacar, B. Rigler

Univ. Klinik für Chirurgie, Klin. Abt. für Herzchirurgie, Graz, Austria

Introduction

Between 1986 and March 1997 100 patients with coronary artery disease and carotid artery stenosis underwent combined CABG and carotid endarterectomy.

Indication

Patients with stable (n = 60) and unstable (n = 24) angina pectoris according to Braunwald class I and II were included in the study. Sixteen patients had a history of myocardial infarction. Patients in Braunwald class III were excluded due to primarily higher risk. All stenosis of the carotid artery were diagnosed by duplex sonography as well as angiography. The indications for carotid endarterectomy were transient neurological events in 38 patients and in 62 cases highgrade (80% stenosis) but asymptomatic carotid artery stenosis.

Methods

The discussed group represented 4.5% of all CABG operations performed during this period. The surgical procedures were always performed by cardiac and vascular surgeons. In all cases carotid endarterectomy was performed prior to CABG while harvesting the saphanous vein. Patient demographics are given in Tables 1 and 2 (Fig. 1)

Table 1. Patient Demographics

Sex m/f	100/20
Mean age	64.5
Diabetes	99/21
Hyperchol.	85
Hypertonus	90
Unstable AP	35
Myocardial Infarc.	63
CAD (I/II/III/LM)	12/24/94/8

Table 2. Patient Demographics

Bilat. Carotis Sten	64
Preoperative Neuro.	
Asymptomtic	82
Prev. Stroke	5
Symptomatic	33
Postoperative Neuro.	
Stroke	2
IIIb	3
EF	60.8%

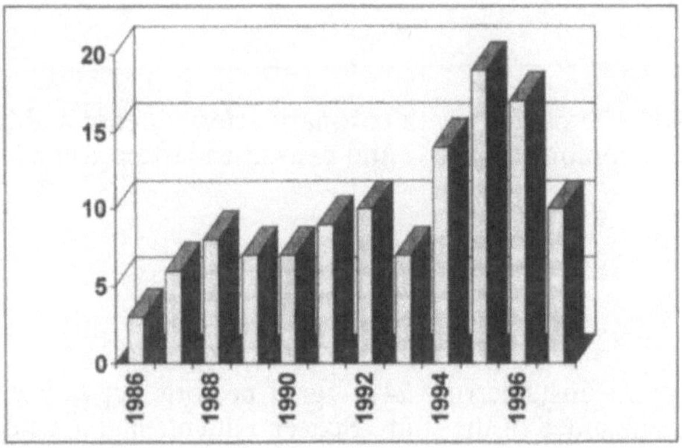

Fig. 1. Operations 1986 – march 1997

Results

The thirty-day mortality was 3% (n = 3). Two on died on the first postoperative day because of cardiac failure. One of them the 18th postoperative day because of pneumonia. Two patients had postoperative transient neurological events (Table 3).

Table 3. Morbidity and 30 day mortality

Morbidity:	
– Stroke	6.0% (n = 5)
– Trans. neurol. events	3.6% (n = 3)
– IABP	2.4% (n = 2)
Mortality (30 day):	
– 3.6% (n = 3), 2 pts because of cardiac failure and 1 pt. because of multi-organ-failure	

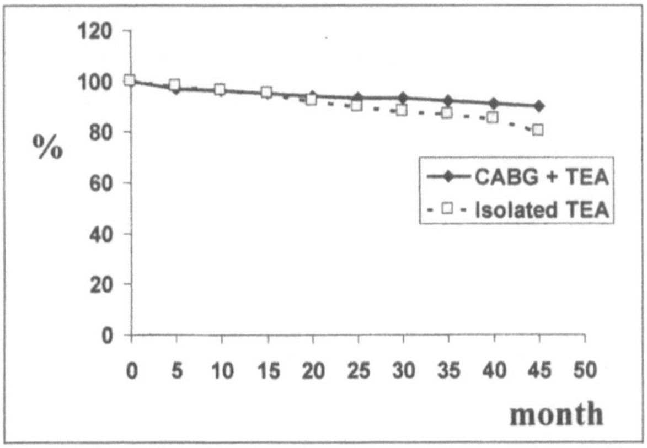

Fig. 2. Survival rate after combined CABG and CEA versus isolated CEA

Conclusion

The results are similiar to those of isolated TEA procedures. Thus, we conclude that combined surgery for severe coronary artery and carotid artery disease (performed by an experienced surgeon) is a safe procedure and can be performed with low mortality and morbidity (Fig. 2).

Author's address:
Luay Salaymeh, M.D.
Univ. Klinik für Chirurgie
Klin. Abt. für Herzchirurgie
Auenbruggerplatz 29
8036 Graz, Austria

Retrospective analysis of simultaenous carotid endarterectomy and coronary artery bypass grafting

M. K. H. Fritz, B. Rosada, T. Weiß[1], A. M. Laczkovics

Department of Thoracic and Cardiovascular Surgery, [1]Departement of Anesthesiology, Ruhr-University, Bergmannsheil Bochum, Germany

Introduction

The coexistence of carotid artery stenosis with coronary artery disease occurs in a small percentage of patients requiring open heart surgical procedures. These patients are individuals at high risk for myocardial infarction and stroke. Whether the combined surgical approach favorably influences the outcome of patients requiring major cardiac operations remains controversial.

The aim of this study is to compare the neurological outcome after simultaneous carotid endarterectomy and coronary heart disease and after cardiac surgery alone in patients with carotid artery stenosis of more than 70%.

Material and methods, Results

75 patients were examined. Simultaneous carotid and cardiac surgery was done in 43 patients (examination group). The other 32 patients underwent cardiac operation only (control group). Both groups were similar in symptoms and signs.

There were 16 unilateral and 27 bilateral carotid stenosis in the examination group, of these 8 patients were symptomatic. Eight patients (18%) had postoperative stroke or neurological deficiency.

In the control group we found 19 patients with unilateral and 13 patients with bilateral carotid stenosis. Only 2 patients (6%) developed neurologic complications or suffered from stroke.

Conclusion

We, therefore, advise simultaneous cardiac and carotid artery surgery only in symptomatic patients or in patients with 90% stenosis or more.

Author's address:
M. K. H. Fritz, M.D.
Klinik für Herz- und Thoraxchirurgie
Berufsgenossenschaftliche Kliniken Bergmannsheil
Bürkle-De-La-Camp-Platz 1
44789 Bochum, Germany

Intraaortic balloon pump assist in patients with peripheral arterial disease

S. Beholz, H. Grubitzsch, K. Ansorge, H.-G. Wollert, L. Eckel

Department of Thoracic and Cardiovascular Surgery, Klinikum Karlsburg, Germany

Introduction

Peripheral vascular disease is known to be one of the most frequent concomitant diseases in patients undergoing open heart surgery, especially coronary artery bypass grafting. Perioperative morbidity is influenced by the age, the preoperative status, and the pattern of concomitant diseases.

In the last 30 years the intra-aortic balloon pump has proven to be a helpful tool in the treatment of patients with left ventricular heart failure due to myocardial infarction or after cardiac surgery since the first clinical application by Kantrowitz and colleagues [7]. Nowadays implantation is performed earlier, even preoperatively to prevent myocardial stunning in patients suffering from unstable angina [9]. Reviewing the literature, an implantation rate of 1.5 to 6.2% after coronary artery bypass grafting can be obtained [4–6, 8] with an emphasis on re-do and emergency procedures [4]. The most frequent complication due to the most often used transfemoral approach is lower limb ischemia; the risk for this is reported to be elevated in patients with peripheral vascular disease [3]. We retrospectively investigated our patients to see if intraaortic balloon pumping using the transfemoral percutaneous approach is influenced by the presence of significant peripheral vascular disease.

Material and methods

From April 1995 to September 1997, 1856 patients underwent open heart procedures in our institution. These procedures included all kinds of aquired heart diseases in adults, most of them coronary artery bypass grafting procedures, aortic and mitral valve replacement or reconstruction, and combined procedures. Due to low output syndrome postoperatively, 81 patients (4.4%) required intraaortic balloon pump assisst, two of them a second time in the postoperative course due to recurrent left ventricular failure. Additionally 6 patients required IABP-assist due to left heart failure in myocardial infarction or unstable angina without undergoing cardiac surgery. In total 89 balloon pump assists were performed in 87 patients. Mean age was 64.7 ± 8.4 years. Sixteen of the patients (18.4%) suffered from peripheral vascular disease preoperatively. In 4 (25%) of these implantation was performed using the transthoracic approach due to extensive calcification of the femoral vessels. Transfemoral approach was performed in 87.6% of all implantations. Assist was performed for 47.1 (1–209) hours.

Lower limb ischemia did not occur in patients using the transfemoral approach but in 5.9% of the patients without significant arteriosclerosis (Table 1). This required balloon removal in 2 patients. Femoral artery thrombembolectomy was not

Table 1. Vascular complications with and without peripheral vascular disease

	Percutaneous transfemoral implantation of intraaortic balloon pump				
	Peripheral vascular disease				total
	with		without		
	n	%	n	%	
lower limb ischemia	0	0	4	5.9	5.1
major amputation	0	0	0	0	0
bleeding	0	0	1	1.5	1.3
infection	0	0	0	0	0
groin haematoma	0	0	0	0	0
ballon entrappment	0	0	2	2.9	2.6
gas loss	0	0	1	1.5	1.3

necessary in any patients. One patient without peripheral vascular disease suffered from repetitive thromboembolism in the femoral artery after balloon removal, requiring major amputation in spite of multiple revascularizations. Balloon entrappment by dried blood due to chronic and silent aspiration required an open technique for removal in two patients without peripheral vascular disease. Bleeding from the punction site occured in one patient without arteriosclerosis. One balloon had to be changed due to gas loss.

In patients requiring transthoracic implantations (n = 10) two severe complications were observed as reported earlier: in one patient a guide wire of the balloon coiled in the aortic arch, requiring another surgical intervention for removal including extracorporeal circulation and aortotomy [1]; in another patient a complete paraplegia due to dissection of the descending aorta with partial thrombosis occured [2]. No further complications were observed.

Total complication rate of intraaortic balloon pump assist was 11.2% in all patients. Mortality in all patients was 52.8%, in the patients requiring the transthoracal approach mortality was 70%.

Discussion

The intraaortic balloon pump is a helpful tool in patients suffering from left ventricular failure following procedures in open heart surgery and myocardial infarction. It reduces afterload of the left ventricle, improves mean arterial pressure by diastolic augmentation, and thereby improves myocardial perfusion in diastole. Perioperative mortality in patients with low cardiac output can be reduced by early implantation [9]. Transthoracic implantation can be performed in patients after procedures in open heart surgery; this sometimes requires one to leave the chest or at least the sternum open. Then a second intervention for closure of the sternum and/or explantation of the balloon is necessary and associated with rare but severe complications as mediastinitis, balloon rupture, and stroke [8]. Therefore, transfemoral implantation should be performed whenever possible. In our patients we found no significant difference between patients with or without peripheral vascular disease concerning the rate of vascular complications. Even the most severe complications occurred in patients without any signs of peripheral vascular disease.

Conclusions

In our experience moderate peripheral vascular disease seems not to be a contraindication for transfemoral intraaortic balloon pump assist. A careful attempt should be done for percutaneous insertion using the usual Seldinger technique avoiding transthoracic implantation which is associated with even more severe complications. Only in cases of severe peripheral vascular disease, e.g. Leriche-Syndrome or aortic aneurysms with thrombotic areas a primary transthoracic approach should be used. Exact physical examination and routinely non-invasive vascular examination as doppler examination are recommended.

References

1. Beholz S, Ansorge K, Wollert HG, Eckel L Rare complications in intra-aortic balloon pump assist – three case reports. Eur J Cardio-thoracic Surg. submitted for public
2. Beholz S, Braun J, Ansorge K, Wollert HG, Eckel L Paraplegia caused by aortic dissection after intraaortic balloon pump assist [Letter]. Ann Thor Surg in press
3. Busch T, Sîrbu H, Zenker D, Dalichau H (1997) Vascular complications related to intraaortic balloon Counterpulsation: An analysis of then years experience. Thorac Cardiovasc Surg 45: 55–59
4. Christenson JT, Buswell L, Velebit V, Maurice J, Simonet F, Schmuziger M (1995) The intraaortic balloon pump for postcardiotomy heart failure. Experience with 169 intraaortic balloon pumps. Thorac Cardiovasc 43: 129–133
5. Del-Rizzo DF, Fremes SE, Christakis GT, Sever J, Goldmann BS (1996)
6. Hedenmark J, Ahn H, Henze A, Nystrom SO, Svedjeholm R, Tyden H (1988) Complications of intra-aortic balloon counterpulsation, with special reference to limb ischemia. Scand J Thorac Cardiovasc Surg 22: 123–125
7. Kantrowitz A, Tjonneland S, Freed PS, Phillips SJ, Butner AN, Sherman JL Jr (1968) Initial clinical experience with intraaortic balloon pumping in cardiogenic shock. JAMA 203: 113–118
8. McGeehin W, Sheikh F, Donahoo JS (1987) Transthoracic intraaortic balloon support: Experience in 39 patients. Ann Thorac Surg 44: 26–30
9. Torchiana DF, Hirsch G, Buckley MJ, Hahn C, Allyn JW, Akins CW, Drake JF, Newell JB, Austen GW (1997) Intraaortic balloon pumping for cardiac support: Trends in practice and outcome, 1968 to 1995. J Thorac Cardiovasc Surg 113: 758–769

Author's address:
Sven Beholz, M.D.
Department of Cardiovascular Surgery
Klinikum Karlsburg
Greifswalder Str. 11A
17495 Karlsburg, Germany

Role of total arterial revascularization in the concomitant disease

A. M. Calafiore, G. Vitolla

Department of Cardiac Surgery, "G. D'Annunzio" University, Chieti, Italy

Introduction

There is no doubt that grafting the left internal mammary artery (LIMA) on the left anterior descending (LAD) artery is the single most important surgical aspect for the long-term survival and for a longer event free survival (5) of patients that undergo myocardial revascularization. This artery, due to its structural properties, (lack of fenestrations in the lamina interna, tunica media basically elastic) showed anatomical instability with time and a resistance to atherosclerosis that made this conduit unique. However, there is no clear evidence that more than an arterial anastomoses (on the LAD) can improve survival or increase the event free interval after surgery. Nevetheless, in the last 10 years multiple arterial grafting became a trend in myocardial revascularization. Bilateral mammary artery grafting became often a routine practice, and the use of other arterial conduits were explored to increase the possibility of arterial revascularization. These conduits, however, are definitively different from IMA, because of basically muscular media and the presence of fenestrations in the lamina interna. On the other side the widespread diffusion of coronary angioplasty, due to improved results with stenting, increased the percentage of patients with so-called high risk factors for coronary surgery. A subgroup of these patients is the one that includes surgical candidates with organ dysfunction that, by itself, can limit the life expectancy and can increase at least the postoperative morbidity and, sometimes, the 30 day mortality. Before analyzing this cohort of patients, we will briefly describe the arterial conduits currently used and the strategy we used.

Arterial conduits

Harvesting technique

Internal mammary artery

This graft is usually harvested as a pedicle from its origin (or more) up to its bifurcation. The cautery is widely used to cut the muscle and the branches are burned or clipped. The fascia, the satellite veins, and a generous portion of muscle is harvested with the IMA. The artery is then injected with 5 ml of the same papaverine solution, and its distal tip occluded with an homoclip (1). Any bleeding from small collaterals is explored.

Since 1994 we changed our technique and harvested the IMA skeletonized. The graft is carefully dissected and the branches are isolated, clipped, and divided with the fine scissors. The IMA is completely lacking of the fascia and any surrounding tissue. This allows one to obtain a longer graft (after papaverine injection there is a mean increase of length of 15–20%) and, furthermore, to reduce the sternal devascularization that follows bilateral IMA harvesting. De Jesus and Acland (4) demonstrated that the three side branches of the IMA (sternal, muscular, and intercostal) have often a common origin. If we do not use the cautery and use the hemoclip and scissors, the sternal vascularization will be reduced only of about 1/3, instead of 3/4 as in the IMA harvesting as a pedicle. This technical aspect is crucial, as not only we have two long conduits, but also many classic contraindications to the use of BIMA (diabetes, obesity, COPD) lose their importance.

Right gastroepiploic artery (RGEA)

This in situ graft, introduced in the 1980s (7), is gaining popularity because its position is ideal for right coronary artery (RCA) system arterial revascularization; as the less diseased vessel, the posterior descending artery (PDA), is easy to reach. As the tunica media is basically muscular, this graft is prone to spasm. During the surgery, all the techniques that can limit this phenomenon (intraluminal injection of papaverine or verapamil, normothermia, etc.) have to be used.

Radial artery (RA)

Introduced in the 1970s, this conduit was renewed in the late 1980s, as the first experience was unsatisfying (2, 3). As this conduit is muscular, to optimize its use, a high flow situation has to be provided (occluded or severely stenotic territory). A reduced flow in the graft means a string sign or an occlusion, as the graft adapts to the amount of flow modifying its internal size. The proximal anastomosis can be performed on the ascending aorta or on a mammary artery.

Inferior epigastric artery (IEA)

This conduit, introduced in the late 1980s, is the ideal prolongation of a branch of the mammary artery (6). However the IEA, if harvested for the whole length, is not ideal, as the distal size is small. We only use the proximal portion (up to the 1st muscular branch to the rectus muscle), where the diameter is about 2 mm. Because the length is about 6–8 cm, we use the IEA as a side branch or an elongation of the mammary artery. As all the muscular conduits, this conduit has to be used in territories with an expected high run off. However, its small length limits its surgical interest.

Surgical strategy

We do believe that both IMA have to be utilized in every patient and that the proper use of BIMA is the key point of a correct myocardial revascularization. The two conduits have to be grafted to the left system, in situ if possible (RIMA to LAD and LIMA to the marginal branches) or as a Y graft, if the RIMA is not long enough or both conduit have to be used for sequential grafting.

The RIMA can be used also in the circumflex territory, passing beneath or over the aorta, but its use to a diagonal branch or the main right coronary artery has to be limited to selected cases (diagonal branch that is, really, a high marginal branch or very soft and not diseased RCA).

The radial artery is a compulsory free graft and the conduit of choice if the RIMA is not used. This conduit is long and has a good size, can be easily managed, and, from the technical point of view, is more similar to the saphenous vein than to the IMA. We recommend to use this graft as a Y graft from the LIMA, performing the proximal anastomosis as the first step. We believe that the proximal anastomosis to the ascending aorta has potential problems. In fact the ascending aorta can be diseased there is always a mismatch between the two walls, and the proximal size of the free graft in generally small. There are also some philosophical consideration, not easy to demonstrate, but suggestive. The arterial free gratt, anastomosed to the aorta, is exposed to a dP/dT different than in the native circulation; moreover the wall stress (proportional to the cube of the radius) in the ascending aorta is higher than the one to which the graft is normally exposed.

These two factors can be at the basis of early or midterm graft failure, reported clearly in the literature at least for the IMA (8). For all these reasons we prefer to anastomose the free graft to the IMA, with the idea of better preserving the native environment. From the technical point of view this anastomosis is easier than the one to the aorta (bench surgery) and can be carefully checked before continuing with the operation.

The use of the IEA is similar to that of the RA; however, the limited length (1/3 of the RA) avoids a widespread use of this conduit; its use is limited as a Y graft to a diagonal branch or to a small marginal. The use of skeletonized IMA allowed us to perform any kind of sequential graft; the use of IEA becomes interesting if, for philosophical reasons, sequential grafting is considered potentially dangerous.

The use of RGEA, in our opinion, has to be limited to the RCA system, mainly the PDA. There is no rationale in using this conduit for other coronary vessel, except if other conduits are not available. However, there is a general principle that has to be followed when an alternate arterial conduit is used. Being all muscular grafts, they have to be used when a high flow situation is expected: severe stenosis or occlusion of the target vessel without an expected high run off. Any other situation (basically moderate stenosis of the target vessel or high resistance in the grafted territory) with an expected low flow in the graft will cause an adaptation to the flow, that is a string sign, up to the occlusion of the graft. This is an important issue and has to be considered when a strategy for the single patient is planned.

Clinical experience

Patients with concomitant disease can be divided in two groups: A, disease increases the mortality and/or the morbidity risk; B, the disease will affected only the long-term outcome of the patient.

Group A includes patients with severe COPD, chronic renal failure or dialysis, diffuse peripheral or cerebral vasculopathy, epathic cirrhosis, and coagulation disorders.

Group B includes patients with malignancy, or immunologic disorders.

Other chronic disease, like diabetes, cannot be considered in any group.

There is no doubt that, independent of the underlying disease, a left internal mammary artery is the graft of choice for the LAD. The use of more arterial conduits is not contraindicated in any patients and depends only on the preferred strategy of the surgeon, who is performing the operation. However, strategic issues have to be taken into account.

In patients with chronic renal failure the use of radial and gastroepiploic arteries has to be avoided. The RA can be necessary in the future for dyalisis and a connection between the abdomen and the pericardial cavity; adherences can be potentially dangerous as well if a peritoneal dialysis has to be considered in the future.

If diffuse peripheral vasculopathy is present, attention has to be pad to any disease that involves the origin of the in situ graft (IMAs and RGEA). A severe stenosis of the subclavian artery will advise the use of the IMA as a free graft. If the subclavian artery is occluded, the RA, in our opinion, is not to be used because the reduction of the driving pressure can reduce the amount of collateral circulation in the muscular territory depending by the harvested RA. In the same situation, the IMA has to be explored before being used as free graft, because in many occasions, the internal size is smaller than usual due to underperfusion.

On the contrary in case of diffuse disease of the ascending aorta the use of multiple arterial grafting is mandatory, provided a peripheral disease is not associated. In these cases one or more saphenous vein graft can be anastomosed to one or two IMAs.

In the presence of severe coagulatin defects the use of the saphenous vein should often to be avoided. In these patients the greatest risk factor is, however, the extracorporeal circulation: in this subgrouup, as well as in patients with malignancy and immunologic disorders, myocardial revascularization on a beating heart is the strategy of choice.

From October 1991 to April 1998, 1305 patients underwent total arterial myocardial revascularization. Concomitant disease were present in 390 patients (group A n = 382, group B n = 8). In Table 1 in hospital mortality is shown (23 patients 1.7%). Six year survival and event free survival are shown in Figs. 1 and 2.

Table 1. Total arterial revascularization in patients with severe concomitant disease

	No.	deaths	%	p
Total arterial revascularization Without concomitant disease	965	19	2.0	ns
With concomitant disease	390	4	1.4	

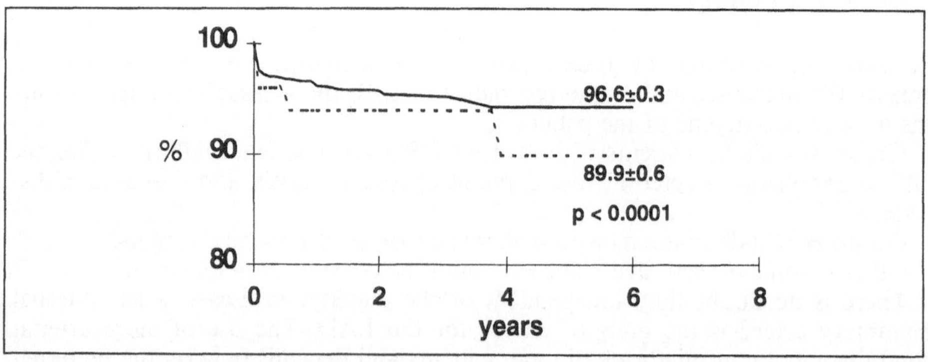

Fig. 1. Six year survival with (········) and without (———) concomitant disease.

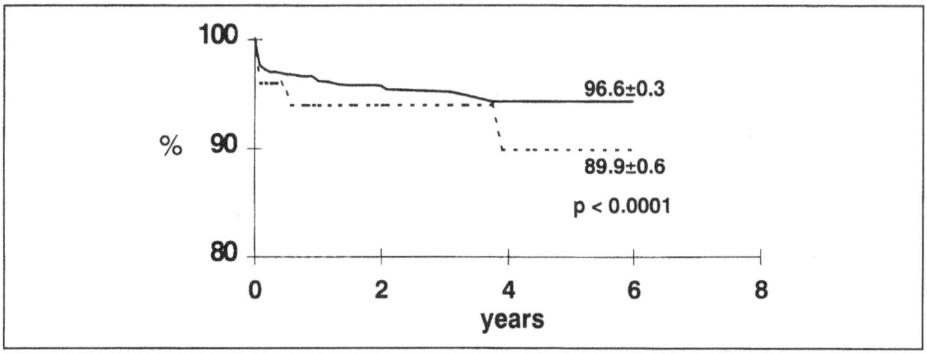

Fig. 2. Six year event free survival with (········) and without (———) concomitant disease.

Conclusions

In this series the presence of a concomitant disease has no influence on early outcome after myocardial revascularization. However, the late survival and long-term survival is significantly worse in this group of patients if compared with patients without concomitant disease. In our opinion, even if the maximum follow up is only 78 months, it is possible that these patientes will not benefit in the long-term of the benefit of the total arterial myocardial revascularization. However, as the early mortality is not increased, the possibility of using only arteries has to be taken into account, as the survival and event free survival curves are nearly coincident. This means that death is the most diffuse event in this group of patients and that those who remain alive have no return of angina, myocardial infarction or repeate revascularization. This is a satisfying target in patients that have, often, reduced life expectancy.

In conclusion, total arterial revascularization in patients with concomitant disease gives good results, improving the quality of life of the patients who survive their disease.

References

1. Calafiore AM, Di Giammarco G, Luciani N, Maddestra N, Di Nardo E, Angelini R (1994) Composite arterial conduits for a wider arterial myocardial revascularization. Ann Thorac Surg 58: 185–190
2. Calafiore AM, Di Giammarco G, Teodori G et al. (1995) Radial artery and inferior epigastric artery in composite grafts: Improved midterm angiographic results. Ann Thorac Surg 60: 517–524
3. Calafiore AM, Teodori G, Di Giammarco G, D'Annunzio E, Angelini R, Vitolla G, Maddestra N (1995) coronary revascularization with the radial artery: New interest for an old conduit. J Card Surg 10: 140–146
4. De Jesus RA and Acland RD (1995) Anatomic Study of the Collateral Supply of the Sternum. Ann Thorac Surg 59: 163–168
5. Loop FD, Lytle BW, Cosgrove DM et al. (1986) Influence of the internal mammary artery graft on 10-year survival and other cardiac events. N Engl J Med 314: 1–6
6. Puig LB, Ciongolli W, Cividanes GVL et al. (1990) Inferior epigastric artery as a free graft for myocardial revascularization. J Thorac Cardiovasc Surg 99: 251–255

7. Suma H, Wanibuchi Y, Terada Y, Fukuda S, Takayama T, Furuta S (1993) The right gastroepiploic artery graft. Clinical and angiographic midterm results in 200 patients. J Thorac Cardiovasc Surg 105: 615–623
8. Verhelst R, Etienne PY, El Koury G, Noirhomme P, Rubay J, Dion R (1996) Free internal mammary artery graft in myocardial revascularization. Cardiovasc Surg 4: 212–216

Author's address:
Antonio Maria Calafiore, MD
Department of Cardiac Surgery
"G. D'Annunzio" University
S. Camillo de' Lellis Hospital
Via C. Forlanini 50
66100 Chieti, Italy

Minimally invasive procedures in patients with severe concomitant disease

J. Cremer, T. Wittwer, M. Strüber, O.E. Teebken, A. Böning, M. Anssar, P. Kim, J. Zuk[1], D. Mehler[1], A. Haverich

Division of Thoracic and Cardiovascular Surgery and [1]Department of Anesthesiology, Hannover Medical School, Hannover, Germany

Introduction

Minimally invasive coronary surgery represents a rapidly developing field strongly influenced by the introduction of new technologies. Some basic principles of these procedures, such as access by minithoracotomies (7), and avoidance of cardiopulmonary bypass (1), were introduced several years ago. But a major breakthrough of such procedures has been attributed to the availability of specific stabilization devices (5), modified retractors (2), video assistance (8), and adapted heart lung machine equipment (10). Although particular approaches of minimally invasive direct coronary artery bypass (MIDCAB) grafting have already been performed in reasonable numbers (3, 12), contraindications and limitations are not yet clearly defined. To get a more precise impression of borderline indications and limitations of MIDCAB revascularization, we evaluated the outcome and complications in patients with comorbidity or anatomic abnormalities.

Material and methods

Surgical technique

Surgical access was gained by use of an anterolateral or anterior minithoracotomy through the 4th or 5th intercostal space following a submammary skin incision (6 to 11 cm). An especially designed retractor system allowed for adequate IMA exposure without resection or subluxation of any part of the ribs (CardioThoracic Systems, Cupertino, California, USA). The left pedicled IMA was isolated at a distance between 8 and 16 cm to facilitate tension-free grafting of anterior (left anterior descending = LAD, diagonal = D) epicardial vessels without the use of video assistance. The anastomoses were performed under mechanical stabilization using one 8-0 running polypropylene suture under systemic heparinization (100 I.U./kg).

Patients

Out of 150 patients who underwent MIDCAB grafting to anterior myocardial vessels since June of 1996 the majority (n = 87) suffered from severe concomitant diseases or presented with abnormal anatomic conditions.

Cardiac findings in these patients also included two vessel (n = 23) and three vessel disease (n = 23) beyond the 41 cases with one vessel disease. Previous myocardial infarction had occurred in 41 patients and 14 revealed unstable angina upon admission. Significant pulmonary hypertension was found in 5 cases of whom 4 had reduced left ventricular ejection fractions below 30%. Interventional approaches were attempted in 18 patients. Moreover, one multi-morbid female with left main stem stenosis (> 70%) had been accepted as interventional treatment appeared unreasonable and conventional surgery was refused (Table 1).

Concomitant diseases

Organ dysfunction

Chronic obstructive pulmonary disease (COPD) was the most frequent preexisting organ dysfunction (n = 20), which required steroid treatment in 7 cases. In addition, lung fibrosis (n = 1) and sarcoidosis (n = 2) were observed. In another 10 patients, the renal function was severely impaired necessitating chronic dialysis in 6 of them. Beyond that, neurologic deficits (n = 16) were occasionally seen resulting from

Table 1. Cardiac findings in 87 patients with comorbidity (PTCA = percutaneous transluminal coronary angioplasty

one vessel disease	41
two vessel disease	23
three vessel disease	23
unstable angina	14
mean ejection fraction ≤ 30%	4
previous myocardial infarction	41
pulmonary hypertension	5
left main stem stenosis	1
previous PTCA/stenting	18

Table 2. MIDCAB and organ dysfunction (COPD = chronic obstructive pulmonary disease)

pulmonary diseases	23
COPD	20
lung fibrosis	1
sarcoidosis	2
renal insufficiency	10
on dialysis	6
neurological deficits	16
previous stroke	11
Parkinson's disease	1
epilepsy	2
previous subdural hematoma	1
dementia	1
hepatic insufficiency	1

Table 3. MIDCAB and vascular disease

• calcification of the ascending aorta/aortic arch	3
• carotid artery stenosis	12
• abdominal aortic aneurysm	3
• peripheral arterial occlusive disease	9
• previous pulmonary embolism	3
• previous deep vein thrombosis	3
• varicosis/saphenectomy	4

Table 4. MIDCAB and disorders of the endocrine system (IDDM = insulin dependent diabetes mellitus)

• IDDM	14
• hyperparathyroidism	2
• thyroid adenoma	1
• hyperthyroidism	2

Table 5. MIDCAB and tumor disease and immunocompromise

• renal cell carcinoma	1
• medistinal metastasis after left upper lobe resection for bronchial carcinoma	1
• melanoma	1
• prostate cancer	1
• chronic immunosuppression following kidney transplant	1

stroke (n =11) or different etiologies (Table 2). Significant hepatic insufficiency with borderline function was found once.

Vascular Diseases

The broad spectrum of vascular comorbidity (Table 3) included a variety of manifestations headed by carotid artery stenoses and peripheral arterial occlusive disease. Extensive calcification of the ascending or entire thoracic aorta (n = 3) was regarded as a contraindication for conventional coronary surgery. History of deep vein thrombosis and pulmonary embolism (n = 3) was also present.

Disorders of the endocrine system malignancies and immuno compromise

Insulin-dependent diabetes mellitus (IDDM) was prediagnosed in 14 patients, in part being candidates for pancreatic or renal transplant. Moreover, hyperthyroidism (n = 2), thyroid adenoma (n = 1), and hyperparathyroidism (n = 2) belong to this entity of diseases (Table 4).

Tumor disease and immuno compromise due to cytostatic or antirejection treatment were present in just a few cases. These particular patients were scheduled for subsequent tumor surgery (n = 3) or on adjuvant chemotherapy/immunosuppression, or had irresectable lesions (Table 5).

Coagulopathies

Preexisting coagulopathies were assessed in 2 patients consisting of von Willebrand's disease (n = 1) or thrombocytopenia below 100,000/μl.

Deformities of the chest or abnormal anatomic conditions

So far none of the patients referred for MIDCAB grafting have been refused secondary to thoracic deformities. Thus, 3 patients with pectus excavatum and one patient with Bechterew's disease were accepted (Table 6). Moreover, 10 cases with previous thoracic access were approached by minimally invasive techniques as well (Table 7). Thereby, the majority had undergone previous open heart surgery via sternotomy. Significant mediastinal shift occurred in one patient after right-sided surgical treatment of tuberculosis. Left upper lobe resection in another patient did not restrict from MIDCAB grafting as well as previous insertion of multiple drainage tubes necessary in left-sided chest traumatization with serial rib fractures.

Obesity

Within our MIDCAB program even extensive obesity was not regarded as an exclusion criteria. The majority of patients had an increased body mass index (BMI) higher than 25 kg/m^2 (Fig. 1). Even values above 35 kg/m^2 were observed in a few cases. The highest value was found in one male with a BMI of 36.16 kg/m^2 (112 kg, 176 cm).

Table 6. MIDCAB and deformities of the chest

• pectus excavatum	3
• mediastinal shift	1
• Bechterew's disease	1

Table 7. MIDCAB and previous thoracic surgery

• left upper lobe resection (left thoracotomy)	1
• previous open heart surgery (sternotomy)	7
• previous surgery for tuberculosis (right thoracotomy)	1
• previous thoracic traumatization with serial (left) rib fractures (multiple drainage tubes)	1

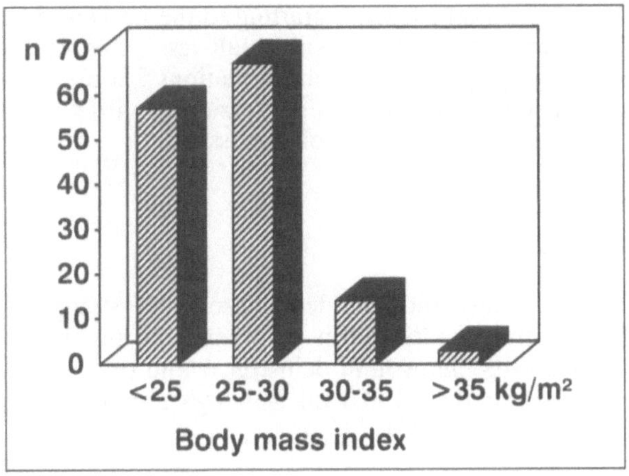

Fig. 1. MIDCAB and obesity

Results

The procedures were usually tolerated well without significant hemodynamic impairment or severe arrhythmias. However, one patient developed ventricular fibrillation while inserting the retractor and was successfully defibrillated allowing for continuation of the procedure.

Mortality

Overall, 3 of the 87 patients died perioperatively. One 68 year old female had a primarily uneventful course despite her complex comorbidity and difficult cardiac situation with three vessel disease, left main stem stenosis, reduced left ventricular ejection fraction, and unstable angina. MIDCAB surgery was requested at any risk as conventional surgery and interventional approaches were refused. She died on postoperative day (POD) 12 due to posterolateral myocardial infarction.

A second male patient, 80 years old, presented with significant COPD and Parkinson's disease associated with compression of the spinal cord after vertebral disc surgery. He too, had an uncomplicated initial course but was found in bronchospasm and hypoxia on POD 3. Thereafter, he did not recover completely and finally died in respiratory failure on POD 52. Another female patient with single vessel disease and calcifica-

Table 8. Postoperative complications (n)

bleeding > 1000 ml/24 h	4
pulmonary atelectasis	2
deterioration of renal function	1
wound dehiscence	1
pericarditis	3
atrial fibrillation	4

tion of the ascending aorta received sequential left IMA grafting to the LAD and D. Extreme vulnerability of the epicardium was combined with small vessel size. In absence of intraoperative complications, she started ventricular fibrillations 5 hours postoperatively. She was taken back to the operating room to get regrafting with venous conduits by conventional means but could not be weaned off bypass.

Postoperative complications

Additional complications (Table 8) were rare and included 2 cases with postoperative atelectasis (requiring bronchoscopy), deterioration of preexisting renal dysfunction, and atrial fibrillation. There was one wound dehiscence, and pericarditis was observed in 3 cases. Bleeding greater than 1,000 ml/24 h was noted 4 times without need for reintervention.

Angiographic results

Early postoperative angiographic control was principally intended except for patients with renal insufficiency. Findings in 56/56 angiographies revealed patent well-functioning grafts in all cases. However, one anastomotic stenosis of about 50% was described. Subsequent interventional procedures according to a hybrid approach were accomplished in 10 of these cases.

Discussion

Among the different minimally invasive approaches in coronary surgery, MIDCAB grafting of the LAD by use of the pedicled LIMA has been widely accepted. Despite the fact that several groups (3, 12) have performed such procedures in reasonable numbers the potential benefit of this procedure in cases of severe comorbidity remains unanswered. This, however, may be of particular importance as especially comorbid patients are exposed to a significantly increased risk when applying extracorporeal circulation (ECC). For example preexisting renal function, cerebral deficits, or COPD have been proven to be associated with a higher a postoperative complication rate (6). Although a statistical analysis was not applied to our patient cohort, the spectrum of complications seems to be different from conventional coronary procedures. In this context it is noteworthy that typical complications of ECC like stroke or other neurological events (9) or systemic inflammation and multiorgan failure (4) were not observed. Even in patients with significant preexisting organ dysfunction, the rate of deterioration or organ specific complications appeared rather low as only 1 of 23 patients had a postoperative critical lung function and one other patient with renal dysfunction and deranged IDDM developed temporary deterioration but did not require dialysis.

Another issue in patient selection and contraindications for MIDCAB procedures deals with chest deformities and abnormal anatomic conditions. Like others (11), it is our experience that chest deformities and previous thoracic surgery have to be individually evaluated. Previous cardiac surgery is not a general contraindication but adequate IMA function has to be assessed preoperatively. In cases with pectus excavatum exposure of the IMA may even be superior.

In the presence of obesity, the procedure becomes obviously more difficult and the required incision length has to be longer but potentially expected complications like wound infections and hematoma were absent in this subgroup.

So far it is concluded that comorbid patients may benefit from MIDCAB procedures avoiding deleterious side effects of ECC. Even in comorbid cases with concomitant disease and multivessel disease, isolated treatment of the culprit lesion or hybrid approaches possess special attraction and can reduce overall complications.

References

1. Benetti FJ, Naselli G, Wood M, Geffner L (1991) Direct myocardial revascularization without extracorporeal circulation. Experience in 700 patients. Chest 100:312–316
2. Boonstra PW, Grandjean JG, Mariani MA (1997) Local immobilization of the left anterior descending artery for minimally invasive coronary bypass grafting. Ann Thorac Surg 63:S76–S78
3. Calafiore AM, Teodori G, Di Giammarco G, Vitolla G, Iaco A, Iovino T, Cirmeni S, Bosco G, Scipioni G, Gallina S (1997) Minimally invasive coronary artery bypass grafting on a beating heart. Ann Thorac Surg 63:S72–S75
4. Cremer J, Martin M, Redl H, Bahrami S, Abraham C, Graeter T, Haverich A, Schlag G, Borst HG (1996) Systemic inflammatory response syndrome after cardiac operations. Ann Thorac Surg 61:1714–1720
5. Cremer J, Strüber M, Wittwer T, Ruhparwar A, Harringer W, Zuk J, Mehler D, Haverich A (1997) Off-bypass coronary bypass grafting via minithoracotomy using mechanical epicardial stabilization. Ann Thorac Surg 63:S79–S83
6. Higgins TL, Estafanous FG, Loop FL, Beck GJ, Blum JM, Paranandi L (1992) Stratification of morbidity and mortality, outcome by preoperative risk factors in coronary artery bypass patients. J Am Med Assoc. 267: 2344–2348
7. Kolessov VI (1967) Mammary artery-coronary artery anastomosis as method of treatment for angina pectoris. J Thorac Cardiovasc Surg 54:535–544
8. Mack M, Acuff T, Young P, Jett GK, Carter D (1997) Minimally invasvie thoracoscopically assisted coronary artery bypass surgery. Eur J Cardio-Thorac Surg 12:20–24
9. Mills SA (1993) Cerebral injury and cardiac operations. Ann Thorac Surg 56:S86–S91
10. Stevens JH, Burdon TA, Peters WS, Siegel LC, Pompili MF, Vierra MA, St Goar FG, Ribakove GH, Mitchell RS, Reitz BA (1996) Port-access coronary artery bypass grafting: a proposed surgical method. J Thorac Cardiovasc Surg 111:567–573
11. Subramanian VA (1996) Clinical experience with minimally invasive reoperative coronary bypass surgery. Eur J Cardio-Thorac Surg 10:1058–1063
12. Subramanian VA (1997) Less invasive arterial CABG on a beating heart. Ann Thorac Surg 63:S68–S71

Authors' address:
PD Dr. Jochen Cremer
Klinik für Thorax-, Herz- und Gefäßchirurgie
Medizinische Hochschule Hannover
D-30623 Hannover

Off-pump coronary surgery in high risk patients

G. Di Giammarco, A. M. Calafiore

Division of Cardiac Surgery, University of Chieti, Chieti, Italy

Introduction

It is generally accepted that the use of extra corporeal circulation (ECC) is related to a variable incidence of postoperative complications, some of them particularly disabling. Among these complications, those involving the central nervous system (CNS) can result even ofter successful coronary surgery.

The risk is related to the preoperative clinical status and is proportional to the age of the patient; this aspect is noticeable as the mean age of the patients recently enrolled for the coronary surgery is increasing.

The aim of this study is to report our experience in off-pump coronary revascularization in high risk patients, show our results, and discuss the benefits related to this technical choice.

Material and methods

Our experience in off-pump coronary surgery started in 1993, but it received a strong impulse from November 1994.

From this date up to September 20, 1997, 1649 patients have been consecutively submitted to myocardial revascularization (MR) in our institution (Fig. 1).

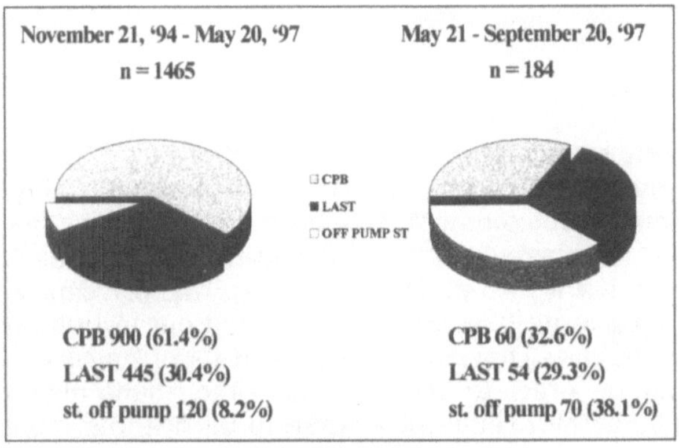

Fig. 1. Trend in CABG technical choice.

Table 1. Off-pump CABG – global experience

year	median stern	LAST	Total	%CABG
'93	9	–	9	
'94	2	11	13	
'95	26	144	170	34.7
'96	74	226	300	43.6
'97 (Sept 20)	88	118	206	46.5
Total	199	499	698	
Deaths	5 (2.5%)	4 (0.8%)	9 (1.3%)	

Table 2. Patients population (May 21–September 20, 1997)

	no CpB n = 70	CPB n = 60	p
age	64.6 ± 10.3	61.4 ± 9.2	< 0.05
≥ 75 y	10	2	ns
female	15	8	ns
EF	53.4 ± 15.5	58.2 ± 15.3	< 0.05
≤ 35%	8	3	ns
urgent	10	8	ns
LM	6	6	ns
redo	2	8	ns
carotid surgery	1	1	ns

Table 3. Major risk factors (May 21–September 20, 1997)

	no CPB n = 70	CPB n = 60	p
diffuse CV disease	5	–	< 0.05
malignancy	3	–	ns
diffuse vasculopathy	4	–	ns
age ≥ 75 y	10	2	< 0.05
chronic renal failure	3	–	ns
COPD	7	1	< 0.05
total	32 (45.7%)	3 (5.0%)	< 0.000

Out of these, 689 patients were revascularized without the aid of ECC. As shown in Table 1, 199 patients were operated through a median sternotomy and 499 were submitted to a left anterior small thoracotomy (LAST operation), receiving in the latter case just the left internal mammary artery (LIMA) to the left anterior descending (LAD) artery; in Table 1 it is also possible to see how the percentage of beating heart operations has progressively increased with time at our institution.

Our purpose is to analyze the data concerning those patients operated on by means of a median sternotomy in order to better compare the results obtained with or without the ECC; we futhermore limit the analysis to the last four months of our experience as in this period the presence of high risk factors to the ECC surgery was the main criteria to assign the patients to the off-pump surgery. Tables 2 and 3 show the demographic characteristics of the patient population and the risk factors distribution, respectively.

The ECC, when utilized, was normothermic and the myocardial protection was achieved by means of the antegrade intermittent warm blood cardioplegia, according to our protocol (6).

The exposure of the anterior vessel (LAD, D) was obtained by putting a swab behind the heart and that of the vessels on the inferior and lateral wall by means of four slings, two behind the inferior vena cava and two through the tranverse sinus; the four slings were settled crossing on the heart surface to limit the site of the anastomosis.

The stabilization of the anastomotical site was in all cases achieved using a mechanical platform. The coronary artery was occluded across the chosen anastomotical site by means of two 4/0 prolene sutures surrounding the artery and tighten with a tourniquet on a small piece of rubber in order to minimize the mechanical truma.

The anastomosis was performed in the majority of cases according to the heel and toe technique, by means of two separate 8/0 or 7/0 prolene sutures passed in continuous fashion. We performed in all cases the quality control of the anastomosis using a Transit Time ultrasound flowmeter.

Concerning the statistical analysis we applied the t-student test to compare continuous variables and the χ^2 test to compare categorical variables. The survival rates were compared by means of z-test. Statistical significance was accepted at $p < 0.05$.

Results

The operative results are shown in Table 4. Along with a lower mean number of distal anastomoses in the off-pump group we registered a prompter awakening, a shorter mechanical ventilation time, and a lower postoperative bleeding in the same group.

The ICU and the in-hospital stay were significantly shorter; we found no difference in operative and late mortality rates (Table 5).

It can be seen that the late mortality in the soubgroup of patients with a low LVEF operated without ECC is higher than in the same subgroup operated with

Table 4. Operative results (May 21–September 20, 1997)

	no CPB n = 70	CPB n = 60	p
anast/patient	2.1 ± 0.7	2.7 ± 0.9	< 0.005
awakening	1.3 ± 1.1	2.0 ± 1.3	< 0.05
mechanical ventilation	5.2 ± 5.1	3.2 ± 2.1	< 0.05
inotropes	5	–	ns
AMI	–	–	ns
bleeding (ml/24 h)	340.9 ± 358.2	675.1 ± 414.5	< 0.005
redo for bleeding	–	1	ns
transfused patients	7	12	ns
CVA	–	1	ns

Table 5. Postoperative results (May 21–September 20, 1997)

	no CPB n = 70	CPB n = 60	p
ICU stay (h)	16.1 ± 12.5	25.4 ± 35.5	< 0.05
in hospital mortality	2 (2.8)	1 [1.6%]	ns
in hospital stay	4.2 ± 1.6	5.0 ± 1.2	< 0.005
late deaths	0	1 [1.6%]	ns

Table 6. Low LVEF patients (January 1, 1995–September 20, 1997)

	no CPB	CPB	p
no. pts	26	45	
age	63.5 ± 10.1	61.6 ± 10.0	ns
≥ 75 y	5	5	ns
EF	27.1 ± 5.0	28.4 ± 4.6	ns
LM	0	4	ns
redo	1	8	ns
anast/patient	1.5 ± 0.8	2.9 ± 0.9	< 0.001
in hospital mortality	1 [3.8%]	2 [4.4%]	ns
late deaths	2 [8.0%]	1 [2.3±)	ns

the aid of ECC (8.0% vs. 2.3%), even if this difference does not reach the statistical significance (Table 6). In the same subgroup the only difference found was in the mean number of distal anastomoses, lower in those patients operated without ECC.

In Fig. 2, the analysis of the actuarial survival rate on the total population is reported; we found no statistical difference (91.1 SD 3.8% with ECC vs. 86.3 SD 3.8% off-pump). In addition, no difference was registered in the event-free survival rate in the same population (Fig. 3).

The same results were observed in the survival rate of patients belonging to the last part of our experience (96.2 SD 2.6% with ECC vs. 93.2 SD 2.7% off-pump) (Fig. 4).

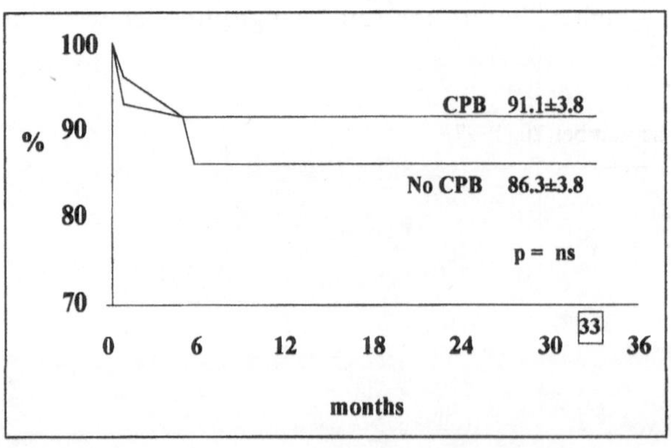

Fig. 2. Actuarial survival (November 14, 1994 – September 20, 1997).

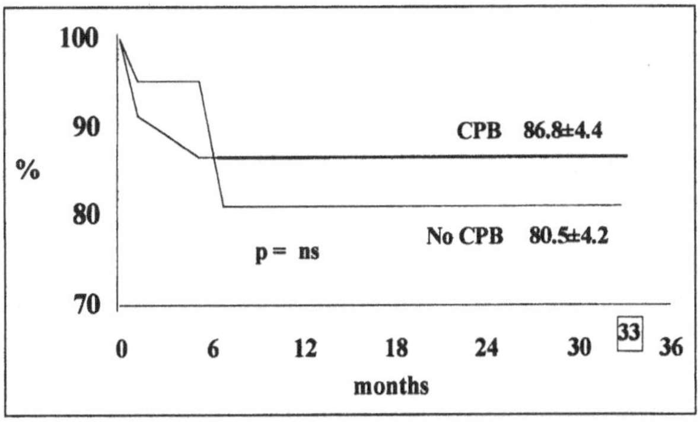

Fig. 3. Event-free survival (November 14, 1994 – September 20, 1997).

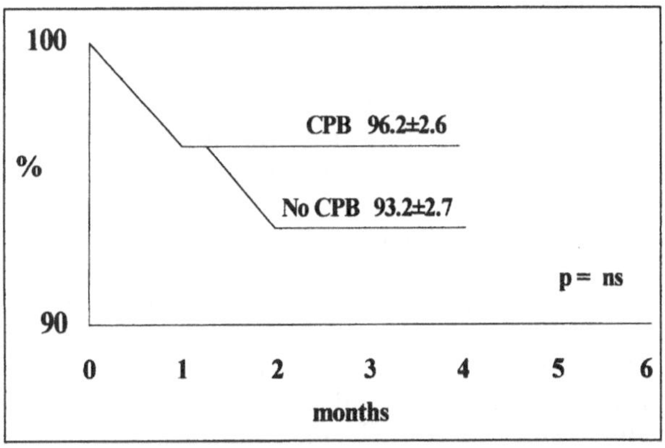

Fig. 4. Actuarial survival (May 21 – September 20, 1997).

Comments

The lack of the ECC at the beginning of the coronary surgery era pushed some pioneering surgeon to accomplish the operation on the beating heart (8). The technical difficulties did not guarantee the diffusion of those methods up to the advent of the ECC and the cardioplegic arrest.

Along with the diffision of the technique of the coronary bypass grafting on ECC, new complications appeared, depending on the ECC itself. The recruitment of even older patients and the related comorbidity represent further risk factors, even if better surgical and anaesthesiological techniques are used.

There is a general agreement concerning the potential damages due to the ECC. Among these complications we should distinguish those involving the CNS from the remaining apparatus. This is why the first ones are sometimes as disabling and minimize a good result obtained in the MR.

The pathogenesis of this damage is related to embolic phenomena (platelets microaggregates, silicon debries, crushing particles due to the manipulation of the aorta) or to hypotension during ECC.

On the clinical point of view they can be evident as somatosensorial or neuropsychological damage. The incidence varies between 3 % if focal damages are considered (12) and up to 30 % including the neuropsychological changes (1). Even if the neuropsychological sequelae after ECC are so frequent they seem to be recovered in 6–12 months after surgery. The prevalent clinical feature is the cognitive deficit (1).

The accuracy of the preoperative screening of the neurological status is of great importance as some of these deficits are evident in the preoperative period.

Blumenthal and coworkers (4) report the results of a comparative study demonstrating the lack of neurological damage in those patients submitted to a PTCA procedure if compared to patients submitted to MR or valve replacement/repair on pump.

Furthermore, the neurological sequelae after ECC seem to be related to the preoperative clinical condition. Newman and coworkers (11) proposed a nomogram in which they assign a score to the preoperative risk factors. The final score is transformed into an odds ratio for neurological damage after ECC.

Along with neurological risk, the ECC may cause any kind of systemical complication. A severe COPD, CRF, hemodialysis, severe liver dysfunction, immunological disorders, and severe coagulopathy are additional preoperative risk factors.

From the technical point of view, some aspects have to be considered. There are anatomical conditions (intramyocardial course of the coronary artery, calcified wall, small vessel calibre) that limit the feasibility of the MR without the cardioplegic arrest.

In addition, the revascularization of the lateral wall is not always possible, and this is particularly true in case of cardiomegaly with low LVEF and/or mitral incompetence without indication of surgical treatment. Furthermore, this technique needs specific training, and the effect of the learning curve on the quality of the results is inevitable.

All these technical considerations along with the lack of clearly defined angiographic results in the literature make the off-pump coronary surgery a technical option that is utilized when ECC is strictly contraindicated.

Apart from some historical experience of extensive use of this method (2, 5), the data reported in the literature concern the use of the off-pump coronary surgery in those patients at a high risk of postoperative complications (3, 7, 10).

In our experience these criteria pushed us to utilized this method in nearly the 50% of cases. In the remaining, we performed an off-pump revascularization as we felt that the operation was feasible and reliable without the ECC.

Those patients showing on the angiogram a low LVEF need special consideration. In our experience the comparison between the two technical choices in this subset of patients revealed a lower number of distal anastomoses in the off-pump group. This uncomplete revascularization can be the cause of recurrence of symptoms. This is why some authors (7) adopted the hybrid approach, completing the revascularization with a PTCA.

In similar cases, if the patient needs a complete revascularization that is not achieveble without the pump, we prefer to use the ECC for a very short period of time to decompress the heart in order to graft just the residual vessel, switching to a hybrid approach with the PTCA only if the arterial cannulation can be dangerous for the patient.

In patients with low LVEF we found no difference in the mortality rates, either inhospital or late; the 8% late mortality registered in the off-pump group was lower than that reported in literature in a similar group of patients (7).

A crucial point is the quality control of the anastomosis in the operating room. T. A. Foliguet and coworkers (7) report a high rate of technical failure discovered at the postoperative angiogram performed on the basis of recurrence of symptoms.

Concerning this issue we believe that the intraoperative check of the anastomosis is mandatory. The Transit-Time ultrasound flow measurement (9) is a reliable method, and it provides useful information about the patency of the anastomosis. It is apt to detect a complete occlusion, either at the proximal or at the distal site of the anastomosis and, if small doses of inotropes are used, it can discover even subcritical stenoses.

Conclusions

The off pump myocardial revascularization is a safe method that allows one to avoid any complications due to the ECC. It is particularly useful in those patients who show a preoperative high risk condition with a normal LVEF, as in these cases an off-pump complete revascularization is easily achievable. The role of this technical choice in low LVEF patients is still to be assessed, requiring further investigation.

The intraoperative check of the quality of the anastomosis is mandatory in order to avoid any unwise and expensive reoperations. Concerning the reduction of the hospital stay, if this technical option is properly adopted, it can contribute to reduce the social cost of the hospital care.

References

1. Benedict RHB (1994) Cognitive function after open-heart surgery: Are postoperative neuropsychological deficits caused by cardiopulmonary bypass? Neuropsychological Review 4: 223–255
2. Benetti FJ, Naselli G, Wood M, Geffner L (1991) Direct myocardial revascularization without extracorporeal circulation. Experience in 700 patients. Chest 100: 312–316
3. Bergsland J, Hasnan S, Lewin AN, et al. (1997) Coronary artery bypass grafting without cardiopulmonary bypass – An attractive alternative in high risk patients. Eur J Cardiothorac Surg 11: 876–880
4. Blumental JA, Madden DJ, Burker EJ, et al. (1991) A preliminary study of the effects of cardiac procedures on cognitive performance. Int J Psychosomatics 38: 13–16
5. Buffolo E, Silva de Andrade JC, Rodrigues Branco JN, et al. (1996) Coronary artery bypass surgery without cardiopulmonary bypass. Ann Thorac Surg 61: 63–66
6. Calafiore AM, Teodori G, Mezzetti A, et al. (1995) Intermittent antegrade warm blood cardioplegia. Ann Thorac Surg 59: 398–402
7. Fulliguet TA, Laborde F, Temkine A, et al. (1997) coronary artery revascularisation without extracorporeal circulation. Indications and results. Eur J Cardiothorac Surg 11: 870–875
8. Kolesov VI (1997) Mammary artery-coronary anastomosis as method of treatment for angina pectoris. J Thorac Cardiovasc Surg 54: 535–544
9. Laustsen J, Pedersen EM, Terp K, et al. (1996) Validation of a new Transit Time ultrasound flowmeter in man. Eur J Vasc Endovasc Surg 12: 91–96
10. Moshkovitz Y, Paz Y, Shabtai E, et al. (1997) Predictors of early and overall outcome in coronary artery bypass without cardiopulmonary bypass. Eur J Cardiothorac Surg 12: 31–39
11. Newman MF, Wolman R, Kanchuger M, et al. (1996) Multicenter preoperative stroke risk index for patients undergoing coronary artery bypass graft surgery. Circulation 94[supplII]: II-74-II-80
12. Roach GW, Kanchuger M, Mangano CM, et al. (1996) Adverse cerebral outcomes after coronary bypass surgery. N Engl J Med 335: 1857–1863

Author's address:
Gabriele Di Giammarco, M.D.
Clinica Cardiochirurgica
Ospedale San Camillo de' Lellis
Via Forlanini, 50
66100 Chieti, ITALY

Aortic valve replacement using a minimal access technique in multimorbid patients – First results

K. Ansorge, H.-G. Wollert, L. Eckel

Department of Thoracic and Cardiovascular Surgery, Karlsburg, Germany

Introduction

Presently trends for minimally invasive procedures are dominating in cardiac surgery. In principle one has to differenciate between "minimally invasive" and "minimal access" techniques. The aims of the new surgical procedures are reduction of perioperative trauma and to provide beneficial effects for patients, such as lower risk of wound infection, fast mobilization, reduced blood loss and need for transfusion. A major point of the high acceptance is the reduced postoperative pain and the cosmetical effect.

To evaluate the minimal access technique in aortic valve replacement we compared 11 patients using the minimal access technique with a conventional treated reference group of 14 patients.

Material and methods

From February to July 1997 the minimal access technique (MAT) was used in 11 patients (6 male / 5 female) in our clinic. All patients suffered from an isolated aortic valve disease. Ten mechanical protheses (9 St. Jude Medical / 1 Medtronic Hall) were implanted, and one commissurotomy was performed. The procedures were carried out using a 6 cm skin incision and a partially upper median sternotomy. The cardiopulmonary bypass was established by cannulation of the ascending aorta and the right atrium. A vent was inserted in the right upper pulmonary vein or the pulmonary trunk. The aortic valve replacement was performed in the usual manner. After weaning from extracorporeal circulation the sternal closure was done with 3–4 cerlages.

The conventional treated reference group (convent: 9 male / 5 female) were operated on by the same surgeon and no differences concerning the demographical and clinical data existed. In this group a St. Jude Medical prothesis was implanted in 13 patients and one patient received a Carpentier-Edwards bioprothesis.

Results

The demographical data and clinical parameters are seen in Table 1.

Table 1. Demographical data and clinical parameters

patients (n/average age)	operation time (min)	clamping time (min)	size of prosthesis (mm average)	blood loss (6 h/total ml)	blood transfusion (units)
MAT (11/62)	200 (155–280)	71 (31–93)	(20.6) 19–25	131/323	1.5 (0–5)
convent (14/63)	173 (150–208)	58 (47–75)	(24.5) 21–29	195/540	1.8 (0–3)

The most important findings were reduced blood loss and reduced need of transfusion in the MAT group. We had no wound infection nor sternum instability in either group. Two patients with partial sternotomy were extubated in the operating theater; a peridural catheter was used in these patients. The duration of stay in the intensive care unit as well at the clinic was similar in both groups.

The aortic clamping time and the duration of operation were prolonged in "minimal access" group.

Discussion

Comparing the data and considering our restricted experience we would like to discuss some advantages but also potential problems in using the minimal access approach for aortic valve replacement.

Advantages:
- lower risk of wound infection
- higher stability of sternum
- faster mobilization (breathing exercises)
- reduced blood loss/transfusion need
- reduced postoperative pain
- closed pericardium in case of rethoracotomy
- high acceptance (cosmetical effect)

Potential problems:
- learning curve
- demanding procedure
- deformation of sternum
- no view on ventricels
- problems in case of resuscitation
- difficult anatomy

Summary

Aortic valve replacement using a "minimal access" technique is a demading approach but in the majority of cases it should be possible to perform the operation in this way. MAT is a procedure with high acceptance and can offer a number of benefits to the patients. The currently existing potential problems will decrease with increasing experience.

References

1. Cosgrove, Delos M et al (1996) Minimally invasive approach for aortic valve operations Ann Thorac Surg 62: 596–597
2. Lytle, B. W. et al. (1996) Minimally invasive cardiac surgery, J Thorac Cardiovasc Surg 111: 554–555
3. Benetti, Frederico J. (1997) Minimally invasive aortic valve replacement, J Thorac Cardiovasc Surg 113: 806–807
4. Konertz, W et al. (1997) Minimal invasiver Aortenklappenersatz, 26. Annual meeting of the German Society of Thoracic and Cardiovascular Surgery, Dresden

Author's address:
Knut Ansorge, M.D.
Department of Thoracic and Cardiovascular Surgery
Greifswalder Straße 11A
17495 Karlsburg, Germany

Minimally invasive heart valve replacement – Benefit for the patient

F. W. Mohr, V. Falk, T. Walther, R. Autschbach, A. Diegeler

Universität Leipzig, Herzzentrum, Klinik für Herzchirurgie, Leipzig, Germany

Introduction

In the last two years there has been a rapid evolution of new surgical techniques for both aortic and mitral valve replacement. Although the term minimally invasive is commonly applied to the various techniques, most operations vary mainly by a different surgical access avoiding median sternotomy. As opposed to minimally or less invasive techniques for myocardial revascularization that in addition to decreasing the surgical access aim at avoiding the use of cardiopulmonary bypass, in less invasive valve surgery extracorporeal circulation is still mandatory. While some authors feel that median sternotomy is potentially harmful in terms of sternal instability and mediastinitis, others argue that it is infact the inflammatory response to cardiopulmonary bypass that causes most of the surgical trauma associated with cardiac surgery (16, 19–20). While the debate is ongoing, this article will focus on the techniques that have been recently developed.

Aortic valve surgery

Traditionally the aortic valve is approached via a median sternotomy. Minor invasive techniques avoiding a median sternotomy were introduced recently to reduce the surgical trauma and, thereby, improve the outcome for the patient at a comparably low risk. When using a minimal invasive approach for aortic valve replacement, good exposure is essential to be able to perform valve replacement procedure as exact as possible. Due to the fact that the ascending aorta anatomically is relatively anterior with little distance from the sternum, an almost perfect exposure can be anticipated from a partial sternotomy. In addition, the pericardium that is not completely opened in less invasive operations keeps the heart and the ascending aorta in an anterior position. A fast and uneventful postoperative recovery resulting from enhanced stability of the thorax is anticipated.

Following a small skin incision various types of partial sternotomy or a parasternal access have been suggested. Cardiopulmonary bypass is usually performed in a standard fashion with cannulation of the ascending aorta and direct cannulation of the right atrium with a two-stage venous cannula. Alternatively the femoral vein can be cannulated percutaneously to drain the right atrium. The ascending aorta is clamped and cardioplegia delivered antegradely, retrogradely or directly into the coronary ostia. A perasternal incision has been initially described by Cosgrove (5). while access to the valve is excellent, the devision and partial resection of two ribs has been criticized (6). Furthermore, the right internal mammary artery has to be sacrificied and cannot be used if coronary revascularization should become necessary. A proximal partial median sternotomy has been suggested by Konertz and colleagues (11). Besides standard aortic valve replacement, implantation of stentless valves and homografts was possible with operating times exceeding those for conventional surgery. A horizontal or transverse sternotomy has also be suggested as well as a T-shaped sternotomy leaving the manubrium intact (21).

A new technique, the S-shaped approach has been developed by our group in order to preserve the continuity of both the upper and the lower bony thoracic circumference (2). In a comparative study the upper partial sternotomy (group 1:16 patients) an S -shaped sternotomy (group 2: 14 patients) and an horizontal sternotomy (group 3: 3 patients) were evaluated. The differences in the sternotomy are shown in Fig. 1. Valve implantation was performed using a standard technique with interrupted pledgeted sutures in a supraannular position for all stented valves. Stentless bioprostheses were implanted in a subcoronary position with interrupted sutures and a running suture line at the top using the freehand technique. Thirty three patients were included, 14 patients were female, none had coronary artery disease. Mean age at operation was 58 ± 13 years. The predominant aortic valve lesion was stenosis in 21 and incompetence in 12 patients. Preoperative ejection fraction was 63 ± 15%. Preoperatively 16 patients were in NYHA class II and 17 patients in NYHA class III. Patients had short-term postoperative ventilation with early extubation and fast-track intensive care therapy if possible. Mobilization was begun immediately after extubation. Postoperative in-hospital stay was attempted to be short and took about one week according to the German standard of early in-hospital rehabilitation. Valve related morbidity and mortality were evaluated according to standard guidelines (2). The surgical exposure of the aortic valve was sufficient in all patients. Three patients had to be converted to a conventional sternotomy (two in group 1 and one in group 2). Conversion was required due to a tear of the ascending aorta, additional venous bypass grafting to the right coronary artery when calcific emboli was suspected and reconstruction of the aortic annulus, respectively. Conversion was easily possible without any additional complications for the patients. Ten patients received a biological aortic valve (conventional =1, stentless biological = 9); 22 Patients had mechanical AVR and one patient received a homograft. Extracorporeal circulation was initiated via the femoral vessels in 9 and by direct thoracal cannulation in 24 patients, respectively. Aortic crossclamp time was 69 ± 15 minutes. Postoperatively, all patients were in a hemodynamically stable condition requiring only minimal doses of inotropic support in the very first postoperative hours. Overall postoperative blood loss was low.

Postoperative complications were as follows: rethoracotomy using the minithoracotomy had to be performed in one patient for excessive bleeding of 950 ml, recovery was uneventful. One patient had to be re-intubated on the third postoperative day for 48 hours due to pneumonia. At one-week postoperative echocardiographic control paravalvular leakage was diagnosed in two patients. Both had a heavily calcified aortic annulus intraoperatively. Reoperation had to be performed in one of these patients with grade 3 valvular incompetence whereas the other patient who had only moderate incompetence and was in NYHA class 1, could be discharged.

A sternal dehiscence was seen in three patients at 5–7 days postoperatively. Two of these patients had a horizontal sternotomy (group 3). Both had no significant clinical symptoms and breathing was not impaired. Therefore, they could be discharged. The third patient had a upper proximal sternotomy (group 1) and had transitional psychosis postoperatively. He was reoperated; later on his course was uneventful.

Postoperative quality of life was comparable to a control group having conventional AVR. On average mobilization was performed half a day earlier after minor invasive

AVR which resulted in a slightly better functional state on the seventh postoperative day. Postoperative pain levels were comparable in both groups (22). Nevertheless, all but one patient were happy with their decision to have minor invasive AVR and would choose the same approach again when asked at follow up.

Other studies as well as our own data underline that less invasive AVR, which has been used for a few months only thus far, is technically feasible at similar results than the conventional approach. Comparably high safety of a new procedure is of utmost importance for the patients and necessary to justify the further use of these techniques.

With both the upper median and the S-shaped partial sternotomy techniques the lower circumference of the bony thorax remains intact. The S-shaped approach is advantageous because the upper bony circumference remains intact as well. Nevertheless, exposure is not as good as with an upper median sternotomy. Due to the smaller access in group 2 half of the patients required femoral cannulation. However this did not lead to any procedure-related complications. At present we recommend the S-shaped approach in patients having a relatively low body weight, whereas the upper median sternotomy should be used in all obese patients and in circumstances where femoral cannulation is contraindicated. The horizontal sternotomy did not yield good exposure; furthermore postoperative bony dehiscence was a rather frequent problem in that group.

As of yet, no differences in postoperative pain were seen in the patients having less invasive AVR in comparison to a group of patients after a conventional operation (22). This could be anticipated because spreading of some ribs might cause the same pain. Nevertheless, earlier mobilization could be achieved in patients after less invasive AVR allowing early recovery.

Mitral valve surgery

As in less invasive aortic valve surgery, cardiopulmonary bypass is required for less invasive mitral valve procedures. Among the different techniques that have been reported, the Port-Access-technique with endoaortic clamping allows a truly minimal access to the mitral valve with an incision not exceeding 4 cm. Patients are positioned in a supine position with the right chest slightly elevated. The right femoral artery and vein are surgically exposed. After systemic heparinisation, a standard 28 Fr venous return cannula (DLP, Grand Rapids, MI) is placed in the femoral vein and advanced to the right atrium under transesophageal echocardiographic (TEE) control. A 21 or 23 Fr Y-shaped arterial return cannula (Heartport) with one arm for arterial return and one arm for placement of the endoaortic clamp is placed in the femoral artery. Venous drainage is enhanced appling moderate suction onto the venous reservoir.

Synchronous with exposure of the femoral vessels, a small horizontal incision is made laterally over the fourth intercostal space. A specially designed rib retractor (Arnold Medizintechnik, Tuttlingen, Germany) is inserted. After initiation of cardiopulmonary bypass the lungs were deflated. The pericardium is opened 3 cm above and parallel to the right phrenic nerve to expose the roof of the left atrium. A 10 mm port is inserted at the second intercostal space in the anterior axillary line to allow placement of a videoscope (Endolive 3D Video Thoracoscope System, Carl Zeiss, Oberkochem, Germany) into the left atrium. Correct placement of the endoaortic clamp is controlled by multiplane transesophageal echocardiography (7). The endoaortic clamp occludes the ascending aorta while the heart is vented through the distal lumen of the endoaortic

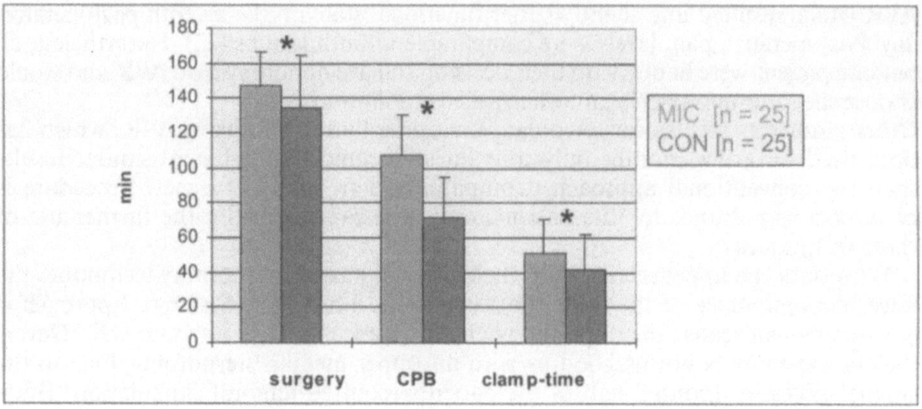

Fig. 1. Comparison of conventional versus minimally invasive mitral valve surgery. CPB = cardiopulmonary bypass time

clamp in the aortic root. Balloon pressure is kept in the range between 250 and 340 mmHg. Cold crystalloid cardioplegic solution is delivered antegradely through the distal endaortic clamp lumen while maintaining aortic root pressure between 50 and 70 mmHg. After cardiac arrest has been established, the left atrium is opened and the mitral valve exposed by an left atrial retractor (Heartport) that is inserted through a second 5mm port at the 6th or 7th right intercostal space parasternally. Mitral valve repair or replacement is performed under three-dimensional videoscopic guidance with specially designed instruments (Heartport). After completion of the procedure the left atrium was closed by a continuous suture. Deairing is performed by inflation of the lungs and simultaneous reduction of venous drainage with the patient placed in Trendelenburg position. Deairing of the aortic root was performed by suction via the distal lumen of the endoaortic clamp. After the left atrium is closed, the endoaortic clamp is deflated leaving the catheter in place for further venting until deairing is completed. The endoaortic clamp is then withdrawn and the chest wound closed. After appropriate reperfusion the arterial and venous cannulas are removed and the femoral vessels reconstructed.

Results

Minimally invasive mitral valve surgery was performed in 75 patients (mean age 60 ± 12 y, mean left ventricular ejection fraction 52 ± 14%) with predominant mitral insufficiency (n = 549 or stenosis (n = 21)). In all patients, injection of an initial volume of 20 to 35 ml (mean inflation volume of 24 ± 6 ml) resulted in sufficient aortic occlusion with a balloon pressure in the desired range of 235 to 360 mmHg. Migration of the balloon during initial placement was observed in 8 patients but could be easily corrected by external manipulation of the catheter under TEE control. Balloon rupture was observed in two patients, surgery was continued with the heart fibrillating.

In all patients, the mitral valve was accessible through the right lateral minithoracotomy. With an incision of less than 5 cm. In 44 patients, the mitral valve was repaired under direct and stereoscopic vision by a combination of repair techniques including quadrangular resection, commissurotomy, sliding plasty, chordal replacement, and partial or complete annuloplasty. As demonstrated by intraoperative TEE, successful repair was achieved in all but three patients. One patient had new moderate mitral stenosis while two patients had residual grade II mitral insufficiency. Mitral valve replacement was subsequentely performed using the same access and surgical technique without enlarging the primary incision. 31 patients (28 primary, 3 after failed repair) underwent mitral valve replacement. Mean duration of operation, cardiopulmonary bypass, and crossclamp times was 180 ± 51 min, 124 ± 46, and 65 ± 26 min, respectively, and longer than with conventional surgery (Fig. 1). In the majority of patients a spontaneous rhythm was present after deflating the endoaortic clamp, whereas 21 patients required one or more external defibrillations of 200 – 360 Joule. In six patients conversion to an enlarged thoracotomy incision (n = 2), a mini-sternotomy (n = 2), or complete sternotomy (n = 2) was neccessary. There were two acute retrograde aortic dissections. In one patient, TEE revealed a rapidly progressing dissection to the level of the aortic valve with the onset of retrograde extracorporeal perfusion. Emergency median sternotomy and supracoronary replacement of the ascending aorta with reconstruction of the aortic arch was performed. The mitral valve was replaced conventionally. In another patient aortic dissection became evident during weaning from CPB. The patient was converted and had replacement of the ascending aorta but finally expired due to persistent low cardiac output.

Primary median intubation time was 19 h (range 5–264 h) with 8 patients requiring ventilation for more than 48 h. Duration of intensive care and hospital stay was 2 d (range 1–36 d) and 12 d (6–36 d), respectively. As compared to matched patients undergoing conventional mitral valve surgery in the last 25 patients a decrease in intubation time, intensive care stay and blood loss was observed (Table 1). In most patients pain medication could be stopped on the second postoperative day. Compared to patients undergoing conventional mitral valve surgery via a medain stereotomy pain as assessed by a visual analogue scale and a daily pain questionnaire was significantly less from postoperative day three onwards (22).

Three patients requiring reexploration for bleeding without enlarging the primary incision. There was only little cardiac related morbidity. Of concern were neurologic complications. Four patients experienced transient hemiparesis. Six patients (8%) died perioperatively or at follow-up. One patient died on postoperative day 12 after of toxic epidermal necrolysis that developed secondary to a superficial skin infection. One patient who had successful mitral valve repair had acute onset of recurrent mitral insufficiency on the third postoperative due to a torn out mitral ring. Mitral valve replacement was performed subsequentely but the patient expired due to irreversible low cardiac output. One patient died from pneumonia, one from multi-organ failure, and one from pulmonary embolism.

Table 1. Comparison of two techniquet for mitral valve surgery. MIC = minimal invasive approach. CON = conventional approach

	MIC (n = 25)	Con (n = 25)	p
blood loss [ml]	588 ± 400	818 ± 780	n.s.
respirator [d]	14 ± 8.8	18.6 ± 15.7	< 0.05
ICU [d]	1 ± 0.5	2 ± 1.2	< 0.005
hospitalization [d]	10 ± 2.4	14.7 ± 4.0	< 0.005
mortality [%]	4	4	n.s.

At discharge, all patients after mitral valve repair showed normal mitral valve function with no or only trivial regurgitation. All implanted valves were functioning normally as shown by postoperative echocardiographic control. At a mean follow-up of 388 ± 29 days, all patients except two had at least returned to their preoperative activity level. NYHA class had improved at least by 1 class in all but 6 patients. Three patients who had mitral valve replacement and normal mitral valve function at their pre-discharge echocardiographic control were readmitted with paravalvular leakage after 5, 7, and 16 weeks, respectively. All patients were reoperated conventionally. One patient with mitral valve repair had new onset of mitral regurgitation and required mitral valve replacement. Two patients had a small residual hematoma and one patient had a lymph fistula in the right groin all of which were treated conservatively.

Discussion

Minimally invasive procedures were introduced in expectation of reduced postoperative pain, recovery time, and cost while providing a favorable cosmetic result as compared with conventional surgery. Using the Port-Access system video assisted mitral valve surgery including complex repair procedures through an incision less than 4 cm has become possible. From our data it is as yet not justified to claim a clinical relevant benefit for the patient from the minimally invasive approach. Clearly, surgical times are still prolonged as compared to the conventional approach. With increasing experience, in this series cardiopulmonary bypass and cross-clamp times became shorter. The length of the thoracotomy incison has steadily decreased, while partial rib-resection is no longer performed. Although the duration of intubation and intensive care treatment are reduced in the last 25 patients as compared to a matched population undergoing median sternotomy mitral valve surgery, the series is to small as to draw definite conclusions. From our daily pain questionnaire, it is obviuos that there is less pain in the minimally invasive group from day four onward. However at this time also patients in the sternotomy group are usually without pain medication. In terms of time to return to work, no data are available as all patients undergo a three week cardiac rehabilitation program.

Serious complications occured. Two retrograde aortic dissections were of major concern. Both events were most likely caused by intimal dissection at the level of the iliac artery induced by the guide wire. Retrograde flow led to complete retrograde aortic dissection. With a change in catheter design the incidence of this complication is currently decreasing. A problem that was infrequently encountered early in this series was incomplete deairing of the heart which might partially explain the high incidence of postoperative confusion. Currently CO_2 insufflation of the surgical field helps to evacuate air thereby decreasing the incidence of air embolisms. Surgical manipulation of the valve and the perivalvular tissue is limited by a decreased range of movement and the use of longer instruments with limited stability. Especially in the presence of annular calcification placement of sutures can be difficult. Knotting is performed outside the chest and knots are placed using a knot-pusher adding 10 minutes of aortic cross clamp time. Refinement of the currently used instruments is, therefore, highly desirable.

The tendency of the balloon to migrate requires continuous observation. Proximal displacement may, in theory, damage the aortic valve, while distal migration may obstruct the brachiocephalic trunk. We observed transient hemiparesis in four patients, a possible cause being temporary translocation of the balloon. There was no change in right radial artery pressure so that monitoring of right radial artery pressure alone can not be considered reliable for exclusion of balloon displacement. Once the left atrium is opened, TEE also fails to locate the balloon properly. Currently transcranial Doppler measurements of the medial cerebral arteries is performed in order to detect misplacement of the balloon (17). With femoral cannulation and retrograde aortic flow there is the potential disadvantage of flushing debris of atheromatous plaques originating from the abdominal or thoracic aorta into the cerebral circulation. It is, therefore, mandatory to examine the aorta prior to endoclamp placement with TEE to identify patients with atheromatous aortic plaques or thrombi and to exclude these patients from an approach that requires retrograde perfusion. In addition, femoral cannulation may cause local complications at the groin as well as ischemic complications of the leg (10). Careful patient selection excluding patients with severe atherosclerosis, kinking or ectasia of the aorta and the peripheral arteries is, therefore, advisable.

The term "minimally invasive" has been applied to a number of different techniques for mitral valve procedures (1, 3–5, 8, 12, 14, 15) but there is still no agreement on what type of procedure should be called minimally invasive (13). There is still a lack of data to proof that the application of minimally or less invasive procedures reduce the surgical trauma and allow for faster recovery. Reports of early extubation and dicharge after minimally invasive valve procedures have to be evaluated carefully as on-table extubation and fast-track intensive care treatment may be applied to these patients besides the surgical approach. Navia and co-workers (15) reported of 25 patients that had a 10 cm right parasternal incision with resection of the 3rd and 4th cartilages and sacrifice of the right internal thoracic artery. Unfortunately, no data to support the conclusion that the smaller incision resulted in a reduction of patient discomfort, a reduction in the incidence and risks of wound infection and blood loss, and in a reduction of recovery time and costs were provided by the authors. To appropriately answer these questions, controlled randomized studies enrolling larger series of patients may be necessary.

References

1. Arom KV, Emery RW (1997) Minimally invasive mitral operations. Ann Thorac Surg 63:1219–20
2. Autschbach R, Walther T, Falk V, Diegeler A, Schilling L, Metz S, Mohr FW (1997) Minimal invasiver Aortenklappenersatz. Z Kardiol 86 (Suppl.2):298
3. Benetti FJ, Rizzardi JL, Pre L, Polanco A (1997) Mitral valve replacement under video assistance through a minithoracotomy. Ann Thorac Surg 63:1150–2
4. Carpentier A, Loulmet D, Carpentier A, Le Bret E, Haugades B, Dassier P et al (1996) Chirurgie a coeur overt par video-chirurgie et mini-thoracotomie. Premier cas (valvuloplastie mitrale) opere avec success. CR Acad Sci III 319:219–23
5. Chitwood WR, Elbeery JR, Chapman WHH, Moran JM, Lust RL, Wooden WA (1996) Video assisted minimally invasive mitral valve surgery: The "Micro-Mitral" Operation. J Thorac Cardiovasc Surg 113:413–420
7. Falk V, Walther T, Diegeler A, Autschbach R, Wendler R, van Son JAM, et al (1996) Echocardiographic Monitoring of minimally invasive mitral valve surgery using an endoaortic clamp. J Heart Valve Dis 5: 630–7
8. Falk V, Walther T, Diegeler A, van Son JAM, Friedrich M, Battelini R, Autschbach R, Mohr FW (1998) Minimal invasive Mitralklappenchirurgie. Acta Chir Aust 30:25–28
9. Falk V, Walther T, Autschbach R, Diegeler A, Battellini R, Mohr FW (1998) Robot Assisted Minimally Invasive Mitral Valve Solo Surgery. J Thorac Cardiovasc Surg 115:470–471
10. Gates JD, Bichell DP, Rizzo RJ, Couper GS, Donaldson MC (1996) Tigh ischemia complicating femoral vessel cannulation for cardiopulmonary bypass Ann Thorac Surg 61:730–3

11. Konertz W, Waldenberger F, Schmutzler M, Ritter J, Liu J (1996) Minimal access valve surgery through superior partial sternotomy: A preliminary study. J Heart Valve Dis 5:638–40
12. Lin PJ, Chang CH, Chu JJ, Liu HP, Tsai FC, Chu PH (1996) Video assisted mitral valve operations. Ann Thorac Surg 61:1781–7
13. Lytle BW. Minimally invasive cardiac surgery (1996) J Thorac Cardiovasc Surg 111:554–5
14. Mohr FW, Falk V, Diegeler A, Walther T, van Son JAM, Autschbach R (1998) Minimally invasive Port-Access mitral valve surgery. J Thorac Cardiovasc Surg 115:567–576
15. Navia JL, Cosgrove DM (1996) Minimally invasive mitral valve operations. Ann Thorac Surg 62:1542–4
16. Pompilli MF, Stevens JH, Burdon TA, Siegel LC, Peters WS, Ribakove GH, et al (1996) Port-Access Mitral valve replacement in dogs. J Thorac Cardiovasc Surg 112:1268–74
17. Schneider F, Falk V, Walther T, Mohr FW (in press) Control of endoclamp position during Port-Access mitral valve surgery using transcranial Doppler. Ann Thorac Surg
18. Schwartz DS, Ribakove GH, Grossi EA, Stevens JH, Siegel LC, Goar F G St, et al (1996) Minimally invasive cardiopulmonary bypass with cardioplegic arrest: A closed chest technique with equivalent myocardial protection. J Thorac Cardiovasc Surg 111:556–66
19. Stevens JH, Burdon TA, Peters WS, Siegel LC, Pompili MF, Vierra MA, et al (1996) Port-Access coronary artery bypass grafting: A proposed surgical method. J Thorac Cardiovasc Surg 111:567–73
20. Stevens JH, Burdon TA, Siegel LC, Peters WS, Pompili MF, Goar F G St, et al (1996) Port-Access coronary Artery Bypass with cardioplegic Arrest: Acute and Chronic canine Studies. Ann Thorac Surg 62:435–41
21. Tam RKW, Almeida AA (1998) Minimally invasive aortic valve replacement via partial sternotomy. Ann Thorac Surg 65:275–6
22. Walther T, Falk V, Metz S, Diegeler A, Battelini R, Autschbach R, Mohr FW (1998) Schmerz und Lebensqualität nach minimal invasiver im Vergleich zu konventioneller Herzoperation. Thorac Cardiovasc Surg 46 (Suppl I):62

Author's address:
Prof. F. W. Mohr
Universität Leipzig
Herzzentrum, Klinik für Herzchirurgie
Russenstr. 19
04289 Leipzig, Germany

Minimally invasive coronary artery bypass grafting in patients with severe concomitant diseases

F.-C. Riess, P. Kremer, K.-P. Kunze[1], C. Loewer, F. Schoeneich, J. Schofer[1], J. Untiedt, N. Bleese

Albertinen-Krankenhaus, Hamburg, [1]Center of Cardiology Hamburg-Othmarschen, Germany

Abstract

Objective: Minimally invasive coronary artery bypass grafting may be superior to the conventional approach in patients with severe concomitant diseases because of less operative traumatization resulting in a better preservation of sternum stability, less postoperative pain, and a better wound healing. The greatest advantage, however, is that operations can be performed without the use of cardiopulmonary bypass (CPB), thus, avoiding multiple adverse effects such as renal, pulmonary, and neurological dysfunctions often associated with CPB. Furthermore, there is no CPB related b cell and t cell depletion, which decreases the risk of infection and the progression of malignant diseases.
Patients and Methods: 15 patients (13 male/2 female, age 58 ± 10 (37–73) y) with coronary 1–3 vessel disease and a left ventricular ejection fraction (EF) of 56 ± 10 (35–79)% were operated on performing a LIMA-to-LAD graft without the use of CPB. In 5 out of these 15 patients concomitant diseases were present (malignant diseases n = 4, diabetes mellitus n = 2, COPD n = 1, renal dysfunction n = 1, previous stroke n = 1). All patients underwent coronary revascularization through an inferior inversed L-shaped mini-sternotomy. The LIMA was harvested up to the 2nd intercostal space under direct vision. Anastomosis to the LAD was performed on the beating heart without use of CPB. In 2 patients with a coronary 3-vessel disease additional coronary stenoses of the RCA and CX could be treated by interventional cardiological techniques after successful LIMA-to-LAD procedure.
Results: All 15 patients underwent a successful LIMA-to-LAD procedure without any intraoperative complications (time of operation: 144 ± 20 (110–180) min, LAD-occlusion time: 22 ± 8 (10–36) min). The postoperative course was uneventful except a re-exploration in 1 patient due to prolonged bleeding (200 ml/h) from the thorax drainages. Postoperatively all patients were free of angina pectoris and coronary angiograms showed a widely patent LIMA graft. No worsening of renal, neurological or respiratory functions occured. All patients could be mobilized on the 1st postoperative day and were discharged on the 6.5 ± 1.5 (4–9) postoperative day in a good condition.
Conclusion: This data indicate that LIMA-to-LAD procedure carried out on the beating heart and without the use of CPB is a secure and effective method in selected patients including coronary 1–3 vessel diseases. Possibly, this minimally invasive approach is advantageous in patients with severe concomitant disease in comparison to conventional coronary bypass operations.

Introduction

Minimally invasive coronary artery bypass operations have recently been introduced into cardiac surgery and has been proven to be an important tool in the cardiac surgeon's armamentarium (2, 3, 5). Obious advantages of the minimally invasive approach are less tissue traumatization and better preserved stability of the sternum, resulting in less postoperative pain and better wound healing. The most important advantage of minimally invasive operations, however, is that CPB with its multiple side effects in virtually any organ system, including the heart,kidneys, lungs, and central nervous system, can be avoided (1). Furthermore CPB-related activation of the complement system, coagulation system, and fibrinolysis system and damage of red cells, leucocytes, and platelets, which may result in bleeding and thromboembolic complications can be avoided as well. The b cell and t cell depletion may increase the risk of infections and could accelerate the progression of malignant diseases.

The CPB apparatus itself is another source of complications such as cannulation-related injuries, gas, and particulate embolism (13), which may result in cerebrovascular events. Especially in elder patients undergoing CPB, strokes occur with a considerable frequency (14) due to aortic atheromas liberated by the perfusion system or hypoperfusion during CPB of cerebral vascular beds because of significant proximal stenotic vascular lesions in the carotid, vertebral or intracranial arteries. Moreover CPB seems to be responsible for a considerable number of neuropsychiatric abnormalitis including depression, confusion, memory loss, decreased cognition, and uncoordination (6), which are not observed in patients undergoing minimally invasive coronary artery bypass grafting. Furthermore the high dose heparin regimen during CPB may increase the risk of perioperative bleeding.

Summarizing, minimally invasive LIMA-to-LAD procedure may result in a better outcome of patients and probably a reduction in costs (7, 9, 12).

Material and methods

Fifteen patients (13 male/2 female) with coronary artery disease (1-vessel n = 8, 2-vessel n = 3, 3-vessel n = 4) were scheduled for a minimally invasive coronary artery bypass operation. In all 15 patients, the LAD was the dominant vessel of good caliber. Thirteen LAD's showed a high-grade proximal lesion; 2 LAD's were proximally occluded. The mean age of the patients was 58 ± 10 (37–73) y, weight 78.8 ± 11.5 (63–97) kg, and left ventricular ejection fraction 56 ± 10 (35–79)%. In 14 patients a sinus rhythm was found and in one patient a chronic supraventricular arrhythmia. In 5 out of these 15 patients concomitant diseases were present (Table 1). Anesthesia was maintained with the intravenous infusion of Propofol and Sufentanyl or Remifentanyl continously and a single bolus injection of Pancuronium bromide. Standard monitoring of cardiac surgery was performed including automatic ST segment analysis and Swan Ganz catheter monitoring. After an inversed L-shaped mini-sternotomy up to the 3rd intercostal space the LIMA was harvested up to the 2nd intercostal space under direct vision and maximal vasodilatation was achieved by injection of Papaverin. After administration of heparin (100 U/kg body weight) the LAD was snared twice in the mid level using silicon loops. After a 5 min period of LAD occlusion followed by a 5 min period of reperfusion, the LAD

Table 1. Preoperative data of patients with severe concomitant disease undergoing minimally invasive LIMA-to-LAD procedure (n = 5)

Patient no.	1	2	3	4	5
Age	69	64	68	60	73
Sex	m	m	m	m	m
EF (%)	40	50	35	60	60
CAD (vessels)	3	3	2	1	3
Stenoses (%)	LAD 80 M1 50 RCA 100, small	LAD 90 D1 60, small M1 90, small RCA 100, calcified	LAD 80 CX 100, small	LAD 85	LAD 100 CX 95 RCA 80
Concomitant diseases	– prostatic cancer – renal dysfunction – diabetes mellitus	– diabetes mellitus – renal tumor	– COPD	– prostatic cancer	– previous partial resection of the colon (carcinoma) and of the liver (metastasis)
Hemoglobin (mg/dl)	13.4	14.1	13.7	12.2	11.8
Creatinine (mg/dl)	2.1	1.1	1.0	1.0	1.1

EF = left ventricular ejection fraction, CAD = coronary artery disease, COPD = chronic obstructive pulmonary disease

was snared again and anastomosis between LIMA and LAD was performed with a running 8–0 monofilic sucture on a locally stabilized anastomosis area on the beating heart without the use of CPB. In the case of retrograde coronary flow through the arteriotomy field, blood was displaced by a CO_2-blower device. No preconditioning was used. When anastomosis had been completed, the silicon loops were taken away and the pedicle was fixed with a fibrin glue in order to avoid kinking of the mammary artery pedicle and the pericardium was closed. A retrosternal drainage as well as a drainage into the left pleural cavity was inserted. Mini-sternotomy was refixed by wires and wound was occluded. In 2 patients with a coronary 3-vessel disease, coronary stenoses of the RCA and the CX could be treated by interventional cardiological techniques after successful LIMA-to-LAD procedure. The quality of the LIMA anastomosis was controlled in a coronary angiogram.

Results

All operations were performed without any intraoperative complications. The period of coronary occlusion of 22 ± 8 (10–36) min was well tolerated by all patients, even by the one with low left ventricular ejection fraction. Patients remai-

Table 2. Intraoperative and postoperative data of patients with severe concomitant diseases undergoing the minimally invasive LIMA-to-LAD procedure (n = 5)

Patient no.	1	2	3	4	5
LAD occlusion time (min)	24	14	20	10	27
Time of operation (min)	115	125	150	145	165
ST elevation during LAD occlusion	–	–	–	–	–
CK (U/L) 4 h postoperatively	28	122	77	82	75
Postoperative ventilation (h)	7	2	2	0	4.5
Hospital stay (days)	8	6	6	8	4
Creatinine (mg/dl) at discharge	12.0	11.1	12.9	11.8	8.9
Hemoglobin (mg/dl) at discharge	2.1	1.1	1.1	0.9	1.1
Complications	–	–	–	–	–
PTCA, postoperatively ("hybrid" procedure)	–	–	–	–	RCA, CX

ned hemodynamically stable without pharmacological support. No arrhythmias occured in any patients. Only slight ST elevations (0.7 ± 0.6 (0.3–1.7) mV) were present in 5 patients. In the other 10 patients, ECG remained completely unchanged during LAD occlusion. After declamping of the LIMA-to-LAD bypass in 8 patients Protamin (3750 ± 1000 U/kg body weight) was administered to reverse the anticoagulatory effect of heparin. The other 7 patients were not antagonized by Protamin. Operation time was 144 ± 20 (110–180) min. The patients were transferred to the ICU and extubated 2.7 ± 2.7 (0–7) h after the end of surgery (Table 2). Creatinine kinase, measured 4 h postoperatively, was 75 ± 30 U/l. No increase of myocardial band creatinine kinase was observed. The postoperative course was uneventful in all patients, except a re-exploration in one patient 3 h after surgery due to prolonged bleeding (200 ml/h) through the thorax drainages. During re-exploration bleeding from the sternum was found, which was treated with diathermia. No transfusion was necessary in any of the 15 patients and the mean hemoglobin value on discharge was 12.0 ± 1.5 (8.8–15.7) mg/dl. No respiratory insufficiency and no diaphragm dysfunction occured. In none of the patients was a worsening of preexistent organ dysfunction (Table 1) observed. All patients were free of angina pectoris, postoperatively, and coronary angiograms showed a patent LIMA-to-LAD anastomosis. Postoperative echocardiography revealed no pathological finding in any patient. During the postoperative course no new episode of supraventricular arrhythmia occured. No cerebrovascular events and no neuropsychiatric abnormalities were observed in any of the 15 patients. Patients were discharged 6.5 ± 1.5 (4–9) days after surgery in a good condition. In 2 patients with a coronary 3-vessel disease, additional coronary stenoses in the RCA and CX were treated by interventional cardiological techniques (4 days/25 days) after successful LIMA-to-LAD procedure.

Discussion

LIMA-to-LAD procedures were performed in a group of selected patients with coronary 1–3 vessel disease and proved to be a safe and effective approach, even in a patient with decreased left ventricular ejection fraction. In all cases a secure anastomosis could be done by local stabilization and the use of a CO_2-blower device. No ventricular arrhythmias occured during coronary occlusion and patients remained hemodynamically stable (6). No preconditioning was used (8). Despite of this fact and a mean LAD occlusion time of 22 ± 8 min no increase of myocardial band creatinine kinase was observed after a minimally invasive LIMA-to-LAD procedure in any patient (11, 16).

In 7 patients with coronary 2- or 3-vessel disease, the LIMA-to-LAD procedure was performed either alone (n = 5) or in combination with postoperative coronary angioplasty of the RCA and CX (n = 2). In all 7 cases the LAD was the dominant vessel. The other coronary vessels were either small or diffuse calcified (n = 3), had stenoses of < 70% (n = 2) or significant stenoses (> 70%), which were treated by angioplasty postoperatively (n = 2). Anastomoses patency rates after minimally invasive LIMA-to-LAD procedure are report to be about 90% (4, 15). In our small group all postoperative angiograms showed a patent LIMA-to-LAD anstomosis. The quality of anastomoses appeared to be the same as the one achieved via the conventional coronary bypass technique. Patients were free of angina pectoris and did not show signs of ischemia in ECG. Routine postoperative angiogram is invasive and expensive. Subramamanian found that echodardiography correlates well with angiography and switched to less-invasive doppler-echocardiography (15).

The avoidance of cerebrovascular strokes and neuropsychiatric abnormalities by elimination of the use of the heart-lung machine is one of the great advantages of the minimally invasive LIMA-to-LAD procedure in contrast to conventional coronary artery bypass surgery. Despite of risk factors (diabetes mellitus, previous stroke) in some patients no cerebrovascular event was observed in our small group of patients.

Less traumatization of tissue and avoiding of the high-dose heparinization and hemodilution of standard CPB are further benefits of the minimally invasive LIMA-to-LAD procedure resulting in a less amount of postoperative bleeding and less demand of transfusion (12). In our group no patient required a transfusion. Interstingly, we did not observe any postoperative new episode of supraventricular arrhyhtmia, which is in contrast to other authors (6, 11, 16).

Respiratory insufficiency and diaphragm dysfunction could not be observed in any patient. In contrast, diaphragm dysfunction occures in 10–80% of patients undergoing conventional coronary artery bypass surgery (7). Having only a limited experience with the postoperative recovery of patients having undergone this new minimally invasive approach, postoperative hospital stay in our group was 6.5 ± 1.5 days, which will be certainly reduced in the future (12).

Conclusion

The results show that LIMA-to-LAD procedure on the beating heart without the use of CPB is a safe and effective method in selected patients with coronary 1–3 vessel disease as well as in patients with severe concomitant diseases. The described minimally invasive LIMA-to-LAD procedure seemed to be a suitable approach especially for patients with severe concomitant diseases in contrast to conventional coronary bypass grafting because preoperative organ dysfunction was not worsened by the use of CPB. In patients with coronary 1–3 vessel diseases the LIMA-to-LAD procedure can be combined with coronary angioplasty. This less invasive approach propably results in a better patient outcome and a reduction of costs.

References

1. Anderson DR, Stephenson LW, Edmunds LH (1991) Management of complications of cardiopulmonary bypass: Complications of organ systems, In: Waldhausen JA, Orringer MB (eds) Complications in Cardiothoracic Surgery. St. Louis, Mo. Mosby Year Book, pp 45–59
2. Benetti FJ, Naselli G, Wood M, Geffner L (1991) Direct myocardial revascularization without extracorporeal circulation. Experience in 700 patients. Chest 100: 312–316
3. Buffolo E, de Andrade JCS, Branco JNR, Teles CA, Aguiar LF, Gomes WJ (1996) Coronary artery bypass grafting without cardiopulmonary bypass. Ann Thorac Surg 61: 63–66
4. Calafiore AM, Angelini GD (1996) Left anterior small thoracotomy (LAST) for coronary artery revascularization. Lancet 347: 263–264
5. Calafiore AM, Giammarco GD, Teodori G, Bosco G, D'Annunzio E, Barsotti A, Maddestra N, Paloscia L, Vitolla G, Sciarra A, Fino C, Contini M (1996) Left anterior descending coronary grafting via left anterior small thoracotomy without cardiopulmonary bypass. Ann Thorac Surg 61: 1658–1665
6. Elefteriades JA (1997) Mini-CABG: A step forward or backward? The "Pro" Point of View. J Cardiothorac Vasc Anesth 11 (5): 661–668
7. Elefteriades JA, Weese-Mayer DE (1996) The diaphragm: Dysfunction and induced pacing, In: Glenn WWL, Baue AE, Geha AS, et al (eds) Glenn's Thoracic and Cardiovascular Surgery (ed 6). Stamford CT, Appleton & Lange pp 623–642
8. Engelman DT, Chen CZ, Watanabe M, Engelman RM, Rousou JA, Flack JE 3rd, Deaton DW, Maulik N, Das DK (1995) Improved 4- and 6-hour myocardial preservation by hypoxic preconditioning. Circulation 92: 1417–1422 (suppl 9)
9. Fonger JD, Nicholson CF, Sussman MS, Salomon NW (1996) Cost analysis of current therapies for limited coronary artery revascularization. Circulation 94: I–51 (suppl)
10. Gundry S, Anees JR, Bailey LL (1996) Coronary artery bypass with and without the heart-lung machine: A case-matched 6-year follow-up. Circulation 94: I–52 (suppl)
11. Jansen EWL, Grundemann PF, Borst C, Eefting FFD, Wesenhagen HH, Diephuis J, Reijnvaan AF, Mansvelt Beck H, O Robles de Medina E, Bredee JJ (1996) Less invasive coronary artery bypass grafting on the beating heart: Initial clinical experience with the Utrecht "Octopus" method for regional cardiac wall immobilization. Circulation 94: I–52 (suppl)
12. Magovern JA, Mack MJ, Ladreneau RJ, Acuff TE, Benckart DH, Hunter TJ, Magovern GJ Jr (1996) The minimally invasive approach reduces the morbidity of coronary artery bypass. Circulation 94: I–52 (suppl)
13. Pae WE, Williams DR, Troncelliti EK, Waldhausen JA (1991) Prevention of complications during cardiopulmonary bypass, In: Waldhausen JA, Orringer MB (eds) Complications in Cardiothoracic Surgery. St. Louis, MO, Mosby-Year Book, pp 39–45
14. Salasidis GC, Latter DA, Steinmetz OK, Blair, JF, Graham AM (1995) Carotid artery duplex scanning in preoperative assessment for coronary artery revascularization: The association between peripheral vascular disease, carotid artery stenosis, and stroke. J Vasc Surg 21: 154–160
15. Subramanian VA (1996) Minimally invasive direct coronary artery bypass surgery via a small left anterior thoracotomy. Video Journal of Cardiothoracic Surg X: 2
16. Tellides G, Maragh M, Smith JM (in press) Minimally invasive coronary artery bypass grafting: Initial Connecticut experience. Connecticut Medicine

Author's address:
Friedrich-Christian Riess, M.D.
Albertinen-Krankenhaus
Abteilung für Herzchirurgie
Suentelstraße 11a
22457 Hamburg, Germany

Cardiac surgery and concomitant thoracic aortic disease

J. S. Coselli and P. J. Oberwalder

Baylor College of Medicine / The Methodist Hospital, Houston, USA

Introduction

In congenital cardiac surgery, the pathology treated frequently presents as a diverse condition with a broad spectrum of manifestations arising from involvement of both the heart and the aorta. Therefore, combined operations on the heart and the aorta are consequently quite often performed in neonates or children. However, cardiac surgery and concomitant surgical interventions of the thoracic aorta as a primary operative procedure in adults is a relatively rare entity. This report focuses on clinical presentations in the adult patient, which require simultaneous procedures, whether they result from a separate pathology or from intraoperative situations, which necessitate concomitant surgery.

Indications for concomitant cardiac and aortic surgery

Management of congenital cardiac pathology in adults

Currently the trend in congenital heart disease is toward a primary surgical correction during infancy; adult, continue to present for both primary and reoperative surgery for congenital heart disease. Indications for surgery may result either from former palliation, residual defects, or sequelae from a previous repair. Furthermore, a few of these manifestations may reach their clinical relevance in the mature patient only (i.e., bicuspid aortic valve with coarctation of the aorta), which then require combined cardiac and aortic surgery.

Special considerations are necessary in patients with Marfan syndrome. The cardiovascular manifestations of this heritable connective tissue disorder are common and deleterious if untreated (18). These include aortic root dilatation, aortic valve regurgitation, aneurysm and/or dissection of the ascending aorta, the aortic arch, the descending and occasionally the thoracoabdominal aorta. All of which are immediate and long-term threats to the survival of these patients. In contradistinction to adult patients with Marfan syndrome, mitral valve disease is the most common cause of morbidity and mortality in infants with the syndrome (21). A variety of anatomic changes affect the mitral valve apparatus. In three-quarters of such patients mitral valve prolapse is present, which is usually benign in its earlier stages. Nevertheless, the rate of progression is unpredictable and serious mitral valve regurgitation may occur: the chorda stretch and may occasionally rupture and lead to the sudden onset of severe mitral regurgitation and congestive heart failure. Other recognized complications include ventricular arrhythmias, sudden death, infective endocarditis, and calcification of the mitral ring. Diagnosis of the severity of mitral valve disease has been significantly improved with the routine intraoperative use of transesophageal echocardiography (TEE). Most of the mitral valve operations in adult Marfan patients are concomitant procedures during their aortic surgery. Intraoperative TEE in these patients should always be used to evaluate the severity of mitral valve regurgitation and left ventricular function. Furthermore, the diameter of the aortic root, the sinotubular junction, and the ascending aorta can be determined precisely. In cases of acute/chronic type I and type II aortic dissection, the surgeon is able to obtain important information regarding the "flap," which separates the true lumen from the false lumen, as well as involvement of the aortic valve or coronary ostia in the proximal extent of the dissection. Gillinow et al. recommend concomitant mitral valve surgery in all patients undergoing aortic surgery (commonly aortic root replacement) if the mitral regurgitation is > 2+ / 3+ (11).

Association of bicuspid aortic valve with aortic abnormalities

Bicuspid aortic valve is one of the most common congenital heart anomalies found in adults (22). Coarctation of the aorta, dissecting aneurysm, and aortic root dilatation may be associated with a functionally normal, stenotic or incompetent bicuspid aortic valve (1, 9, 10, 13). A retrospective study by Hahn et al. (13) revealed a high prevalence of aortic root dilatation in patients with a hemodynamically normal bicuspid aortic valve. This aortic root disease can express itself in older adults as an aneurysm with aortic regurgitation or appear even more dramatic in younger adults as aortic dissection. The risk of aortic dissection in individuals with congenitally bicuspid and unicommissural aortic valves is 9–18 times higher than in patients with tricuspid aortic valves (9).

Takayasu's disease

Takayasu's disease is a chronic inflammatory disease of unknown etiology involving the aorta and its major branches with an incidence of 1.2 to 2.6 per million per year within the North American and European population (14). It most commonly involves the aortic arch and its major branches (type I) with changes that are usually marked at branch points in the aorta. Type II affects the thoracoabdominal aorta and particularly the renal arteries. Type III combines features of both types I and II. The pulmonary artery and its branches may also be involved (type IV) (23). The arterial lesions are purely stenotic in the majority of patients and purely aneurysmatic in only 2% of cases. Aortic regurgitation as a consequence of disease of the proximal ascending aorta is seen in about 25% of cases. Coronary artery involvement may cause angina or myocardial infarction. Surgical tratment is indicated to relieve cerebral ischemia, resolve aortic coarctation, repair aortic or arterial aneurysms, correct renovascular hypertension, treat aortic regurgitation, respectively, and chronic heart failure. Aortic valve replacement is usually performed with aortic repair or bypass grafts to affected arch branches. Otheki et al. (20) reported their experience of concomitant aortic valve replacement and other aortic procedures in 12 patients with Takayasu's arteritis (4 male and 8 female patients, with a mean age of 48 years, range 24 to 67 years). Stenotic lesions were present in the aortic arch branch in nine (75%) and in the pulmonary artery in seven (58%) patients. Aneurysmal dilation in the ascending aorta of more than 6 cm was found in four (33%), coronary lesion in four (33%), thoracic aortic lesion in six (50%), and a lesion in the abdominal aorta and its visceral branch in six (50%) patients. Simple aortic valve replacement alone was performed in two patients. Concomitant aortic valve replacement was carried out in ten patients: aortic root reconstruction in two, ascending aortic plication in three, coronary artery bypass grafting in two, aortic arch branch bypass grafting in one, aortic arch branch bypass grafting and coronary ostium endarterectomy in one, and mitral valve replacement and ascending aortic plication in one patient. There were no operative deaths, and only one patient died later, 18 months after the operation, because of secondary amyloidosis.

Intraoperative complications

Acute intraoperative aortic dissection

With the progressively increasing age of patients submitted to cardiac cardiac surgery, calcified and friable aortas susceptible to possible intraoperative injuries are likley to be more frequently encountered. The site of aortic cannulation and the aortic cross-clamping are recognized as to be prone to the development of intraoperative aortic dissection. Additionally, poorly closed aortotomy sites, as with aortic valve replacement or proximal aortic vein graft anastomosis, may be associated with such a problem. Congenital syndromes associated with an abnormal aortic wall, severe initimal atherosclerosis, mural calcification, and poststenotic aneurysmal dilatation with thinning predisposes for "iatrogenic dissections". Furthermore, femoral arterial cannulation with retrograde arterial perfusion, or the insertion and placement of an intra-aortic balloon are known to, on occasion, result in the development of retrograde aortic dissection. The incidence of acute intraoperative aortic dissection ranges from 0.03 to 0.35% with a hospital mortality of 14.8% (25). Prompt recognition is fundamental to successful management. The use of transesophageal echocardiography can be helpful in determining the extent of involvement of the dissection process. Treatment depends on the extent of the dissection; if localized and involving only a small aortic segment, plication may be sufficient. Occasionally, excision of a small affected aortic segment with reconstitution of the aortic edges and closure using a Dacron patch may be of use. Extensive dissections are best treated by resection and graft replacement of the proximal aorta. If the arch is involved, deep hypothermic circulatory arrest is used for partial or total arch replacement. In rare cases, if the aortic root, or the coronary ostia or even the aortic valve are involved, a composite valve graft may be necessary. Prevention should include complete incision of the intimal layer for aortic cannulation, application and removal of clamps during brief periods of reduced flow and pressure, avoidance of multiple aortic clamp applications, and careful inclusion of all aortic layers in suture lines. Arterial cannulation over a guide wire in suspicious femoral arteries is also very helpful (12, 19).

Atherosclerotic disease of the ascending aorta

Significant atherosclerotic disease involving the ascending aorta occurs in 5–13% of patients with open heart surgery and may cause stroke or embolization to the coronary, visceral, and renal arteries during the manipulation of the aorta. An autopsy study of 221 patients who underwent myocardial revascularization or valve operations revealed a high correlation of atheroemboli with severe atherosclerosis of the ascending aorta. 46 of 48 pts (95.8%) who had evidence of atheroemboli had severe atherosclerosis of the ascending aorta (3). The degree of atherosclerotic disease is classified as mild aortic disease with a localized thickening (≤ 3 mm) of the ascending aorta, moderate aortic disease with focal areas of moderate or severe atherosclerosis (> 3 mm intimal thickening) and severe aortic disease with multiple areas of severe atherosclerosis or circumferential involvement. Intraoperative inspection of the outside of the aorta does not provide clues to the degree of atheromatous involvement. However, the disease is most common in patients with symptomatic disease of other major arteries, smoking, hypertension, and increasing age (Table 1). Intraoperative epiaortic or transesophageal echocardiography remains the "gold standard" in the evaluation of suspicious segments of the aorta. This technique was used intraoperatively in 500 consecutive patients undergoing cardiac surgery and revealed a 14–29% incidence of significant ascending aortic atherosclerosis (25). Manipulation, cannulation or clamping of the diseased aorta are the most common maneuvers resulting in distal embolization and stroke. Prevention of embolic complications of an atherosclerotic aorta can be achieved by 1) screening (preoperative and intraoperative) of the ascending aorta, 2) identification of high-risk patients, and 3) aggressive surgical treatment of moderate or severe atherosclerotic aorta. Once the extent of disease is evident, further steps toward reducing the risk of atherosclerotic emboli are necessary (Table 2). Severe atherosclerotic aortic disease may require resection and replacement of the aorta with a tube graft. Deep hypothemic circulatory arrest may be necessary to replace an affected aortic arch. The use of retrograde cerebral perfusion is an excellent adjunct to flush out embolic material from the cerebral vessels in such cases. In coronary artery revascularization procedures, the risk for atheromatous emboli can be reduced by using 1) Single clamp technique, or 2) "Non touch-technique" (Proximal vein anastomoses are performed end-to-side to internal mammary artery grafts or innominate artery; arterial revascularization only). Proper technical management of the problem has

Table 1. Characteristics of patients with ascending aorta atherosclerosis – modified from [16]

Characteristics	No Atherosclerosis (n = 969)	Atherosclerosis (n = 213)	p-value
Age, years; mean (range)	67.7% ± 8.5 (50–90)	71.1 ± 8.0 (50–70)	< 0.0001
Left main disease, %	21.3	25.6	0.159
Extent of coronary disease	2.76 ± 1.4	3.02 ± 1.3	0.012
Hypertension	61.7	66.7	0.160
Smoking	46.4	61.3	< 0.0001
Peripheral vascular disease	6.8	19.5	< 0.0001

Table 2. Techniques to reduce the risk of atheromatous emboli in atherosclerotic aorta disease

Arterial cannulation of the aciliary artery
distal aortic arch
femoral artery
Hyperthermic fibrillatory arrest
Patch aortoplasty
Aortic endarterectomy
Replacement of the ascending aorta

been shown to substantially reduce the morbidity and mortality in the treatment of affected patients (16, 25).

Aortic valve insufficiency and concomitant ascending aortic Aneurysm/dissection

The correct treatment of ascending aortic aneurysm or dissection with aortic valve insufficiency is still a challenging controversy for all cardiac surgeons. A variety of surgical methods has evolved through the years but still precise guidelines have not yet been defined. In general, the surgical procedures consist of two basic techniques: 1) separate valve and graft replacement (26) and 2) composite valve graft replacement (2). Since their introduction, both techniques have undergone a number of modifications.

Yun et al., compared all currently available information from a number of different centers and found that early and late results of separate versus composite valve graft replacement seem to be quiet similar (29). Recently, aortic valve-sparing procedures, first described by Yacoub et al. (27) and subsequently modified by David et al. (5–7), have become popular in the treatment of annuloaortic ectasia with aortic regurgitation. However, proper patient selection and precise operative technique remain crucial in achieving excellent early and long-term results for patients with fusiform ascending aortic aneurysm or dissection with aortic valve regurgitation. The following guidelines for management of concomitant ascending aortic aneurysm/dissection and aortic valve regurgitation have been proposed by Yun et al. (29): 1) separate valve and graft replacement (SVG) is considered in older patients with relatively preserved sinuses and if the aortic valve cannot be repaired or in those with atherosclerotic aneurysms. Care should be taken to resect most of the sinuses to prevent late aneurysmal degeneration of the residual aortic root. SVG is also an option in non-Marfan patients with relatively normal aortic root anatomy. Second, composite valve graft replacement (CVG) is the method of choice in Marfan patients and in patients with destroyed sinuses by aortic dissection or pronounced dilatation of the aortic annulus. If the aortic valve leaflets are normal and the aortic annulus is not excessively dilated, a valve-sparing procedure might be a good alternative in selected patients. Third, CVG homograft root replacement or a synthetic CVG procedure is advisable in patients with complex prosthetic valve endocarditis or multiple paravalvular leaks. With all CVG procedures a "modified" technique of reimplantation of the coronary arteries should be used to avoid the potential for late false aneurysm formation (4, 24).

Coronary artery disease and aortic dissection

Today, less invasive diagnostic tools, such as transesophageal echocardiography, computed tomography, and magnetic resonance imaging are widely used for the diagnosis of acute/chronic aortic dissections. However, they are unable to reliably provide adequate information about concomitant coronary artery disease in patients with aortic dissection. The advanced age of the patient population affected by aortic dissection makes severe coexisting coronary artery disease a significant consideration. Therefore, an effort to reduce perioperative mortality or morbidity caused by myocardial infarction has to be made with an evaluation of the coronary artery anatomy at the time of presentation, particularly in those patients with multiple risk factors. Creswell et al. (4) reviewed 62 patients with aortic dissection type A (42 acute and 20 chronic). Among the patients with acute dissection, 23 underwent coronary arteriography and in 8 patients (34.8%) one or more coronary lesions > 50% narrowing were found. Among the patients with chronic dissection, 6 patients (42.9%) of 14 who underwent coronary arteriography had one or more stenotic lesions > 50% of their coronary arteries. Consequently, they, carried out simultaneous coronary bypass grafting in 4 patients with acute and in 6 patients with chronic type A aortic dissection. There were no intraoperative deaths. The authors consequently recommended all patients with an acute type A dissection who were in a stable clinical and hemodynamic condition and all patients with a chronic type A dissection undergo preoperative coronary arteriography.

In an earlier series of 302 patients, JR Young et al. (28) looked at the presence of coronary artery disease (CAD) in patients with infrarenal (289) and thoracoabdominal aortic aneurysms (13). Prior to elective aortic reconstruction, coronary arteriography was performed in all patients and, in addition, myocardial revascularization was carried out when indicated. 36% of all patients were identified as having CAD. Compared to an evaluation of patients suspicious of CAD by means of standard clinical criteria, CAD was identified in 42% of patients suspected to have CAD and in 19% of those in whom CAD was not expected.

Even in patients with impaired left ventricular function, Mohr and colleagues were able to present excellent results in combined procedures of coronary artery bypass grafting and abdominal aortic aneurysm (AAA) resection. 25 patients with a mean age of 69.4 years (range 55–80 years) underwent AAA resectiom either with a tube graft (12 patients) or bifurcation graft (13 patients). 30-day mortality was 12% (3 patients) and 1-year actuarial survival was 88% (17).

During the period between January 11, 1986 and August 18, 1997 the senior author treated 1,000 surgically for pathology involving the thoracoabdominal aorta. These included 586 male patients (58.6%) and 414 female patients (41.4%).

Table 3. Ascending and aortic arch aneurysms with concomitant cardiac surgery – results of operation

Complication	Concurrent CAB	p-value	Concurrent valve	p-Value	Concurrent CAB & valve	p-value
	(n = 186)		(n = 404)		(n = 110)	
Stroke	8 (4.3%)	0.310	7 (1.7%)	0.010	3 (2.7%)	1.000
Cardiac	35 (18.8%)	0.004	59 (14.6%)	0.080	24 (21.8%)	0.002
Bleeding	9 (4.8%)	0.234	15 (3.7%)	0.683	7 (6.4%)	0.086

Table 4. Thoracoabdominal aortic aneurysms with concomitant cardiac disease – results of operation

Complication	Coronary artery disease	p-value	Prior CAB and/or angioplasty	p-value
Renal failure	30 (8.6%)	0.087	12 (7.7%)	0.600
PAR/PLG	20 (5.8%)	0.404	10 (6.5%)	0.342
Bleeding	8 (2.3%)	0.299	2 (1.3%)	1.000
Cardiac	40 (11.4%)	0.041	14 (9.0%)	0.972

The mean age was 65.6 years. There were 257 patients (25.7%) with aortic dissection and 743 patients with nondissection pathology. The over all early survival was 95.2% (690 patients). Of these 1000 patients treated surgically for thoracoabdominal aortic aneurysm, 35.1% (351 patients) had concomitant coronary artery disease. Postoperative cardiac related complications in these patients occurred in 11.4% (40 pts) and in 9.0% (14 pts) in those patients who had a previous myocardial revascularization or coronary angioplasty (Table 3). During the time period between January 1987 and September 1997, 691 patients underwent surgical repair of an ascending aorta and/or transverse aortic arch aneurysm. Of these, 262 patients (37.9%) presented with coronary artery disease at the time of their aortic surgical procedure, and in 186 patients (71%) simultaneously coronary bypass grafting was performed. The postoperative cardiac related complications occurrred in 24 of 110 patients (21.8%) undergoing concomitant coronary artery bypass grafting and aortic valve replacement at the time of proximal aortic replacement (Table 4).

References

1. Becker AE, Becker MJ, Edwards JE (1970) Anomalies associated with coarctation of the aorta. Circulation 41: 1067–1076
2. Bentall HH, De Bono A (1968 A technique for complete replacement of the ascending aorta. Thorax 23: 338–339
3. Blauth CI, Cosgrove DM, Webb BW et al. (1992) Atheroembolism from the ascending aorta. An emerging problem in cardiac surgery. J Thorac Cardiovasc Surg 103: 1104–1111
4. Creswell LL, Kouchoukos NT, Cox JL et al. (1950) Coronary artery disease in patients with type A aortic dissection, Ann Thorac Surg 59: 585–590
5. David TE, Feindel CM (1992) An aortic valve-sparing operation for patients with aortic incompetence and aneurysm of the ascending aorta. J Thorac Cardiovasc Surg 103: 617–622
6. David and C. M. Feindel (1995) Repair of the aortic valve in patients with aortic insufficiency and aortic root aneurysm. J Thorac Cardiovasc Surg 109: 345–352
7. David TE (1996) Remodeling of the aortic root and presentation of the native aortic valve. Operative Tech Cardiac Thorac Surg 1: 44–56
8. Davila-Roman VG, Barzilai B, Kouchoukos NT et al. (1994) Atherosclerosis of the ascending aorta. Stroke 25: 2010–2016
9. Edwards WD, Leaf DS, Edwards JE (1978) Dissecting aortic aneurysms associated with congenital bicuspidaortic valve. Circulation 57: 1022–1025
10. Fenoglio JJ, McAllister HA, DeCastro CM et al. (1977) Congenital bicuspid aortic valve after age 20. Am J Cardiol 39: 164–169
11. Gillinow MA, Hulyalkar A, Cameron DE et al. (1994) Mitral valve operation in patients with the Marfan's syndrome. J Thorac Cardiovasc Surg 107: 724–731
12. Gott JP, Cohen CL, Jones EL (1990) Management of ascending aortic dissections and aneurysm early and late following cardiac operations. J Card Surg 5: 2–14
13. Hahn RT, Roman MJ, Maftader AH et al. (1992) Association of aortic dilatation with regurgitant, stenotic and functionally normal bicuspid aortic valves. J Am Coll Cardiol 19: 283–287
14. Kerr GS, Hallahan CW, Giordano J et al. (1994) Takayasu arteritis. Ann Intern Med 120: 919–929
15. Kouchoukos NT, Wareing TH, Murphy SF et al. (1991) Sixteen year experience with aortic root replacement: Results of 172 operations. Ann Surg 214: 308–320
16. Mills NL; Everson CT (1991) Atherosclerosis of the ascending aorta and coronary artery bypass. J Thorac Cardiovasc Surg 102: 546–553
17. Mohr FW, Falk V, Autschbach R et al. (1995) One-stage surgery of coronary arteries and abdominal aorta in patients with impaired left ventricular function. Circulation 91: 379–385
18. Murdoch JL, Walker BA, Halpern BL. et al. (1972) Life expectancy and causes of death in the Marfan syndrome. N Engl J Med 286: 804–808

19. Murphy DA, Craver JA, Jone EI et al. (1983) Recognition and management of ascending aortic dissection complicating cardiac surgical operations. J Thorac Cardiovasc Surg 85: 247–256
20. Ohteki H, Itoh T, Natsuaki M et al. Aortic valve replacement for Takayasu's arteritis (1992) J Thorac Cardiovasc Surg 104: 482–486
21. Pyeritz RE, Wappel MA (1983) Mitral valve dysfunction in the Marfan syndrome. Am J Med 74: 797–807
22. Roberts WC The congenitally bicuspid aortic valve: a study of 85 autopsy cases. (1970) Am J Cardiol 26: 72–83
23. Svensson LG, Crawford ES (1983) Aortic dissection and aortic aneurysm surgery: clinical observations, experimental investigations, and statistical analyses. Curr Probl Surg 30: 33–35
24. Svensson LG, Crawford ES, Hess KR et al. (1992) Composite valve graft replacement of the proximal aorta: Comparison of techniques in 348 patients. Ann Thorac Surg 54: 427–439
25. Wareing TH, Davila-Roman VG, Kouchoukos NT et al. (1992) Management of the severely atherosclerotic ascending aorta during cardiac operations. J Thorac Cardiovasc Surg 103: 453–462
26. Wheat MW Jr, Wilson JR, Bartley TD (1964) Successful replacement of the entire ascending aorta and aortic valve. JAMA 188: 717–719
27. Yacoub M, Fagan A, Stassno P et al. (1983) Result of valve conserving operations for aortic regurgitation. Circulation 68: III–321 (abstr.)
28. Young JR, Hertzer NR, Beven EG et al. (1986) Coronary artery disease in patients with aortic aneurysm: a classification of 302 coronary angiograms and results of surgical management. Ann Vasc Surg 1: 36–42
29. Yun KL, Miller DC (1997) Ascending aortic aneurysm and aortic valve disease: What is the most optimal surgical technique? Sem Thorac Cardiovasc Surg 9: 233–245

Author's address:
Joseph S. Coselli, M.D.
6560 Fannin, #1100
Houston, TX 77030, USA

The timing of aortic root replacement in the Marfan syndrome: Computerised decision support

T. Treasure, C. Reynolds[1], O. Valencia, A. Child[2], S. Gallivan[1]

Cardiothoracic Unit, St George's Hospital, Blackshaw Road, London SW17 0QT, [1]Clinical Operational Research Unit, Department of Statistical Science, University College London, Gower Street, WC1E 6BT, [2]Department of Cardiological Sciences, St George's Hospital Medical School, Cranmer Terrace, London, SW17 0RE England

Introduction

Among Marfan syndrome patients (1) the most common cause of premature death is aortic dissection. The natural history of the disease has been well studied. In the classical study of McKusick's group at John Hopkins, age at death was 32 years ±16.4 years (5). Already, the use of betablocker therapy, and elective aortic root surgery have prolonged life on average by greater than 25% (6). Increased awareness has enhanced diagnostic ability of clinicians and patients alike, but still, there is much discussion about the optimum time to operate to replace the aortic root (4, 7).

The surgical dilemma

Patients with Marfan syndrome have substantial risk of aortic dissection resulting in death in early adulthood. Timely replacement of the aortic root is specifically intended to pre-empt this event and save life. There are data to suggest that life expectancy amongst Marfan patients has increased (5, 6), and the inference is that surgery has contributed to this whilst also preventing aortic regurgitation. However, even in the most experienced and best hands, this operation has a 30 day mortality of 5% (3). It also results in life-long anticoagulation therapy and catastrophes such as endocarditis in the graft (2), thrombosis of the valve, devastating cerebral embolism, and anticoagulant related haemorrhage. Root replacement early in an individual's life, if successful, may result in many additional years of life. Conversely, many potential years of life would be lost if the operation is unsuccessful. In terms of expected life years, with or without aortic root replacement, the pros and cons of the decision depend very much on the patient's age and actuarial effects. Aortic Root Diameter (ARD) amongst Marfan syndrome patients is also known to be related to height and age. In spite of all these many factors that relate to the decision whether to opt for aortic root replacement, the best advice at present is that the decision be based on a single 'critical' aortic root diameter of 5.0 cm. There are surely better grounds for making this very difficult decision.

Initial studies

Measurement of aortic root diameter is the basis for deciding whether to opt for surgery to replace the aortic root. With increasing surgical confidence, the 'critical' aortic root diameter thought to indicate the need for surgery has reduced from 6 cm to 5.5 cm, to 5 cm (4). However, 5.0 cm is too late to save some patients who have already dissected and probably would lead to some older patients with stable aortic dimensions undergoing unnecessary surgery. Indeed, analysis of records from our own database suggest that it is inappropriate to have a single 'critical' aortic diameter for all patients and that account should be taken of age and height. Perhaps other factors should also be considered.

We aim to improve decision making in relation to Marfan syndrome. We have worked on computerised decision aids to assist the interpretation of serial echocardiograph measurements and, taking account of individual patient features, to give recommendations concerning the timing of aortic replacement. Towards this end, our first steps have been to develop a computer system that can display an individual's aortic root measurements and where they lie in relation to a reference range standardised for the patient's age and height.

In order to derive preliminary reference ranges, we have gathered data concerning 81 classically diagnosed Marfan syndrome patients, aged between 18 and 70 years old. All of these patients had undergone echocardiograph examinations of the aortic root which was measured at level B (see Fig. 1) just above the aortic valve cusp. In order to obtain a statistically independent set of data, the analysis made use of only one aortic root measurement for each patient. This was chosen to be the first available. Choice of the second or subsequent measurement would have indicated a decision not to operate, and hence introduced potential selection bias. Multiple linear regression was used to investigate relationships between the aortic root diameter and height, age and sex. A multiple linear regression was performed.

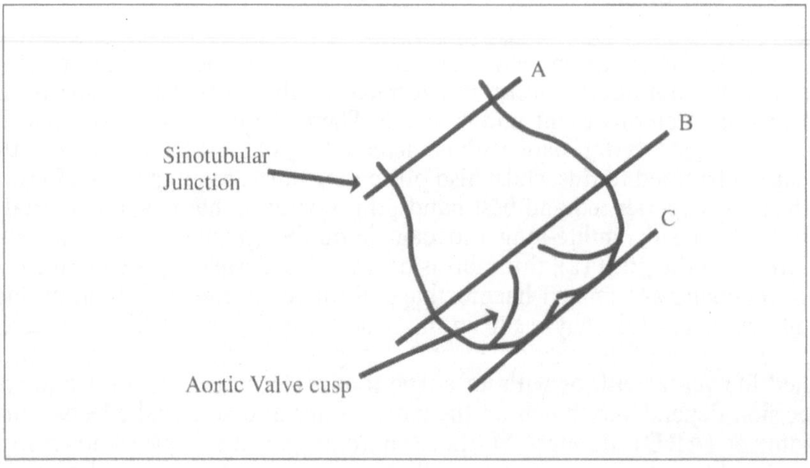

Fig. 1. Echo measurement sites

Results of multivariate analysis

The analysis identified height and age as being variables significantly associated with aortic root diameter. Gender was not independently associated with aortic root diameter except insofar as it is related to height. A scatterplot of aortic root diameter against height, and an associated regression line is shown in Fig. 2.

Based on this multivariate analysis, an equation (see below) was derived for adult Marfan syndrome patients that gives the relationship between the mean aortic root diameter and the patients' height and age. In order to identify typical ranges of aortic root diameters, dependent on age and height, estimates were also calculated for the 5th and 95th percentiles.

Development of the prototype decision support system

As a first step in the development of tools to improve decision making in Marfan syndrome, a computer system has been written that can be used to provide clinicians with a graphical summary of the history of an individual's echocardiograph assessments. This displays a serial plot of a patient's aortic root diameter. The display also makes use of the results of the multivariate analysis described above. Ranges are displayed that indicate where the patient's measurements lie in relation to what would be expected for a group of Marfan syndrome patients of that height

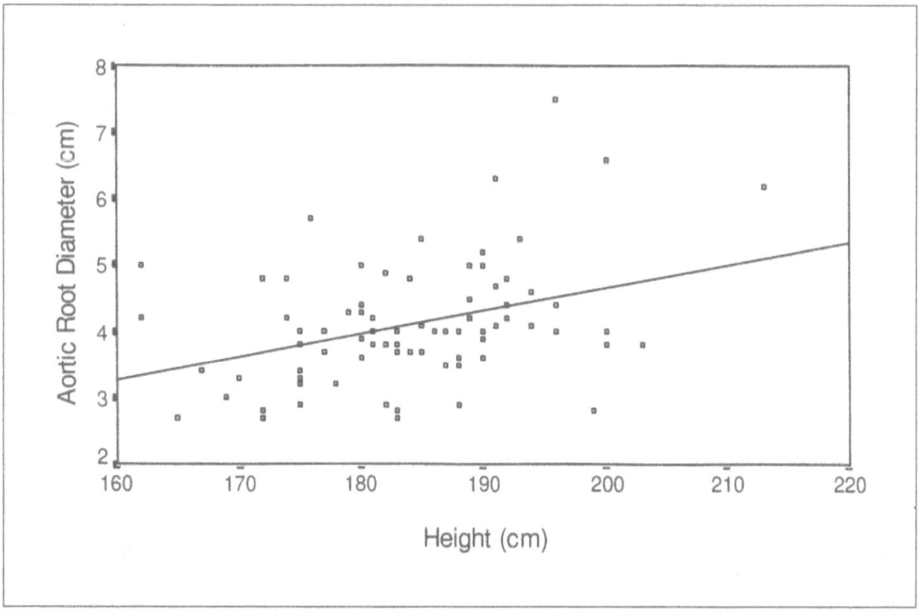

Fig. 2. Height vs ARD

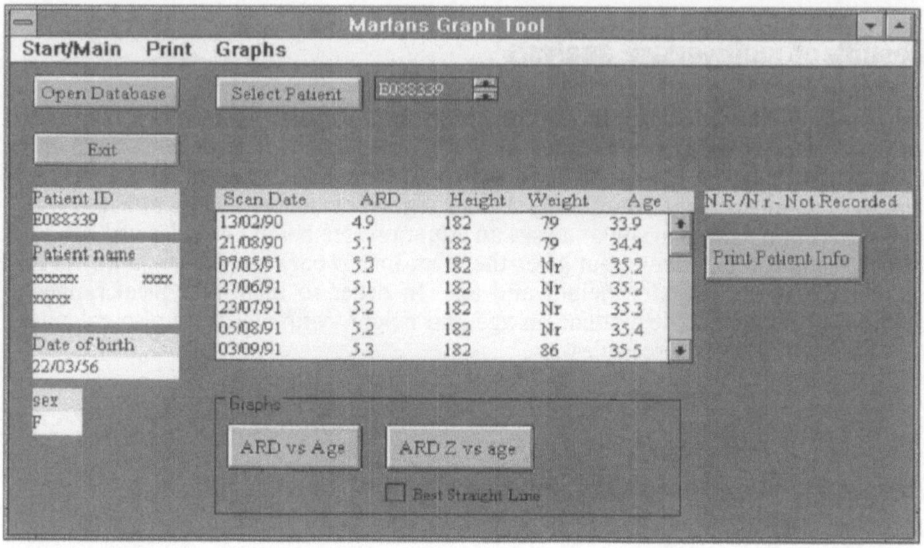

Fig. 3. User Interface

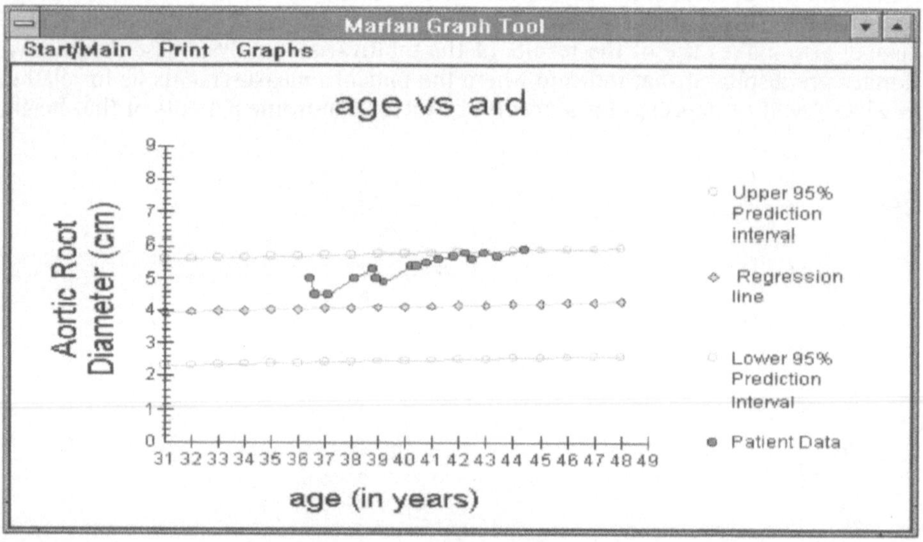

Fig. 4. Patients ARD is steadily increasing

and age. Based on this, the clinician can examine trends in the data and determine whether a particular patient is following an expected course or whether there are worrying departures from the usual dimensions for Marfan patients.

The software is user friendly making use of a menu system that allows the user to examine raw data for patients (see Fig. 3) or to display graphical summaries (see Figs. 4–7) showing serial plots of a patients' echocardiograph results and reference ranges dependent on the patient's age and height. The system also displays the occurrence of major events such as the dates of any operation or dissection.

Figs. 4–7 illustrate serial echocardiograph plots for different patients. These are not typical, involving lengthy follow up, but they have been chosen to illustrate the use of the computer system. Figs. 4 and 5 illustrate the history of patients whose aortas were steadily dilating and, consequently, aortic root replacement was carried out. Fig. 4 illustrates that patient data may be expected to show a relatively high degree of variability.

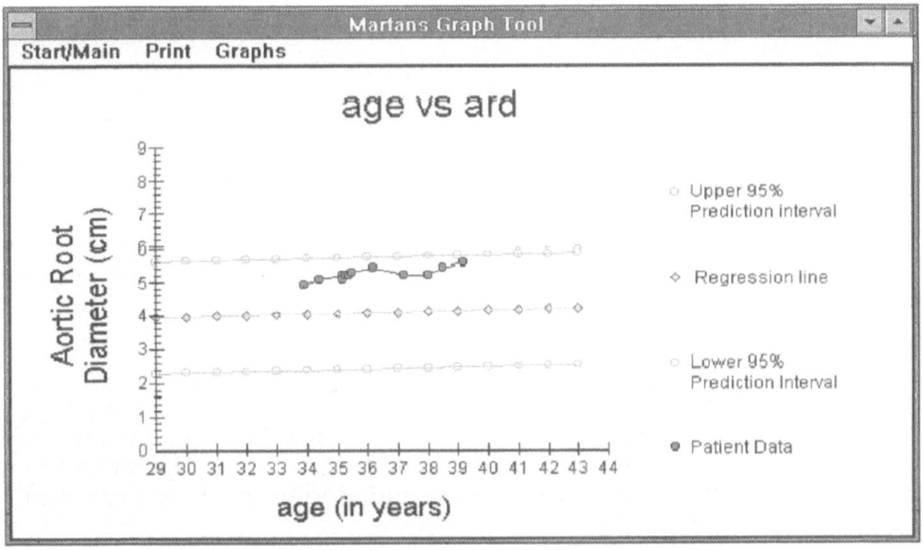

Fig. 5. Patients ARD is increasing

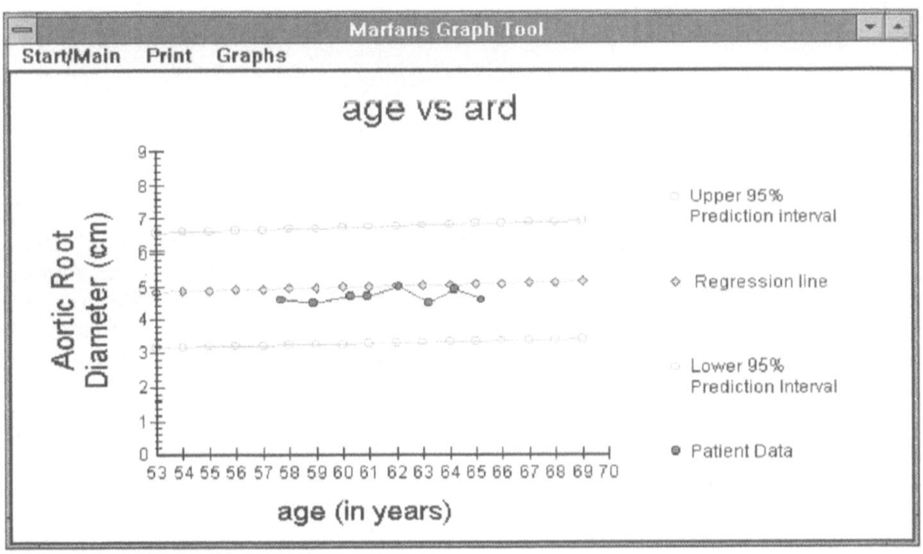

Fig. 6. Older patients may need a different reference range

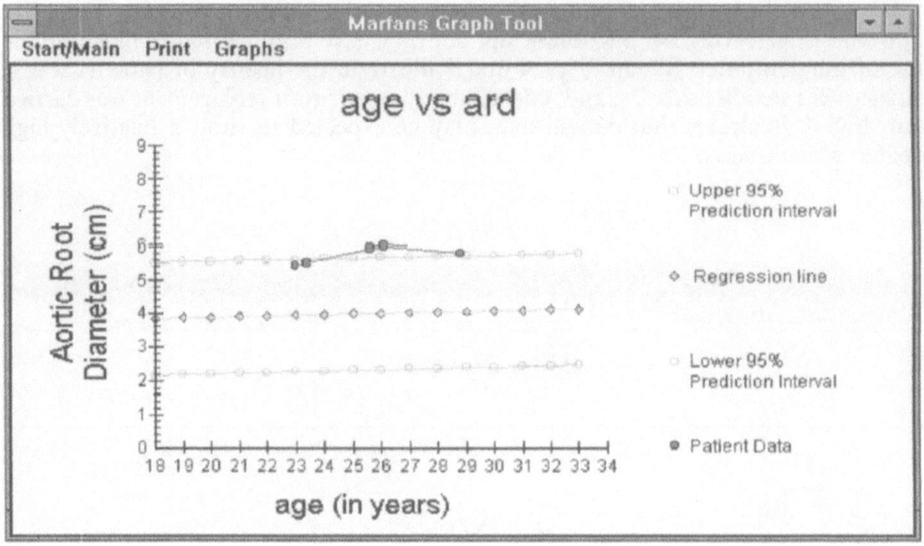

Fig. 7. Patients ARD is on the limit of the reference range

Fig. 6 illustrates an older and taller patient, reflected by an adjusted reference range. This patient has an average aortic root diameter, for a Marfan patient of that age and height, but this is close to the critical value of 5.0 cm often used to indicate the need for surgery.

Fig. 7 shows a patient who has been undergoing conservative treatment and not yet dissected even though they have reached the estimate for the upper 95% percentile for the Marfan population. Here is a case where we would recommend operation on what we know to date but the patient has been followed for 6 years without referral for surgery.

Conclusions

The display has several advantages. It has been developed in consultation with the clinicians who will be using it and so is responsive to their needs. The display allows the user to judge where a particular patient's root diameter places them in relation to the whole Marfan population. The display of a patient's echo data over time shows how echo measurements can vary and highlights the difficulties in relying on a single cut-off point for what is usually a variable echo history. The development of a reference range based on the 95% percentiles allows a Marfan patient to be compared with a general Marfan population who have a similar aortic morphology. Comparison with a normal population gives little insight.

Future Work

The prototype computer system that has been developed displays serial aortic root measurements, standardised for height and age. Further development is planned to add facilities to aid clinical decision making. Although the system has considerable potential, it is as yet unproven. We intend to assemble serial echocardiogram data on 500 Marfan syndrome patients from several centres. We will use these data to calibrate and test the system's performance in determining when patients are at imminent risk of aortic dissection and in urgent need of surgery. As part of this programme of research, there will be a need to improve the precision and scope of the reference ranges used to adjust for age and height. Other potential factors affecting aortic root diameter may need to be taken into account. As yet our analysis has made no allowance for factors such as family history and calibration of our system has been carried out only for adult Marfan patients.

There is also scope for investigating mathematical techniques for analysing the decisions associated with the option of aortic root replacement. At present, our hypothesis is that decision making would be improved by judging how far a patient's aortic root diameter departs from the mean, corrected for age and height. We hypothesise that patients whose aortic diameter lies beyond the 95th percentile for a Marfan population have a high risk of aortic dissection. While this is probably the case, there is a deeper question associated with the critical value for aortic diameter that warrants surgery. If a decision is deferred until the diameter is beyond the upper 95th percentile, then it may often be made too late.

Other potential decision rules might improve decision making still further. If one could reach a stage whereby reasonably accurate forecasts can be made of the probability that dissection would occur within six months, then very powerful decision analytic methods are available that might assist the surgeon. Decision making associated with Marfan Syndrome often relies on an implicit judgement of the short term risk that a patient will dissect unless surgery is performed. Indeed, the decision to opt for surgery may follow from a belief that the risk of perioperative death is less than the probability of dissection and death before the next ultrasound assessment. While at first sight this appears to be a rational strategy, it takes no account of patients' age, their life expectancy nor the longer term view and it is not clear that such a decision rule should be expected to be optimal. An alternative is to use decision analytical methods to combine risk estimates with actuarial data. Data gathered will serve the secondary function of providing a basis for examining whether such an alternative decision making framework is worth investigating.

References

1. Beighton P, et al. (1988) International nosology of heritable disorders of connective tissue. Berlin AM J Med Genet 29: 581–94
2. Cameron DE, Gott VL (1993) Composite Aortic Valve Replacement and Graft Replacement of the ascending Aorta Plus Coronary Ostial Reimplantation: How I do It. Semin-Thorac-Cardiovasc-Surg 5(1): 63–5
3. Gott VL et al (1996) The Marfan syndrome and the cardiovascular surgeon. Eur J Cardiothorac Surg 10: 149–158
4. Afternoon panel session (1995) In: Hetzer R, Gehle P, Ennker J (eds) Cardiovascular aspects of Marfan syndrome Darmstadt, Steinkopff 125–126

5. Murdoch JL, Walker BA, Halpern BL, Kuzma JW, Mckusick VA (1972) Life expectancy and causes of death in Marfan syndrome. N Engl J Med 286: 804–808
6. Silverman DI, Burton KJ, Gray J, Bosner MS, Kouchoukos NT, Roman MJ, Boxer M, Devereux RB, Tsipouras P (1995) Life expectancy in Marfan syndrome. Am J Card 75(2): 157–60
7. Treasure T (1993) Elective replacement of the aortic root in Marfan's syndrome. Br Heart J 69: 101–3

Author's address:
Professor Tom Treasure
Cardiothoracic Unit
St George's Hospital
Blackshaw Road, Tooting, London SW17 0QT

Cardiac surgery and connective tissue disorders

U. P. Rosendahl, J. Ennker

Heart Institute Lahr/Baden, Lahr, Germany

Introduction

Connective tissue disorders are mostly systemic diseases with involvement of several organs or organsystems. Disease processes that entail abnormalities of the connective tissue are polymorphic in their manifestations because of the widespread and crucial function that connective tissue serves in the body (11).

The connective tissue of the heart is created by highly differentiated cardiac myocytes, which create not only the connective tissue of this organ but the parenchyma as well. High fibrillar collagen turnover in the heart and its valve leaflets in particular, is dynamic and essential to tissue repair. Connective tissue supports of the heart and the vascular structures play an comprehensive part in usual cardiovascular performance, and it is therefore not supprising that many connective tissue disorders produce important pathophysiologic processes that affect cardiac and vascular elements.

The prevalance of connective tissue diseases differs with a wide range from common diseases like rheumatoid arthritis to rare diseases like Behcets's syndrome as is shown in Tables 1 and 2.

Collagen disorders and vasculitis syndromes

Involvement of the cardio-vascular system is commonly found in connective tissue diseases like collagen disorders and vasculitis syndromes or congenital disorders as the Marfans, Ehlers Danlos syndrome, and Osteogenesis imperfecta (14, 21, 24,

Table 1. Connective tissue disease prevalance: inflammatory diseases and vasculitis syndromes

Disease	Prevalance
Rheumatoid arthritis	0.3–2.1: 100
Systemic lupus erythematosus	15–50: 100000
Ankylosing spondylitis (M. Bechterew)	0.5–4: 1000/0.05–0.5: 1000
Behcets's syndrome	Japan 1: 1000 – NA/Eur 1: 1000 1: 500000

Table 2. Connective tissue disease prevalence: congenital disorders

Disease	Prevalance
Marfan's syndrome	1: 10000 – 1: 20000
Osteogenesis imperfecta	1: 30000

Table 3. Connective tissue diseases: collagen disorders/inflammatory diseases

Rheumatoid arthritis
Systemic lupus erythematosus
Progressive systemic sclerosis (diffuse scleroderma)
Mixed connective tissue disease
Sjoegren's disease
Ankylosing spondylitis (M. Bechterew)
Behcets's syndrome
Reiter's syndrome

Table 4. Connective tissue diseases: vasculitis syndromes

Temporal arteritis
Takayasu arteritis
Mucocutaneous lymph node syndrome (Kawasaki's disease)
Systemic necrotizing vasculitis (Polyarteritis nodosa)

Table 5. Connective tissue diseases: congenital disorders

Marfan's syndrome (15 q)
Ehlers-Danlos syndrome
Osteogenesis imperfecta

33). Collagen diseases (e.g., systemic lupus erythematosus, rheumatic arthritis, progressive systemic sclerosis, mixed connective tissue disease, Sjoegren's disease) give rise to a range of systemic manifestations and involve the heart to a different degree (Table 3).

Common, often clinically not evident, and rather rarely a lifethreatening complication of the underlying disease are pericarditis (12, 21, 33), cardiomyopathy, and aortic- or mitralvalve disease.

Even cardiovascular manifestation of rheumatic or collagen diseases necessitating cardiac surgery are only found in a rather small subgroup of affected patients; there is an increasing number of reports during recent years on patients requiring cardiac surgery for cardiac complications of connective tissue diseases, either as a result of longer survival of affected patients and/or due to corticosteroid treatment [2, 12, 14, 21, 24, 33).

Patients with underlying connective tissue diseases are of high risk for complications in spite of an uneventful surgical procedure due to renal, pulmonary, gastrointestinal, and hematological alterations. Continuous high dose anti-inflammatory drug treatment often leads to fragile tissue, increasing the risk of surgical failure.

Cardiac involvement in connective tissue diseases

Echocardiographic studies aimed at the cardiac involvement in connective tissue diseases in correlation with antiphospholipid antibodies in patients with systemic lupus erythematosus, rheumatoid arthritis, and primary antiphospholipid syndrome have shown that cardiac involvement is frequent in patients with connective tissue diseases but unrelated to serum markers (12, 16, 24, 33).

Valvular lesions

Echocardiographically about 40% of systemic lupus erythematosus patients, 17% of progressive systemic sclerosis patients, and 25% of rheumatoid arthritis patients have valvular lesions. Abnormal left ventricular filling index and decreased left ventricular performance are found in about 15% of systemic lupus erythematosus patients, 30% of progressive systemic sclerosis patients, and 40 % of rheumatoid arthritis patients (16).

Pericardial disorders

Pericardial disorders occurring in connective tissue diseases are not uncommon and may present as acute or chronic pericarditis with or without an effusion. It is most frequently found in scleroderma (59%), followed by systemic lupus erythematosus (44%), mixed connective tissue disease (30%), rheumatoid arthritis (24%), and polymyositis/dermatomyositis (11%). Nevertheless, in most circumstances, the diagnosis of pericardial involvement is not found until autopsy as cardiac tamponade or constriction is rare in these diseases (13, 31).

Cardiovascular manifestations in Rheumatoid arthritis, Systemic lupus erythematosus (SLE) and Ankylosing spondylitis (Morbus Bechterew) (Table 6)

Rheumatoid arthritis

The most prevalent systemic rheumatic disease is rheumatoid arthritis, affecting about 1 % of the population (33). Various cardiovascular manifestations have been described including pericarditis, valvular disease, coronary artery disease, myocarditis conduction disorders, aortic disease, and pulmonary hypertension. Pleuropulmonary manifestations as pulmonary fibrosis or renal insufficiency due to diffuse vasculitis increase the risk of major surgery in these patients. Long-term systemic corticosteroid therapy with doses over the cushing threshold of 7.5 mg/d need to be considered while planing cardiac surgery to avoid major complications. Liver function abnormalities must be anticipated in about 20% of patients treated with intermittent Methotrexate therapy (30).

Table 6. Connective tissue diseases: cardiovascular manifestations of systemic lupus erythematosus

Pericarditis
Constrictive pericarditis
Cardiomyopathy
Valvular disease
Libman-Sacks endocarditis
Aortic and Mitral insufficiency/stenosis
Coronary artery disease

Pericarditis

Pericarditis is the most common cardiac lesion seen in patients with rheumatoid arthritis. It occurs in around 11–50% of RA patients with chest pain being the chief complaint. Peripheral oedema and orthopnoea sometime accomplish the clinical diagnosis of pericardial constriction. Still, clinically evident rheumatoid pericarditis is infrequent.

Pericarditis usually resolves with aggressive treatment of the underlying arthritis with corticosteroids, nonsteroidal anti-inflammatory drugs, or disease modifying drugs like Methotrexate. However, pericarditis may lead to constrictive pericarditis and cardiac compression and, therefore, necessitate cardiac surgery.

Constrictive pericarditis

Constrictive pericarditis in rheumatoid arthritis is a rather rare condition with a prevalence of less than 1% (32). It should be treated surgically as therapy with corticosteroids or Methotrexate is not indicated (15). Cardiac tamponade appears to be extremely rare.

Escalonte and Beardmore 1990 investigated the incidence and the outcome in patients with rheumatoid arthritis and pericardial compression. In their series of 960 patients with rheumatoid arthritis, 12 patients had clinical pericarditis of whom 5 had signs of pericardial compression (15).

Once the diagnosis of constrictive pericarditis with compression of the heart is made, the treatment is almost uniformly surgical through decortication of the heart.

Pericardiocentesis should only be performed as a life-saving procedure and may be followed by intrapericardial injection of corticosteroids, but this does not prevent recurrence. The two year mortality in patients with cardiac compression in their series was nevertheless 100% (15).

Valvular disease

Echocardiographic studies observed valvular lesions in almost 25% of patients with rheumatic arthritis (16).Valvular lesions in rheumatoid arthritis involve the valve leaflets and valve rings and may be pathologically identical to rheumatoid nodules. Valves may be affected by non-granulomatous valve inflammation resulting in fibrosis and thickening of valve leaflets. Mostly the mitral and/or the aortic valve are affected, rarely the tricuspid or pulmonary valve.

Only a small number of patients require aortic or mitral valve replacement due to valvular disease on the foundation of rheumatoid arthritis. If surgical valve replacement is needed, it is often made difficult due to fragile annular tissue in view of chronic inflammation and continuous corticosteroid treatment.

Coronary artery disease

Autopsy studies detected in up to 20 percent of patients with rheumatic arthritis involvement of the coronary arteries in the form of coronary vasculitis (22). Histopathological studies of endocardial biopsies in patients with rheumatoid arthritis IgM revealed deposits in small blood vessels resulting in small vessel arteritis (1, 28). Arteritis in rheumatoid arthritis tends to be restricted to smaller endo and intramyocardial vessels but is also found in larger coronary arteries (22).

The treatment of symptomatic coronary vasculitis due to rheumatoid arthritis should be according to the treatment of the underlying disease with aggressive corticosteroid and immunosuppressive therapy. Localized stenoses warranting a surgical approach may require coronary artery bypass grafting. Data with respect to long-term results are presently not available.

Myocardial dysfunction

Myocarditis in rheumatoid arthritis is mostly nonspecific and rarely causes clinical significant myocardial dysfunction (22). The necessity of heart transplantation due to cardiomyopathy on the base of myocarditis in rheumatoid arthritis patients has not yet been described.

Conduction disturbances

Ten percent of patients with rheumatic arthritis will develop some degree of conduction disturbances (22). Most prevalent is a first degree atrio-ventricular block, but fascicular blocks and other arrhythmias have been described (11).

Higher degree system conduction abnormalities are rare but might necessitate implantation of a permanent pacemaker (11).

Aortitis

Aortitis might occur in rheumatoid arthritis in about 5% of patients (18). It may lead to aneurysmal enlargement of the aorta and aortic valvular incompetence necessitating aortic valve replacement or aneurysmal repair.

Aortitis is characterized by a dense adventitial inflammatory fibrosis involving the sinuses of valsalva and the proximal aorta, particular adjacent to the commissures. The process may extend below the base of the aortic valve and may involve the base of the anterior mitral leaflet or even the adjacent ventricular septum causing conduction disturbances.

Although involvement of the thoracic aorta is most common, in some cases the abdominal aorta might be affected as well (18). Rarely congestive heart failure secondary to thoracic aortitis and aortic valvulitis can be found (18).

Systemic lupus erythematosus

Cardiac manifestations of systemic lupus erythematosus are rare. More commonly they are found during the autopsy than clinically (11, 13). Echocardiographically more than 50% of SLE patients have irregularities including valvular abnormalities, pericardial disease, and myocardial abnormalities (9, 14, 24).

Pericarditis

Over 30% of patients with active disease present with pericarditis (14, 20). Symptomatic patients have pericardial effusions; pericardial tamponade may occur, but is, with an incidence of 1%, rather rare (14, 20).

Pericarditis is usually treated with corticosteroids and non steroidal anti-inflammatory drugs. If cardiac-tamponade occurs, most patients will require pericardiotomy or a pericardial window for long-term relief (11, 21).

Myocarditis

Myocarditis is found clinically in about 10% of patients. The treatment is similar to that of other cardiomyopathies (6, 14).

Endocarditis

The socalled Libman-Sacks endocarditis was first described in 1924 (23).

Although endocarditis commonly complicates the course of systemic lupus erythematosus, there are only a handful of reports about endocardial lesions causing valvular dysfunction resulting in valve replacement (17, 29).

Up to 1994 only 14 cases of mitral valve replacement due to valvulitis in systemic lupus erythematosus had been reported (27), until 1996 there were already 25 reported cases (24). The frequency of valvular dysfunction has increased over the years, either as a result of longer survival of patients or due to corticoid therapy (14, 24). Recent reports showed that valvulopathy in SLE can affect bioprosthetic valves, a finding that has significant implications as to the type of valve replacement in these patients.

Mitral valve replacement after initial mitral valve reconstruction in a patient with systemic lupus erythematosus was first reported in 1995 (10). The patient had to undergo a redo-operation because of recurrent mitral valve stenosis due to progression of valve thickening and calcification one year after the initial operation. Therefore, it has to be considered that conservative operation techniques in the way of reconstructive valve surgery do not alter the natural history of the disease and should be cautiously used in Patients with SLE (10).

Coronary artery disease

Until the beginning of the era of continuous steroid treatment, coronary artery disease was rare in patients with systemic lupus erythematosus (11). The incidence of coronary artery disease in patients suffering from systemic lupus erythematosus treated with steroids continuously for more than one year has increased to over 40% since then (27). Management usually aims for decreasing corticosteroid therapy and control of common risk factors. The phenomenon of increased atherogenesis might be related to continuous steroid treatment leading to longer survival of patients and furthermore increased incidence of hypertension and hyperlipidemia (19, 26). Only a few reports about coronary artery bypass grafting in these patient have since been published in the literature.

Cardiac surgery in SLE

Clotting disturbances due to binding of the lupus anticoagulant to the prothrombin complex can lead to severe clotting abnormalities, which under the circumstances of cardiopulmonary bypass might result in severe bleeding complications. Additionally, most chronic SLE patients are anaemic and have thrombocytopenia, consequently increasing the risk of surgical intervention.

Since close to 50 % of SLE patients will develop glomerulonephritis during their life, the risk of developing renal failure in the circumstances of cardiac surgery is high and might be a major cause of morbidity and mortality in these patients.

Ankylosing spondylitis (Morbus Bechterew)

Bulkley et al. in 1973 was the first to describe the characteristic cardiovascular lesions in patients with ancylosing spondylitis and aortic regurgitation (8). Up to 10 % of patients with ancylosing spondylitis have echocardiographically proven but clinically silent aortic valve disease (25). Increasing shortening and thickening of the aortic valve cusps as well as dilatation of the aortic root may lead to aortic regurgitation and subsequent left ventricular dysfunction due to dilation necessitating valve replacement. Mitral valve insufficiency secondary to mitral valve prolapse is uncommon (3).

Asymptomatic left ventricular dysfunction even in the absence of valvular disease has been found in up to 53% of patients with ancylosing spondylitis (7).

Due to changes in the conductive tissue, different conduction disturbances, from first to third degree atrio-ventricular block to WPW syndrome, are quite frequent in patients with ancylosing spondylitis (5), sometimes necessitating permanent pacemaker implantation.

Cardiac surgery in patients with connective tissue disorders at the Heart Center Lahr/Baden from January to September 1997

From the 01 Jan 1997 to the 31 Aug 1997, we performed cardiac surgery in over 1400 patients using cardio-pulmonary bypass.

Thirteen of these patients were on continuous steroid and/or Methotrexate treatment for symptomatic connective tissue diseases. Ten patients had a collagen disorder, three patients a vasculitis syndrome. Nine of the ten patients with a collagen disorder were diagnosed with rheumatoid arthritis (RA). One patient had Sjögrens syndrome. The three remaining patients had the diagnosis of a vasculitis syndrome;

two of them suffering from arteritis temporalis and one diagnosed with a p-ANCA positive vasculitis. Three patients were diagnosed of ancylosing spondylitis and were not on continuous but intermittent steroid treatment.

The majority of these patients (84.7%) were referred for coronary artery bypass grafting due to severe coronary artery disease; the remainder (15.3%) were referred for aortic- or mitral valve replacement due to severe valve disease.

Six of the nine patients with Rheumatoid arthritis were referred for coronary artery bypass grafting (CABG) because of severe coronary artery disease (CAD). Two patients were referred for aortic valve replacement because of aortic stenosis of which one patient had concomitant CAD. One patient had mitral valve insufficiency and CAD and was referred for mitral valve replacement and CABG.

Two of the three patients with vasculitis syndromes were referred for CABG on the basis of severe CAD; one patient was referred for mitral valve replacement due to mitral valve stenosis; who was free of coronary artery disease. All three patients with ancylosing spondylitis were referred for coronary bypass procedures on the basis of severe coronary artery disease.

Left ventricular function was preoperatively evaluated in all patients either through echocardiography or left ventricular angiography. The average LV-function in this group of patients was normal (LV-EF: 54.6%). Only one patient had severely impaired left ventricular function (LV-EF: 25%). This patient with rheumatoid arthritis was referred for Mitral valve replacement and CABG on the base of severe Mitral insufficiency and CAD.

None of the patients had clinical or echocardiographically (if performed) signs of pericarditis or severe pericardial effusion. Half of the patients in this group had a normal pulmonary function test. Severe impairment of the pulmonary function was found in only two patients. Both patients had rheumatoid arthritis, were referred for valve replacement, and had a significant longer postoperative ventilation time than the average in this group. (22 h / average 11.5 h).

The majority of patients had normal renal function. Nevertheless, in three patients (23%) renal function was severely impaired. One patient with p-ANCA positive vasculitis was on chronic hemodialysis due renal involvement of the underlying disease.

All but the three patients with ancylosing spondylitis received continuous prednisolon therapy. One patient with rheumatoid arthritis and one patient with Sjörgren‘s disease received additional Methotrexate treatment. Only one patient in the rheumatoid arthritis group was, in addition to steroids treated with Salazasulfidine. The oral corticosteroid treatment ranged from 4–30 mg prednisolon daily.

Operative data

Peri- and postoperative data were collected retrospectively. Perioperative bloodloss was measured until the last chest-tube was removed, usually on the second postoperative day. Postoperative ventilation time was measured as the time from arrival of the patient in ICU until the moment the patient was taken off mechanical ventilation. Total length of ICU – or Hospital stay was measured in days, with any time a patient stayed longer than 12.00 p.m. accounting for a full day.

Statistic evaluation of data in the form of statistic tests was not suitable due to the small number of patients in total and particularly in the subgroups. Nevertheless, the analysis of perioperative data with regard to the performed procedure yielded differences regarding bypass-time, perioperative bloodloss (Table 9), postoperative ventilation time and total length of hospital-stay (Table 10). But

Table 7. Preoperative data: Patients with connective tissue diseases on continious cortico-steroid treatment undergoing cardiac surgery at the Heart Center Lahr 1997

No.	Connectivetis-sue disease	Cardiac diagnosis	LV-function LV-EF (%)	Pulmonary function test	Renal-function serum – creatinin (i.U.)	Prednisolon/ Methotrexate Tx
1	Rheumatoid arthritis	CAD	55	normal	2.7	10 mg
2	Rheumatoid arthritis	CAD	50	normal	0.9	30 mg
3	Rheumatoid arthritis	AS + CAD	60	normal	1.2	5 mg
4	Rheumatoid arthritis	CAD	67	normal	0.9	5 mg
5	Rheumatoid arthritis	CAD	65	restrictive lung-disease	1.0	4 mg + Methotrexate
6	Rheumatoid arthritis	CAD	70	normal	0.8	10 mg
7	Rheumatoid arthritis	AS	55	restrictive + obstructive	0.8	5 mg
8	Rheumatoid arthritis	CAD	68	normal	0.9	5 mg
9	Rheumatoid arthritis	MI + CAD	25	restrictive + obstructive	1.6	4 mg + Salazasulfidine
10	Arteritis temporalis	CAD	55	obstructive lung-disease	1.2	12.5 mg
11	Arteritis temporalis	MS	45	restrictive lung-disease	0.9	5 mg
12	Sjögren syndrome	CAD	46	restrictive lung-disease	2.3	25 mg + Meth. 10 mg
13	p-ANCA pos. vasculitis	CAD	50	normal	7.7	15 mg
14	Ancylosing spondylitis	CAD	50	obstructive lung-disease	1.0	/
15	Ancylosing spondylitis	CAD	68	restrictive lung-disease	1.4	/
16	Ancylosing spondylitis	CAD	45	normal	1.1	/

Table 8. Postoperative data: Patients with connective tissue diseases on continiuos cortico-steroid treatment undergoing cardiac surgery at the Heart Center Lahr 1997

No.	Procedure	Bypass/ clamp time	Postoperative bloodloss (ml)	Post operative ventila- tion time	ICU stay (days)	Complications	Hos- pital stay (days)
1	Redo 2 + 1 CABG/IABP	211/84	1250	15 h	24	low cardic- output	25
2	CABG 3 + 1	141/80	765	8 h	2	none	11
3	CABG 2 + 1/ AVR	115/75	1150	8 h	1	none	6
4	CABG 2 + 1	121/74	240	12 h	3	supraventricu- lar arrhythmia	7
5	CABG 3 + 1	97/55	1000	6 h	4	supraventricu- lar arryhthmia	8
6	CABG 3 + 1	51/79	1100	7 h	1	none	4
7	AVR	130/81	550	22 h	2	none	6
8	CABG 2 + 1	55/33	435	9 h + 48 h	1 + 2	generalized Fit	9
9	CABG 3 + 1 MVR	201/131	1915	22 h	7	pulmonary failure	16
10	CABG 3 + 1	78/49	220	15 h	1	none	6
11	MVR	83/48	1405	11 h	8	pulmonary failure	8
12	Redo CABG 1 + 1	93/63	210	12 h	2	none	7
13	CABG 1 + 2	120/71	550	8 h	1	none	6
14	CABG 3 + 0	98/61	500	5 h	4	pulmonary failure	6
15	CABG 2+ 2	78/44	1500	15 h	11	pulmonary failure/pleural effusions	21
16	CABG 2+ 2	88/52	1195	5 h	1	none	7

these findings did not correlate with the specific underlying connective tissue diseases.

The number of applied bypass-grafts whether arterial or not did not differ significantly. Aortic cross-clamping time, total bypass-time and postoperative ventilation time did increase according to the complexity of the performed procedure. However, this finding did not correspond with the postoperative course, regarding bloodloss, ICU – or total length of hospital-stay. Preoperative lung function-test results seemed to be related to postoperative ventilation time if the

Table 9. Procedure and operative data

	Bypass-time (min)	Clamp-time (min)	No. grafts	No. arterial grafts	Bloodloss (ml)
CABG	92	59	3.6	1.2	750.5
REDO-CABG	152	73	2.5	1.0	730.0
VALVE + CABG	132	83	3.5	1.0	1255.0

Table 10. Procedure and postoperative data (median values)

	Post-operative ventilation time (hours)	ICU intermediate care (days)	Hospital-stay (days)
CABG	9.0	3.1	8.5
REDO-CABG	13.5	13	16.0
VALVE + CABG	15.75	4.5	9.0

Table 11. Preoperative lung-function and postoperative ventilation time (median values)

Lung function-test results	Ventilation-time (hours)
normal	9
restrictive or obstructive pulmonary disease	8.8
combined restrictive and obstructive pulmonary disease	22

patient had severe combined obstructive and restrictive pulmonary disease (Table 11) yet with only two patients in this subgroup, one would not draw any conclusion from this finding.

Corticosteroids and perioperative course

To evaluate a questionable relationship between the daily corticosteroid dose and the perioperative course we compared data of patients who took less than 5 mg corticosteroids daily (n = 7) with data of patients who took more than 5 mg corticosteroids daily (n = 6).

This comparison did not reveal any differences between both groups' ventilation time, number of days in ICU or total length of hospital stay (Table 12). The group of patients with a daily dose of less than 5 mg corticosteroids orally showed a slightly higher (956.4 ml) average perioperative bloodloss than the group of patients who took a higher daily dose of corticosteroids (682.5 ml) (Table 13). This particular finding, in combination with the overall findings in our group of patients con-

Table 12. Preoperative cortisteroid treatment and postoperative ventilation time, ICU, and hospital stay (median values)

Preoperative corticosteroid Tx	Ventilation time (hours)	ICU stay (days)	Hospitals stay (days)
< 5 mg/day	12.8	3.7	8.5
> 5 mg/day	10.8	5.1	9.8

Table 13. Corticosteroid treatment and perioperative bloodloss (median values)

Preoperative corticosteroid Tx	Perioperative bloodloss (2 days)
< 5 mg/day	956.4 ml
> 5 mg/day	682.5 ml

tradicted the already above mentioned theory that patients, who are on continuous steroid treatment have a higher risk if they have to undergo cardiac surgery.

References

1. Ahern M, Lever JV, Cosh J (1983) Complete heart block in rheumatoid arthritis. Ann Rheum Dis 42: 389
2. Alpert MA, Pressly TA, Mukerji V, Lambert CR, Mukerji B (1992) Short- and long-term hemodynamic effects of captopril in patients with pulmonary hypertension and selected connective tissue disease. Chest 102: 1407
3. Alves MG, Espirito-Santo J, Queiroz MV, et al. (1988) Cardiac alterations in ancylosing spondylitis. Angiology 39: 567
4. Bergfeldt L, Edhay O, Rajs J (1984) HLA - B27 associated heart disease: Clinicopathologigic study of three cases. Am J Med 77:961
5. Bergfeldt L, Vallin H, Edhay O (1984) Complete heart block in HLA-B27 associated disease: Electrophysiological and clinical characteristics. Br Heart J 51. 184
6. Bornstein DG, Fye WB, Arnett FC, Stevens MB (1978) The myocarditis of systemic lupus erythematosus: Association with myositis. Ann Intern Med 89: 619
7. Brewerton DA, Goddard DH, Moore RB, et al. (1987) The myocardium in ancylosing spondylitis: A clinical echocardiographic and histopathologic study. Lancet 1-8540: 995
8. Bulkley BH, Roberts WC (1973) Ankylosing sondylitis and aortic regurgitation: Description of the characteristic cardiovascular lesion from study of eight necropsy patients. Circulation 48: 1014
9. Cervera R, Font J, Paré C, et al. (1992) Cardiac disease in systemic lupus erythematosus: Prospective study of 70 patients. Ann Rheum Dis 51: 156
10. Chauvad SM, Kalangos A, Berrebi AJ, Gaer AR, et al. (1995) Systemic lupus erythematosus valvulitis: mitral valve replacement with a homograft. Ann Thorac Surg 60 1803
11. Coblyn JS, Weinblatt ME (1997) Rheumatic diseases and the heart. In: E. Braunwald (ed) Heart Disease p 1776 Philadelphia, Sannders
12. Corrao S, Salli L, Arnone S, Scaglione R et al. (1995) Cardiac involvement in rheumatoid arthritis: Evidence of silent heart disease. Eur Heart J 16: 253
13. D'Angelo WA, Fries JF, Masi AT, Shulman LE (1969) Pathologic observations in systemic sclerosis (scleroderma). A study of 58 autopsy cases and 58 matched controls. Am J Med 46: 428
14. Doherty NE, Siegel RJ (1985) Cardiovascular manifestations of systemic lupus erythematosus. Am Heart J 110: 1257

15. Escalonte A, Kaufmann RL, Quimorio FP, Beardmore TD (1990) Cardiac compression in rheumatoid pericarditis. Semin Arthritis Rheum 20: 148
16. Gabrielli F, Alcini E, Prima MA, Lucifero A, Masala C (1996) Cardiac involvement in connective tissue diseases and primary antiphospholipid syndrome: Echocardiographic assessment and correlation with antiphospholipid antibodies. Acta Cardiol (Belgium) 51: 425
17. Galve E, Condill-Riera J, Pigrau C et al. (1988) Prevalance, morphologic types and evolution of cardiac valvular disease in systemic lupus erythematosus. N Engl J Med 319: 817
18. Gravallese E, Corson J, Coblyn JS, et al (1989) Rheumatoid aortitis: A rarely recognized but clinically significant entity. Medicine 68: 95
19. Haidir YS, Roberts WC (1981) Coronary arterial disease in systemic lupus erythematosus: Quantification of degrees of narrowing in 22 necropsy patients (21 women) aged 16 to 37 years. Am J Med 70: 775
20. Kahl L (1992) The spectrum of pericardial tamponade in systemic lupus erythematosus. Arthritis Rheum 35 1343
21. Langley RL, Traedwell EL (1994) Cardiac tamponade and pericardial disorders in connective tissue diseases: Case report and literature review. J Natl Med Assoc 86: 149
22. Leibowitz WB (1963) The heart in rheumatoid arthritis. Ann Intern Med 58: 102
23. Libman E, Sacks B (1924) A hithero undescribed form of valvular and mural endocarditis. Arch Intern Med 33: 701
24. Morin AM, Boyer AS, Nataf P, Gandjbakhch I (1996) Mitral insufficiency caused by systemic lupus erythematosus requiring valve replacement: Three case reports and a review of the literature. Thorac cardiovasc Surgeon 44: 313
25. O'Neill TW (1992) The heart in ancylosing spondylitis. Ann Rheum Dis 51: 705
26. Petri M, Spence D, Bone L, Hochberg MC (1992) Coronary artery disease risk factors in the Johns Hopkins Lupus Cohort: Prevalance, recognition by patients and preventive practice. Medicine 71: 291
27. Roberts WC, Bulkley BH (1975) The heart in systemic lupus erythematosus and the changes induced in it by corticosteroid therapy: A study 36 necropsy patients. Am J Med 58: 243
28. Slack JD, Waller B (1986) Acute congestive heart failure due to the arteritis of rheumatoid arthritis. Early diagnosis by endocardial biopsy: A case report. Angiology 37: 477
29. Straaton KV, Chatham WW, Reveille JD, et al. (1988) Clinically significant valvular heart disease in systemic lupus erythematosus. Am J Med 85: 645
30. Takahashi T, de-la Garza L, Ponce-de-Leon S, Palacios-Macedo et al. (1995) Risk factors for operative morbidity in patients with systemic lupus erythematosus: an analysis of 63 surgical procedures. Am Surg 61: 260
31. Thadani U, Iveson JM, Wright V (1975) Cardiac tamponade, constrictive pericarditis and pericardial resection in rheumatoid arthritis. Medicine 54: 261
32. Thould AK (1986) Constrictive pericarditis in rheumatoid arthritis. Ann Rheum Dis 45: 89
33. Toumandis ST, Papamichael LG, Antoniades MI, Pantelia MI et al. (1995) Cardiac involvement in collagen diseases. Eur Heart J 16: 257

Author's address:
U. P. Rosendahl, MD
Department of Cardio-Thoracic-Surgery
Heart Institute Lahr/Baden
Hohbergweg 2
77933 Lahr, Germany

Cardiac surgery and the influence of endocrine disorders

K. H. Usadel

Medizinische Klinik I, University of Frankfurt/Main, Germany

Patients with known or unknown endocrine diseases need special care under stressful situations, e.g., surgical procedures. Due to this reason the following diseases must be pointed out:

- Hypofunction of the adrenal cortex
- Hypoparathyroidism
- Functional alterations of the thyroid
- Diabetes mellitus

Hypofunction of the adrenal cortex

Hypofunction of the adrenal cortex with the consequence of an absence of reagibility to stress like infections, any surgical operation, etc., often lead to all signs of acute hypocortisolism (i.e., Addision's disease). It does not matter on the pathophysiology of the adrenal insufficiency but the consequences as increased mortality, reduced wound healing, and reduced recovery comparable. Adrenal insuffciency is either caused by absence of functioning adrenal cortical cells (zona glomerulosa producing mineral corticoids and zona fasciculata producing mainly cortisol) due to autoimmune adrenalitis, tuberculosis or adrenalectomy or by the lack of hypothalamo-pituitary stimulation by CRH and ACTH (hypothalamopituitary tumors). An unclear pre- or postoperative situation should be quickly diagnosed by the i.v. ACTH stimulation test (Synacthen®). Serum cortisol levels at 0' and 30' prove an existing problem which should lead immediately to therapeutic consequences which would be the same as under already known adrenal cortisol insufficiency. Recommended therapy should be as follows: 100 mg hydrocortisone (water soluble) i.v. parenteral as continous i.v. infusion per 8–12 h. Depending on blood pressure additional mineralocorticoid medication need also to be parenterally given (i.e., Aldocorten®, Astonin-H®) under intensive care conditions. Depending on the postoperatively recovery oralization of the medication can be managed within the first days with the aim of slowly reducing the medication to a permanent therapeutical dose. Interdisciplinary management including management of occuring increase of blood glucose levels which might also lead to therapeutical consequences is strictly indicated, and lifelong, controlled treatment with glucocorticoids and if necessary including mineralocorticoids is necessary. Only a perfectly educated patient is able to self-manage stress induced relative or absolute adrenocortical insufficiency. This also includes self-injection of hydrocortisone in situations with diarrhea and vomiting.

Hypoparathyroidism

Hypoparathyroidism might exist due to autoimmune pathogenesis or as a permanent complication due to parathyroidectomy or thyroidectomy mediated hypofunction, respectively. The normal preoperatively known situation which is often treated by vitamine D hormones and calcium substitution might lead to hypocalciemia in perioperative phases. This should not happen in carefully treated patients since the long half-life of vitamine D hormones keeps calcium levels constant. In other cases continous calcium infusion should overcome acute hypopituitarism. Calcium and electrolyte control is regularly managed in cardiosurgical precedures anyhow.

In any disorder of the parathyroid function either hyper- or/and hypofunction, the preoperative bone status should be evaluated. Severe osteoporosis and osteopenia might lead to bone fractures even in the thorax after surgical management.

Functional alterations of the thyroid

Hypofunction of the thyroid has regularily led to continous substitution therapy before cardiac surgery. Unknown and actually diagnosed hypofunction due to autoimmune thyroiditis Hashimoto should be carefully treated with thyroid hormones, since thickening of coronary artery subendothelial areas can be reversible by hormone treatment and might be initiate by increased pulse rate to cardiac ischemias in the inital phase of hormonal replacement therapy. Known and correctly managed treatment of hypofunction of the thyroid (also caused by operative reduction of the organ) will need no parenteral perioperative hormone substitution and oral treatment can be continued as soon as possible after surgery.

Thyreotoxicosis: Overt hyperfunction of the thyroid reveals many symptoms like sweatening, tachycardia, nervousness, tremor, loss of body weight, etc. Euthyreosis should be achieved before cardiac surgery if possible. Latent hyperfunction which is defined by suppressed TSH and normal levels of thyroid hormones in the blood may also reveal discrete symptoms like tremor and arrhythmias. In any case latent or overt hyperthyreosis is regularily aggravated by exogenous application of iodine, e.g., diagnostic procedures using contrast media by angiography. Hyperthyreosis is mainly caused by "Graves' disease" or in the majority of older people by toxic adenomas or disseminated autonomies. A major problem of older people with latent or overt hyperthyreosis is the lack of classical symptoms. This means that hyperthyreosis very often is oligosymptomatic so that a great number of these patients remain undiagnosed. Relevant symptoms in these patients often are depressiveness, tachycardia, and cardiac arrhythmias. Often these unclear cardiac symptoms initiate angiography with the necessity of the application of iodine containing contrast media. As a consequence to this transformation from latent to overt, hyperthyreosis can occur and undiagnosed existing hyperthyreosis will be aggravated. For older patients undergoing cardiac surgery, preoperative screening for thyroidal hyperfunction is indicated. For economic reasons clinical examination of TSH is strictly recommended. If TSH is suppressed additional determination of fT4, fT3, ultrasound of the thyroid, and additional diagnosis, e.g., scintiscanning, dermination of antibodies, is indicated. If thyreotoxicosis has been diagnosed and time for treatment before cardiac surgery is available, treatment with thyreostatica, i.e., methimazole, thiouracile, is indicated.

If actual surgery or application of iodine by angiography is strictly indicated, therapeutical induced blockade of iodine uptake must be performed.

Prophylaxis of iodine induced thyreotoxicosis by the use of iodine containing contrast media.

If latent or overt hyperfunction of the thyroid is suspected and if immediate angiography is necessary, blockade of iodine uptake has to be initiated. This means that before any angiography is performed at least clinical investigation of the thyroid has to be done and clinical symptoms should be evaluated. Initially a blood sample should be analyzed for TSH and if supressed then additionally for fT4, fT3, and TSH-receptor antibodies. Additionally, ultrasound and scintiscanning is indicated.

Prophylaxis

Suspected thyreotoxicosis: 2 days or the latest 1 hour before angiography 1200 mg/day of perchlorate p.o. The therapy must be continued for an additional 2 weeks with a dose of 3 × 600 mg/day.

Overt thyreotoxicosis: Initially 3 × 80 mg/day of methimazole (Favistan®) i.v. and additioinally 40 mg/day p.o. In additional perchlorate in the same dose as mentioned above has to be given but prolonged for 8 weeks.

Diabetes mellitus

Diabetic patients are frequent candidates for surgery because many of them are of older age in which the incidence of operations is greater. Diabetes mellitus is associated with an increased prevalence of macrovascular disease affecting coronary and cerebral arteries as well as peripheral arterial supply. Preoperative recognition of this altered carbohydrate metabolism is essential to prevent complications during the perioperative period. Any surgical stress will adversely affect the metabolic status of the diabetic patient through the influence of counter-regulatory hormones with an increase of the demand for insulin. Preoperative medical evaluation requires analysis of the total patient. Beside analysis of the metabolic status, including nutrition and levels of blood glucose control is important to establish optimal conditions for management during surgery. Any diabetic patient should be admitted 1–2 days prior to the scheduled operation to provide a final adjustment and stabilization. Interdisciplinary treatment including diabetologists is required. For intraoperative management two technics for insulin administration are recommended. Preference is given to the use of regular insulin added to the intravenous glucose solutions. No subcutaneous insulin is used preoperatively. The amount of insulin ordered for each liter of 5% dextrose ranges from 10–20 U. For those whose total daily requirement is 40 U or less 10 U are used; 15 U for those receiving 50–80 U, and 20 U for those with higher insulin requirement. The dosis of regular insulin is ordered for each of 3 l of 5% dextrose solution given during the day of operation.

A second time honored method is that of splitting the usual insulin dose giving 1/3 to 1/2 of the total subcutaneously on the morning of operation. The preoperative feeding is based on 1000 ml of 5% dextrosis solution. Following the operative procedure a similar dose of insulin is administered in the recovery room or upon return to the room. continous blood glucose determination has to be performed during the operation and in the recovery room.

In type II diabetes blood glucose determination should be done continously during the operation and postoperatively every 4 to 6 hours. If blood glucose is higher than 250 mg/dl regular insulin subcutaneously should be given in the postoperative phase. If the blood glucose is not controlled preoperative and perioperative hyperglycemia develops, these patients are given exogenous insulin as discribed for patients with diabetes type I.

References

References are available from the author.

Author's address:
Prof. Dr. med. K.-H. Usadel
Zentrum der Innere Medizin
Medizinische Klinik I
Johann Wolfgang Goethe-Universität
Theodor-Stern-Kai 7
60590 Frankfurt am Main, Germany

Cardiac surgery in diabetic patients

Ø. Risum, M. Abdelnoor

Surgical Department A, Rikshospitalet, Oslo, Norway

Heart disease in patients with diabetes mellitus

Diabetes mellitus can be defined as an elevated plasma glucose level due to insufficient insulin effect. The importance of heart disease in patients with diabetes mellitus did not become apparent until the risk of diabetic coma decreased. Still, it is well documented that diabetes mellitus is associated with increased risk of cardiovascular mortality and morbidity (3, 7, 9).

However, the morphologic appearance and anatomic distribution of arteriosclerotic disease is similar in patients with diabetes mellitus as in non-diabetics, but diabetic patients have a greater prevalence of coronary arteriosclerotic lesions, have more extensive arteriosclerotic disease, and have evidence of coronary heart disease at an earlier stage than non-diabetic patients (13, 18).

Additional cardiac dysfunction may be secondary to complications of diabetes mellitus, such as microangiopathy, neuropathy, and/or myopathy. Therefore, heart disease in a young insulin-dependent individual may be different than in a patient with gestational diabetes. Table 1 lists the type of diabetes associated with different heart abnormalities (16).

Table 1. Classification of diabetes and the principal cardiovascular abnormalities at increased risk

Classification of diabetes	Principal cardiovascular abnormalities at increased risk
Type I (IDDM)	Cardiomyopathy, ASCVD, autonomic neuropathy
Type II (NIDDM)	ASCVD
Gestational	Cardiomyopathy, fetal hypertrophy subaortic stenosis
Impaired glucose control	ASCVD

IDDM: Insulin-dependent diabetes mellitus; NIDDM: non-dependent diabetes mellitus; ASCVD: Arteriosclerotic cardiovascular disease

The relation between diabetic complications and heart disease

At autopsy, chronic microvascular changes of diabetes clearly occur in the heart. Also, typical microaneurisms, interstitial fibrosis, myocardial degeneration, and fusiform dilatations of in isolated vessels may be present. Today, rigorous glucose control may prevent, or at least reverse, the developement of these pathological findings.

Silent myocardial infarction and painless myocardial ischemia is frequent in diabetic individuals due to neuropathia. Breathlessness and decreased exercise tolerance may be the only symptom of angina pectoris or myocardial infarction. Alterations in heart rate, orthostatic hypotension, and insulin edema are also clinical manifestations, especially in patients with severe neuropathy.

Epidemiology of diabetes mellitus

The Framingham study (9) showed that the relative risk for cardiovascular disease for men was 2.7 for women and 2.1 for men over a 20 year follow-up. The association of diabetes with other risk factors also showed an increased probability of subsequent cardiovascular disease. Other studies (7, 16) have shown that the relative risk may be three to four times higher in diabetic men and five to six times higher in diabetic women than in non-diabetic patients. The average life expectancy in diabetic patients has been shown to be shortened by 8 years (2), and the increased risk of female diabetes could be partially explained by the increased number of accompanying risk factors (9).

Diabetes mellitus and coronary artery bypass surgery

Diabetes mellitus influences all forms of cardiac surgery, but it is of special importance in coronary artery bypass surgery since diabetes is an aethiological factor in the developement of arteriosclerosis.

The three randomized clinical trials, the Veterans Administrative Cooperative Study, the European Prospective Study, and the Coronary Artery Surgery Study (CASS) all included diabetic patients, but the results showed no difference in survival when surgical and medical treatment was compared as far as diabetes mellitus was concerened.

As for early mortality in diabetic patients undergoing coronary artery bypass surgery, the results are conflicting in the literature, as some authors found an increased risk (6, 8, 10, 17) while others reported no increase (3, 5, 11, 14).

Low output syndrome necessitating intraaortic balloon-pumping is a serious condition in CABG surgery. Are the diabetic patients submitted to bypass surgery more prone to low output syndrome than non-diabetics? Relatively little has been published on this specific issue (5, 14). We have already mentioned the increased relative risk of mortality in diabetic patients in general. What effect does CABG

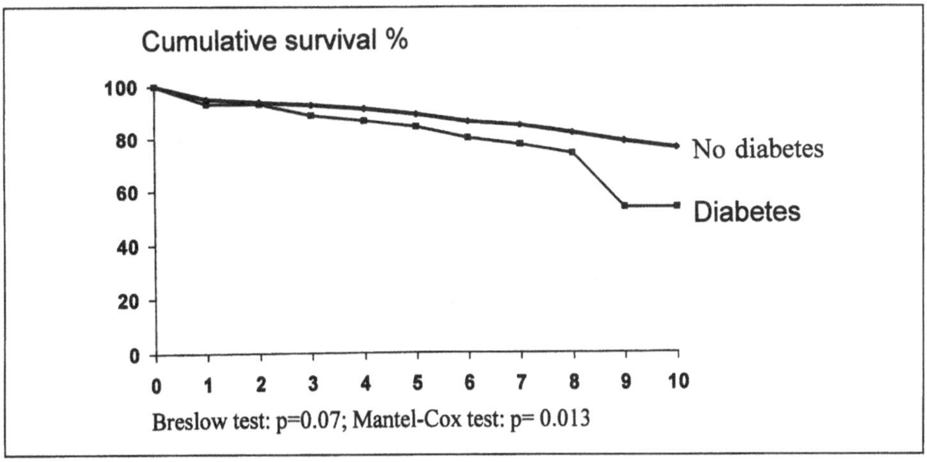

Fig. 1. Survival after CABG

surgery have on long-term survival in diabetic patients? (Fig. 1). Once again, the results in the literature are conflicting (1, 4, 11, 12). In a recent study (14), we showed the difference in relative risk between operated and non-operated diabetic patients in the Norwegian population. Without being conclusive, it may seem is if CABG may have a favorable effect on survival.

Neither the randomized clinical trials nor the results of observational studies have shown any difference in the incidence of myocardial infarction or angina pectoris following coronary artery bypass (11, 14), dispite the well-known aggressive course of arteriosclerotic disease. Does this suggest a protective effect of coronary artery bypass surgery on the diabetic heart?

Research problems of cardiac surgery and diabetes mellitus

Ideally, a randomized clinical trial with enough statistical power, i.e. a sufficient number of patients included in the study, would give the ultimate answer for evaluating the efficacy of cardiac surgery versus medical therapy in patients with diabetes mellitus. However, to perform a clinical trial today on this basis would probably be unethical and certainly impractical and expensive. For this reason, we will have to rely our research on observational studies now and in the future.

Why do the results of different observational studies vary so greatly and why are they apparently inconclusive? The reason may be due to three specific problems: (1) the low prevalence of diabetes mellitus. The prevalence of diabetes mellitus is assumed to be arround 2% in Western populations but usually somewhat higher in patients submitted to surgery (14). (2) A problem of bias and (3) a problem of statistical power. Table 2 shows the number of patients needed to achieve necessary power for the different end-points in our recent study.

Table 2. Number of patients necessary

Early mortality	Low output syndrome (IABP)	Total mortality	Angina pectoris	Late myocardial infarction
4420	2800	900	1120	1400

Sample size of requirement for a type 1 error of 5% and an excess risk (RR = 2) of diabetic patients compared to non-diabetic patientswith a power (1-type 2 error) of 80%

Conclusion

Modern treatment of diabetes mellitus has greatly reduced the serious complications of this disease. We can today say that cardiac surgery in patients with diabetes mellitus is generally favorable. There are also indications of a positve effect on survival of coronary artery bypass surgery compared to non-operated patients with diabetes mellitus. Coronary artery bypass surgery seems to have a protective effect on the myocardium of the diabetic heart.

In the future, research of diabetes mellitus and cardiac surgery must rely on observational studies that eliminate bias and have sufficient statistical power.

References

1. Adler DS, Goldman L, O'Neil A, Cook EF, Mudge GH, Shemin RJ, DiSesa V, Cohn LH, Collins JJ (1986) Long-term survival of more than 2,000 patients after coronary artery bypass grafting. Am J Cardiol 58:195–202
2. Bale CS, Entmacher PS (1977) Estimated life expectancy of diabetics. Diabetes 26:434
3. Clement R., Rousou JA, Engelman RM, Breyer RH (1968) Perioperative morbidity in diabetics requering coronary artery bypass surgery. Ann Thorac Sur 46:321–323
4. Cosgrove DM, Loop FD, Lytle BW, Gill CG, Golding LAR, Gibson C, Stewart RW, Taylor PC, Goormastic M (1986) Determinants of 10 year survival after primary myocardial revascularization. Ann Surg 202:480–90
5. Fietsham Jr, Basett J, Glover JL (1991) Complications of coronary artery surgery in diabetic patients. Am Surg 57:551–7
6. Gersch BJ, Kronmal RA, Frye RL, Schaff HV, Ryan TJ, Gosselin AJ, Kaiser GC, Killip T (1983) Coronary arteriography and coronary artery bypass surgery: Morbidity and mortality in patients ages 65 years or older. Circulation 67:483–91
7. Håheim LL, Holme I, Hjerman I, Leren P (1993) The Oslo Study Abstract. Conference on Diabetic Research, Oct Bergen, Norway
8. Johnsen DW, Pedraza PM, Kayser KL (1981) Mortality and relief of angina in 254 consecutive patients followed four to eight years after coronary bypass surgery. Abstracts Circulation 64: Suppl.IV:IV–92
9. Kannel WB McGee DL (1979) Diabetics and cardiovascular disease: The Framingham Study. JAMA 241:2035–2038
10. Kennedy JW, Kaiser GC, Fisher LD, Maynard C, Fritz JK, Meyers W, Mudd JG, Ryan TJ, Coggin J (1980) Multivariate discriminant analysis of the clinical and angiografic predictors of operative mortality from the Collaborative Study in Coronary Artery Surgery (CASS). J Thorac Cardiovasc Surg 80:876–87
11. Laurie GM, Morris GC, Glaeser DH (1986) Influence of diabetes mellitus on the results of coronary artery bypass surgery. Follow-up of 212 diabetic patients ten to 15 years after surgery. JAMA 256:2967–71

12. Morris JJ, Smith R, Jones RH, Glower DD, Morris PB, Muhlbaier LH, Reves JG, Rankin JS (1991) Influence of diabetes and mammary artery grafting on survival after coronary bypass. Circulation 84: SupplIII:III-275–84
13. National Diabetes Data Group: Classification and diagnosis of diabetes mellitus and other categories of glucose intolerance (1979) Appendix II, Diabetes, 28:64
14. Risum Ø, Abdelnoor, Svennevig JL, Levorstad K, Gullestad L, Bjornarheim R, Simonsen S, Nitter-Hauge S (1996) Diabetes mellitus and morbidity and mortality risks after coronary artery bypass surgery. Scand J Thor Cardiovasc Surg 30:71–75
15. Robertson WB, Strong WP (1968) Atherosclerosis in persons with hypertension and diabetes mellitus. Lab Invest 18:538–51
16. Royal College of Physicians of London and the British Cardiac Society (1976) Diabetes and coronary heart disease. Prevention of coronary heart disease. Report of a joint working party. J R Coll Phys 10:253–255
17. Salomon N, Page US, Okies JE, Stephens J, Krause AH, Begelow JC (1983) Diabetes mellitus and coronary artery bypass:short-term risk and long-term prognosis. J Thorac Cardiovasc Surg 85:264–271
18. Strandness DW, Priest RW, Gibbons GE (1964) Combined clinical and pathological study of diabetic and peripheral arterial disease. Diabetes 13:336–372

Author's address:
Dr. Ø. Risum, PhD
Surgical Department A
University of Oslo
Pilestredet 32
N-0027 Oslo

Influence of blood cardiolegia or crystalloid cardioplegia on serum glucose in diabetic or non-diabetic patients

W. Kallweit, J. Braun, L. Eckel

Clinic for Thoracic and Cardiovascular Surgery, Klinikum Karlsburg, Germany

An increased serum glucose level during cardiopulmonary bypass is due to a decreased utility of glucose by postaggression metabolism, hypothermia, and cardiac depression. Nevertheless, some cardioplegic solutions contain glucose to nutriate the ischemic myocardium. Some entremely high serum glucose levels by diabetic and non-diabetic patients under cardiopulmonary bypass and blood cardioplegia prompted us to investigate different cardioplegic solutions.

In 37 patients undergoing open heart surgery in conventional extracorporal circulation (ECC), cardioplegic arrest, and mild hypothermia, we measured the serum glucose levels at different times (pre-ECC, while cardioplegia was installed, post-ECC, arrival in ICU and 3, 4, 6, 12, 14 hours postoperatively)

We formed two groups: Group I with 10 diabetic patients and group II with 27 non-diabetic patients. Each group was divided and given St Thomas cardioplegia

Table 1. Group I (10 diabetic patients) and group II (27 non-diabetic patients) results

group I

diabetic	pre ECC	cardio-plegia	post ECC	ICU	3 h
STC	134	147	168	184	256
BCP	151	214	218	212	199
p	> 0.05	> 0.05	> 0.05	> 0.05	> 0.05
	4 h	6 h	12 h	14 h	
STC	232	188	215	222	
BCP	170	245	247	156	
p	> 0.05	> 0.05	> 0.05	> 0.05	

group II

non-diabetic	pre ECC	cardio-plegia	post ECC	ICU	3 h
STC	106	103	133	147	184
BCP	118	175	190	185	176
p	> 0.05	< 0.05	< 0.05	> 0.05	> 0.05
	4 h	6 h	12 h	14 h	
STC	184	190	170	150	
BCP	188	171	163	150	
p	> 0.05	> 0.05	> 0.05	> 0.05	

(STC) as crystalloid cardioplegia or blood cardioplegia (BCP) with 25 g/l glucose (Buckberg scheme).

Insulin was not given intraoperatively or during intensive care. The infusion plan was identical in all groups.

As seen in Table 1, in group I no significant difference between both cardioplegic solutions could be found.

On the other hand in the non-diabetic group II significantly higher serum glucose levels were reached during use of the cardioplegic solution and ECC with blood cardioplegia than with St. Thomas solution. Later on no significant difference was found.

There is no evidence of extensive disturbances in glucose metabolism by using glucose containing cardioplegic solutions in diabetic or non-diabetic patients in our investigation. The increased serum glucose level during operation is due to a decreased utility of glucose by post-aggression metabolism, hypothermia, and cardiac depression as proved in the past.

Author's address:
W. Kallweit, M.D.
Clinic for Thoracic and Cardiovascular Surgery
Klinikum Karlsburg
Greifswalderstr. 14
17495 Karlsburg, Germany

Prevention of postoperative atrial tachyarrhythmias by magnesium sulfate after heart surgery in diabetics and non-diabetics

H.-G. Wollert, H. Grossmann, L. Eckel

Department of Thoracic and Cardiovascular Surgery, Klinikum Karlsburg, Germany

Postoperative atrial tachyarrhythmias (PAT) is one of the most common complications after cardiac surgery. From the clinical point of view there is no doubt that magnesium sulfate ($MgSO_4$) postoperatively stabilizes sinus rhythm in cardiac surgery by reducing heart rate, increasing atrioventricular conduction time as well as atrioventricular node refractory period (1, 2, 3). Although we know that magnesium plays an important role in preserving membrane integrity, the mechanism of this effect is not yet well understood.

To assess the prevention of postoperative atrial tachyarrhythmias after coronary artery bypass grafting (CABG), we investigated in a prospective randomized study the effect of postoperative magnesium substitution on diabetic and non-diabetic patients.

Giving 3 g magnesium-5-sulfate in 1000 ml 5% dextrose (100 ml/h = 300 mg/h) over ten h on the first postoperative day we found the results seen in Table 1.

Conclusion

- Postoperative substitution of magnesium is an effective concept for prevention of PAT after cardiac surgery.
- There is no significant difference between subgroups of diabetic or non-diabetic patients concerning the effectiveness of PAT prevention by magnesium.

Table 1. PAT prevention by magnesium sulphate

	Magnesium group (n = 130)		Control group (n = 120)	
	with PAT (n = 20)	without PAT (n = 110)	with PAT (n = 42)	without PAT (n = 78)
Diabetes (n = 35/37)	7 (20.0%)	28 (80.0%)	11 (29.7%)	26 (70.3%)
Non-Diabetics (n = 95/83)	13 (13.7%)	82 (86.3%)	31 (37.4%)	52 (62.6%)
Summary (n = 130/120)	20 (15.4%)	110 (84.6%)	42 (35.0%)	78 (65.0%)

- In adaequate dosages (as we have used) there are no negative side effects in magnesium administration (especially no negative inotropic effects as found in antiarrhythmic drugs).
- One dosage concept on the first postoperative day; no further drug administration for atrial fibrillation.

References

1. England, MR et al. (1992) Magnesium administration and dysrhythmias after cardiac surgery. JAMA 268: 2395–2402
2. Fanning WJ et al. (1991) Prophylaxis of atrial fibrillation with magnesium sulfate after coronary artery bypass grafting Ann Thorac Surg 52: 529–533.
3. Karmy-Jones R et al (1995) Magnesium sulfate prophylaxis after cardiac operations. Ann Thorac Surg 59: 502–507

Author's address:
H.-G. Wollert, M.D.
Department of Thoracic and Cardiovascular Surgery
Klinikum Karlsburg
Greifswalder Str. 11A
17495 Karlsburg, Germany

Hyperlipoproteinemia and cardiac surgery

E. von Hodenberg

Heart Institut Lahr/Baden, Dept. of Internal Medicine and Cardiology

Introduction

The prognosis of coronary artery bypass patients depends not only on the patency of bypass grafts but of course also on the atherosclerotic progression of native coronary vessels. However, the pathology of arteriosclerosis seems to be different in venous grafts, arterial grafts, and native vessels. Epidemiologic and experimental studies have clearly demonstrated that the development and progression of atherosclerosis in both graft and native vessels are influenced by the presence of various risk factors, such as hypercholesterolemia, nicotine, diabetes, hypertension, etc. The present article is focussed on the diagnostic and therapeutic implication of hyperlipidemia in cardiac surgery patients.

Atherosclerosis in bypass grafts

As early bypass closures are mainly the consequence of thrombotic events (11), atherosclerotic changes in venous grafts can be observed not before the end of the first year after bypass operation (1, 2). Atherosclerotic lesions in vein grafts are rich of lipid laden macrophages, so-called foam cells, and resemble the experimentally cholesterol-induced lesions in animal models. Therefore, it may be possible that lipid lowering is very effective in preventing the formation of these lesions.

However, angiographic studies demonstrate that graft stenoses are normally not detectable before 3 years after the operation and are mainly visible between 5 and 10 years after the operation (7, 8). At the end of 10 years after operation about 70% of bypass grafts have significant (>50%) stenosis. In addition patients with bypass graft atherosclerosis have at least twice the risk of bypass occlusions after 10–12 years (4). It seems rather possible that rupture of the lipid rich plaques is responsible for this late thrombotic occlusion. Thus, patients with low cholesterol levels may have a lower risk to develop bypass atherosclerosis and occlusions.

In contrast to vein grafts arterial grafts have a much better patency rate: after 10 years more than 90% of arterial grafts are still patent (5). Histologically atherosclerosis in arterial grafts resemble the one of native vessels. Compared to venous grafts, patients with arterial revascularization have a lower incidence of late clinical events and a better long term survival (6, 18).

Hyperlipidemia and coronary artery disease

The influence of hyperlipidemia on the development of coronary artery disease has been demonstrated by numereous experimental, epidemiologic, and clinical studies. It is clearly proven that elevated serum total cholesterol and low-density lipoprotein cholesterol (LDL-C) are associated with a higher risk of atherosclerotic disease development including coronary heart disease (CHD) (5, 14, 24, 26). Decreasing CHD mortality rates are observed with lower cholesterol levels throughout the distribution of a population. Countries with a very low average cholesterol level such as China have a very low incidence of CHD and myocardial infarctions (10).

There are also several indications that elevated total cholesterol and LDL-C may cause plaque-instability (16). Furthermore there are reports on the effects of cholesterol on endothelial function (25). Elevated LDL-C seem to impair the activity of endothelial cell derived relaxing factor (NO) and therefore affect the vascular tone.

The so-called lipid hypothesis, to demonstrate that lowering plasma cholesterol levels decreases progression of coronary artery disease and even leads to regression of preexisting coronary lesions, was proven in several interventional studies. Clinical trials have consistently demonstrated a decrease in morbidity and mortality from CHD and other atherosclerotic diseases and associated events in hyperlipidemic patients without the clinical evidence of CHD (primary prevention) or in patients with established CHD (secondary prevention).

The West of Scottland (WOS) study demonstrated that lowering cholesterol levels with the HMGCoA reductase inhibitor Pravastatin in individuals without evidence of CHD but with total cholesterol levels of about 260 mg/dl reduces the incidence of serious coronary events, coronary mortality and even total mortality (23). Other primary prevention trials with lipid lowering drugs such as cholestyramine (Lipid Research Clinic Study) and gemfibrocil (Helsinki Heart Study) showed a decrease of coronary mortality but no effect on total mortality (13, 17).

Concerning secondary prevention numerous trials have shown beneficial effects of cholesterol lowering on the incidence of clinical coronary events, coronary but also total mortality. A series of angiographic studies have used quantitative coronary angiography to demonstrate that in patients with CHD aggressive lipid lowering may cause a decrease of CHD progression and in some cases even a regression of preexisting lesions.

The first major secondary prevention study was the Scandinavian Simvastatin Survival Study (4S), a double-blind, placebo-controlled trial in 4,444 patients with angina pectoris or prior myocardial infarction and hypercholesterolemia (baseline LDL-C 188 mg/dl) (22). The active group of patients was treated with Simvastatin to decrease their total-cholesterol below 200 mg/dl. The patients were followed an average of 5.4 years, and in the active treatment group a reduction in LDL-C of 35% was observed. This was associated with a 34% decrease of serious coronary events, a 42% decline of cardiac mortality, and even a 30% decline in total mortality. The active treatment group showed also a 37% decrease of need for new coronary interventions such as PTCA or coronary artery bypass surgery. The reduction of major coronary events was similar for different subgroups classified by age, gender, presence or absence of diabetes, smoking status, and concurrent treatment with beta-blockers or calcium channel-blockers.

The Cholesterol and Recurrent Events (CARE) study was a double-blind, placebo-controlled trial in 4,159 post-myocardial infarction patients with lower cholesterol levels (LDL-C 115-174 mg/dl) (21). The HMG-CoA reductase inhibitor Pravastatin was used as the cholesterol lowering agent. Patients were followed for a median of 5 years. While LDL-C decreased with an average of 32%, a 24% decline of coronary mortality and non-fatal myocardial infarction could be archieved in the drug treatment group. Similar reductions were demonstrated in other coronary endpoints, whereas no statistical effect was observed on reduction of total mortality, which was not designed as a primary endpoint.

The CARE study therefore suggests that lipid lowering therapy in patients with CHD and low to "normal" cholesterol levels is effective in reducing coronary morbidity and mortality.

Lipid lowering therapy and coronary artery bypass surgery

It can be concluded from all secondary prevention studies that patients with CHD and low to normal, as well as elevated cholesterol levels profit from a cholesterol lowering therapy. A few trials specially reviewed the effect of cholesterol reduction on the outcome of patients, who had undergone coronary-artery bypass surgery. The post-coronary artery bypass graft (post-CABG) trial investigated the effect of the lipid lowering agent Lovastatin on angiographic findings and additional revascularization procedures (19). A baseline LDL-C of 155 mg/dl was aggressively reduced to 93 mg/dl in comparison to a moderate reduction (LDL-C of 136 mg/dl). The additional treatment of warfarin was also tested. After a mean follow-up period of 4.3 years, a 29% reduction of Re-revascularization procedures (PTCA, or Re-CABG) was observed in the aggressively treated group. Warfarin had no effect. The decrease of coronary mortality and total mortality was not statistically significant.

One of the first major angiographic studies, the Cholesterol Lowering Atherosclerosis Study (CLAS), was performed in 188 patients, who had undergone coronary bypass surgery at least 3 months before entering the trial (3). Since at the time of the study potent cholesterol lowering drugs such as HMGCoA-reductase inhibitors were not yet available, the patients (average cholesterol 260 mg/dl) were randomized to receive combined colestipol (30 g/day) and niacin (4 g/day) plus diet or placebo plus diet. Entry in the trial occurred an average of 3.3 years after bypass surgery. The follow-up period and second angiogram was 2 years (CLAS I) and 4 years (CLAS II) after the first angiogram. The combined drug treatment caused a 25% reduction of total cholesterol and a 43% decrease of LDL-C. Progression and regression were determined by use of a global change score ranging from –3 to +3. Compared to the placebo group the active drug group showed a 40% reduction of patients with new lesions and with progression in the sapheneous vein grafts. There was also a significant reduction of new lesions in native vessels as well as in the vein grafts in patients treated with the cholesterol lowering agents. However, there was no difference of new graft occlusion between the placebo and the treatment group.

The beneficial effect of cholesterol lowering was maintained after 4 years, as demonstrated in the CLAS II study (9). In the native vessels 52% of the drug treated patients had no progression compared to 15% of the control patients; in addition 18% of the treated patients had regression versus 6% of the placebo patients. New lesions in bypass grafts had developed in 16% of the drug-treated group compared to 38% of the placebo group.

It should be noted, however, that the CLAS study was performed only in men and that only venous grafts were analyzed. Compared to venous grafts, of course, arterial grafts show a rather slow development of atherosclerosis.

Treatment guidelines

Because of the convincing experimental and clinical evidence, treatment guidelines for elevated cholesterol levels have emerged from several authoritative institutions in recent years.

Among others the European Atherosclerosis Society (EAS) (20) and the National Cholesterol Education Program (NCEP) (12) came up with specific recommendations to manage hyperlipidemia. The present article will only focus on secondary prevention guidelines.

According to the NCEP-Adult Treatment Panel II (ATP II) recommendations LDL-C < 100 mg/dl is defined as optimal for patients with CHD. In patients with LDL-C > 130 mg/dl drug treatment is unequivocally recommended, whereas in patients with LDL-C between 100 and 129 mg/dl drug treatment may be suggested according to the physician's clinical judgement.

The EAS guidelines define the target LDL-C level in the range of 115–135 mg/dl.

The basis for a cholesterol-lowering therapy is a healthy diet and physical activity. A normal or ideal weight should be archieved. The AHA gives the following diet suggestion:

fat	< 30% of total calories
saturated fat	< 7% of total calories
polyunsaturated fat	< 10% of total calories
monounsaturated fat	< 15% of total calories
carbohydrates	> 55% of total calories
cholesterol	< 200 mg/day

If drug-treatment is indicated, HMG-CoA reductase inhibitors and resins are the most potent cholesterol lowering agents. The positive effect of Simvastatin in CHD patients was shown in the 4S-study and of Pravastatin in the CARE study. Among other HMGCoA-reductase inhibitors, such as Lovastatin, Fluvastatin and Cerivastatin, Atorvastatin is the most effective cholesterol lowering statin with an additional lowering effect on triglycerides. Currently it is not known, whether Atorvastatin is also more effective in slowing the process of atherosclerosis. Additional interventional trials with this drug in CHD patients are underway.

Fibrates and nicotinic acid have a less potent effect on cholesterol reduction but are effective for the treatment of elevated triglycerides. Therefore, these drugs are recommended in hypertriglyceridemia and combined hyperlipoproteinemia.

In very severe cases of hypercholesterolemia (patients with familial hypercholesterolemia) drug treatment may not be sufficient to lower cholesterol. These very few high-risk patients might be then eligible for lipid-apheresis.

References

1. Atkinson JB, Forman MB, Perry JM (1985) Correlation of saphenous vein bypass graft angiograms with histologic changes at necropsy. Am J Cardiol 55:952–955
2. Atkinson JB, Forman MB, Vaughn WK (1985) Morphologic changes in long-term saphenous vein bypass grafts. Chest 88:341–348
3. Blankenhorn DH, Nessim SA, Johnson RL, Sanmarco ME, Azen SP, Cashin-Hemphill L (1987) Beneficial effects of combined colestipol-niacin therapy on coronary atherosclerosis and coronary venous bypass grafts. J Am Med Assoc 257:3233–3240

4. Bourassa MG, Fisher LD, Campeau L (1985) Long term fate of bypass grafts. The Coronary Artery Surgery Study and Montreal Heart Institute experiences. Circulation 72:V-71-V-78
5. Breslow JL, Plump A, Dammerman M (1996) New mouse models of lipoprotein disorders and atherosclerosis. In: V Fuster, R Ross, E Topel, (Eds.) Atherosclerosis and Coronary Heart Disease. New York: Lippincott-Raven
6. Cameron A, Kemp HG Jr, Green GE (1986) Bypass surgery with the internal mammary artery graft 15 year follow-up. Circulation 74:III-30-III-36
7. Campeau L, Enjalbert M, Lesperance J (1985) The relation of risk factors to the development of atherosclerosis in saphenous vein bypass grafts and the progression of disease in the native circulation. A study 10 years after aortocoronary bypass surgery. N Engl J Med 311:1329–1332
8. Campeau L, Enjalbert M, Lesperance J (1983) Atherosclerosis and late closure of aorto-coronary saphenous vein grafts. Sequential angiographic studies at 2 weeks, 1 year, 5 to 7 years, and 10 to 12 years after surgery. Circulation 68:II-1-II-7
9. Cashin-Hemphill L, Mack WJ, Pogoda JM, Sanmarco ME, Azen SP, Blankenhorn DH (1990) Beneficial effects of colestipol-niacin on coronary atherosclerosis. J Am Med Assoc 264:3013–3017
10. Chen Z, Peto R, Collins R, MacMahon S, Lu J, Li W (1991) Serum cholesterol concentration and coronary heart disease in a population with low cholesterol concentrations. BMJ 303:276–282
11. European Coronary Surgery Study Group (1982) Long-term results of prospective randomized study of coronary artery bypass surgery in stable angina pectoris. Lancet 2:1173–1180
12. Expert Panel on Detection, Evaluation and Treatment of High Blood Cholesterol in Adults (1993) Summary of the second report of the National Cholesterol Education Program (NCEP) Expert Panel on detection, evaluation and treatment of high blood cholesterol in adults (Adult Treatment Panel II). JAMA 269:3015–3023
13. Frick MH, Elo O, Haapa K, et al. (1987) Helsinki Heart Study: primary prevention trial with gemfibrozil in middle-aged men with dyslipidemia. N Engl J Med 317:1237–1245
14. Gordon T, Kannel WB, Castelli WP, Dawber TR (1981): Lipoproteins, cardiovascular disease and death: the Framingham study. Arch Intern Med 141:1128–1131
15. Grondin CM, Campeau L, Lesperance J (1984) Comparison of late changes in internal mammary artery and saphenous vein grafts in two consecutive series of patients 10 years after operation. Circulation 70:208–212
16. Lee RT, Libby P (1997) The unstable atheroma. Arterioscle Thromb Vascul Biol. 17:1–9
17. Lipid Research Clinics Program (1984) The Lipid Research Clinics Coronary Primary Prevention Trial results, I: reduction in incidence of coronary heart disease. JAMA 251:351–364
18. Loop FD, Lytle BW, Cosgrove DM (1986) Influence of the internal mammary-artery graft on 10 year survival and other cardiac events. N Engl J Med 314:1–6
19. The Post Coronary Artery Bypass Graft Trial Investigators (1997) The effect of aggressive lowering of low-density lipoprotein cholesterol levels and low-dose anticoagulation on obstructive changes in saphenous-vein coronary-artery bypass grafts. N Engl J Med 336:153–162
20. Pyorala K, DeBacker G, Graham I, et al. on behalf of the Task Force (1994) Prevention of coronary heart disease in clinical practice. Recommendations of the Task Force of the European Society of Cardiology, European Atherosclerosis Society and European Society of Hypertension. Eur Heart J 15:1300–1331
21. Sachs FM, Pfeffer MA, Maye LA, et al. for the Cholesterol and Recurrent Events Trial Investigators (1996) The effect of pravastatin on coronary events after myocardial infarction in patients with average cholesterol levels. N Engl J Med 335:1001–1009
22. Scandinavian Simvastatin Survival Study Group (1994) Randomized trial of cholesterol lowering in 4444 patients with coronary heart disease: the Scandinavian Simvastatin Survival Study (4S). Lancet 344:1383–1389
23. Shepherd J, Cobbe SM, Ford I, et al. (1995) Prevention of coronary heart disease with pravastatin in men with hypercholesterolemia. N Engl J Med 333:1301–1307
24. Stamler J, Wentworth D, Neaton JD (1986) Is the relationship between serum cholesterol and risk of premature death from coronary heart disease continuous or graded. Findings in 356, 222 primary screenees of the Multiple Risk Factor Intervention Trial (MRFIT). JAMA 256:2823–2828
25. Treasure CB, Klein JL, Weintraub WS, et al. (1995) Beneficial effects of cholesterol-lowering

therapy on the coronary endothelium in patients with coronary artery disease. N Engl J Med 332:481–487

26. Verschuren WM, Jacobs D, Bloemberg BP, et al. (1995) Serum total cholesterol and longterm coronary heart disease in different countries: twenty-five-year follow-up of the Seven Countries Study. JAMA 274:131–136

Author's address:
Priv.-Doz. Dr. Eberhard von Hodenberg
Heart Institute Lahr/Baden
Dept. of Internal Medicine and Cardiology
Hohbergweg 2
77933 Lahr, Germany

Cardiac surgery in patients with renal disease

P. Stelzer

Beth Israel Medical Center New York, USA

The complex relationships between the heart and the kidneys make them essential partners in the ongoing well-being of the healthy individual but also make each susceptible to major consequences when the other is diseased or injured. The activation of the renin-angiotensin system in the setting of renal artery stenosis is a classic example of how the compromised kidney adversely affects the heart. Similarly, the nephrosclerosis associated with hypertensive heart disease destroys kidneys with relentless efficiency. An immune-complex nephropathy can accompany active endocarditis resulting in renal failure or a septic embolus can destroy a kidney even more directly.

As the population of patients coming to cardiac surgery ages and the expectations of what can be accomplished increase, the presence of significant renal disease in this population is increasing as well. This comorbid condition has many implications regarding the risks, treatment strategies, and limits on the success of such operations. Many times the renal problem is a reflection of a more global systemic illness such as Diabetes Mellitus, hypertension or diffuse atherosclerotic disease affecting peripheral, cerebral, and coronary as well as renal vessels. Chronically elevated calcium and phosphorus levels can cause soft tissue calcification involving arteries, valves, and myocardium. Pericardial disease is often seen in patients with renal failure as well. The vascular access devices and fistulas essential for hemodialysis can become infected and lead to endocarditis.

Pre-operative preparation

Standard preoperative screening chemistries should include the BUN and Creatinine levels and as such provide an important warning, if elevated. A high degree of suspicion should be directed to elderly or diabetic patients with only midly elevated creatinine (1.5–2.0 mg/dl). Higher levels of creatinine (2.5–5.0) are an obvious warning sign. Patients on chronic dialysis are obviously easy to identify and are actually easier to manage since there is no concern about trying to preserve renal function. Those on hemodialysis may develop hemodynamic compromise from acute changes in their cardiac disease, making dialysis difficult. Similarly, patients on peritoneal dialysis (PD) may experience respiratory problems when the diaphragm is elevated by large volumes of fluid in the setting of acutely compromised pump function. Clearly, these factors need to be carefully controlled in the preoperative state. Some patients' hearts, however, cannot wait for the kidneys to be optimal. This creates serious problems postoperatively.

Cardiac catheterization precedes most cardiac surgical procedures and, in patients with renal compromise, this can be a significant renal insult. Use of nonionic contrast material may decrease the incidence of allergic reactions, but, unfortunately, does not lessen the renal burden. The patient with a creatinine between 2.5 and 5.0 almost always suffers some degree of renal insult from angiographic procedures. This is particularly true for the diabetic patient. A strategy for optimizing hydration without overloading the heart's ability to handle that fluid may require the aid of invasive hemodynamic monitoring, specifically a pulmonary artery catheter. A urinary drainage catheter is a very simple and effective tool for keeping track of output and avoiding the late discovery of oliguria. Some institutions have advocated a regimen of prophylactic mannitol, renal dopamine, and continuous furosemide infusion along with generous hydration during and immediately after angiography. However, none of these has been conclusively demonstrated to be more effective in preventing renal failure than simple saline infusion. Techniques aimed at minimizing the contrast load should be encouraged. These include elimination of routine ventriculography, leaving the evaluation of ventricular function and mitral valve function to non-invasive modalities such as echocardiography. Use of digital angiographic enhancement can allow lower contrast volumes for each coronary injection, and the number of views should be kept as low as possible.

Timing of surgery can be an awkward matter of walking the tightrope between waiting for renal recovery and avoiding further cardiac compromise. Clearly, there is no justification for delay in the patient with ascending aortic dissection, persistent unstable angina despite maximal medical and balloon pump therapy, or the patient with endocarditis and acute valve failure with pulmonary edema. Life ranks above kidney on the priority list. However, many patients can be stabilized and time allowed for recovery of renal function after contrast load. Clearly, the patient with an acutely rising creatinine after catherization is at high risk for renal failure if taken to surgery before the kidney has a chance to recover. Ideally, the creatinine should be allowed to return all the way to baseline before proceeding with surgery. This should be done even in the absence of oliguria.

The patients already on dialysis should be optimized by appropriate preoperative dialysis. This usually means the day before surgery, but can be immediately before if hyperkalemia is a problem. The goals are to optimize fluid and electrolyte status prior to surgery. Transfusion is usually not necessary as this can be done intraoperatively. Overly aggressive dialysis may prove counter-productive if hemodynamic compromise results. Hypotension, for example, is poorly tolerated by the patient with severe left main coronary stenosis. Peritoneal dialysis continues right up to the time of surgery, at which time the peritoneal cavity should be empty. Some PD patients may require temporary hemodialysis for adequate preparation.

Intra-operative management

In the operating room, the anesthesiologist may be faced with unique technical problems due to previous vascular access procedures on chronic dialysis patients. Arterial lines probably should not be placed in extremities with shunts or fistulas. Similarly, central venous cannulation should avoid sites of permanent access and may be impossible at a site where previous access may have failed or caused thrombosis. Blood pressure should be maintained at a higher than usual level in the patient with compromised renal function and renal dose dopamine (2–5 microgm/kg/min) may help to optimize renal blood flow. A low threshold for loop diuretics should help keep the urine flowing, intermittent or continuous infusion both being options. If not used prophylactically, they should be used liberally.

The same dictum for maintaining perfusion pressure to the kidney is passed to the perfusionist. High flows and neosynephrine are typically used to accomplish this. Mean pressures of 70 mmHg or higher should be sought. High doses of alpha constricting agents may be very harmful in the patient with borderline renal function and appropriate transfusion may help avoid the low resistance problem. Many renal patients are anemic, although the use of erythropoietin has made the average hematocrit close to 30%. Standard hemodilution may drop this below 15%, and there is little point in ending up with a hematocrit of 23% in a patient who has a poor mechanism for restoring his red cell mass. Mannitol is used in the pump prime to add osmotic diuretic effect as well as to serve as a free-radical scavenger. Hemoconcentration devices should be used on any patient with compromised renal function so as to avoid volume problems. Combined with appropriate transfusions, hemoconcentration should be used to allow the patient to come off cardiopulmonary bypass euvolemic with a hematocrit close to 30%.

High potassium solutions used for myocardial protection may require modification to lower concentrations for longer procedures where high volumes are needed. Some potassium can be removed through the hemoconcentration device if additional saline is "rinsed" through the system. The guiding principle for the perfusionist should be to leave the kidney nothing to do for the first twelve hours after bypass.

Specific procedures may have unique aspects in renal failure. Coronary arteries can have a diffuse "graham-cracker crumb" calcification which makes finding an ideal arteriotomy site difficult. The diabetic with end-stage renal disease can prove extremely challenging in this regard and endarterectomy may be required. Even the potential replacement conduits such as the radial artery may be extensively calcified or may have been used for dialysis access.

It may be possible or even desirable to modify the surgical approach in patients with renal dysfunction by avoiding cardiopulmonary bypass altogether. Some patients may be candidates for "beating heart" grafting either through standard sternotomy or less invasive techniques. The diffuse nature of coronary disease in these patients, however, may limit the application of these techniques. Similarly, the temptation to use catheter-based interventions for the renal patients must be discouraged because of the poor results in this group. Up to 80% restenosis has been reported for dialysis patients within six months (3). The exact mechanism for this malignant restenosis is unknown, but Ahmed and Kirshenbaum postulate it to be due to the high incidence of comorbidities in these patients (diabetes, peripheral vascular disease) as wall as enhanced platelet aggregation and adverse lipid profiles (1).

Valvular heart disease can be very different in the patient with renal disease as well. Due to the more rapid rate of tissue calcification in general, the midly stenotic aortic valve, for instance, can be expected to progress at a more rapid rate than other patients, thereby making it advisable to address this lesion earlier in the patient who is undergoing coronary artery bypass grafting (CABG). The early and rapid calcification of bioprosthetic valves in dialysis patients make tissue valves a poor choice. Despite the need for anticoagulation, mechanical valves are preferred if primary valve repair is not possible.

Hemostasis may be more difficult to achieve in the renal patient. Aprotinin can be used in the dialysis patient, but this drug should be avoided in the patient who still has some renal function. Platelets and fresh frozen plasma may occasionally be required, but one must remember the volume price paid for using these in patients whose ability to get rid of excess volume is compromised. Meticulous surgical technique is the primary defense against bleeding.

Post-operative management

Post-operatively, the renal patient requires more careful attention to fluid management. Vasoactive drips may be required but should be concentrated to avoid volume overload. In general, blood loss should be replaced with blood. Some patients may ironically respond to prophylactic furosemide infusions with excessive diuresis. The resulting potential for dehydration of the dysfunctional kidney must be assiduously avoided. A general rule is to replace any urine output in excess of 200 cc/hour with saline. Antibiotic regimens must be modified for renal insufficiency. Serum concentrations can and should be measured for potentially toxic drugs such as aminoglycosides and vancomycin.

Arrhythmias are common after cardiac surgery, especially atrial fibrillation, and their treatment may be different in the face of renal dysfunction. Procaine amide must be used with caution in patients with elevated creatinine levels. The buildup of its n-acetyl metabolite severely limits its use in patients with creatinine over 3.0 mg/dl. Amiodarone, with its primary hepatic excretion, can be a very useful drug for both atrial and ventricular arrhythmias if Beta-blockers fail. Lidocaine, in general, is not a problem except for the volume of dilution. ACE inhibitors should be avoided in general.

Peritoneal dialysis should be resumed within 24 hours of surgery, generally waiting until the patient is extubated with stable respiratory mechanics. Smaller exchange volumes can help to avoid respiratory problems. Tonicity of the dialysate should be adjusted along with potassium concentration depending on serum chemistries and volume status of the patient. Hemodialysis should begin the day after surgery but more frequent treatments with gentler volume removal may be necessary for the first week.

Results

In the state of New York, all cardiac surgical procedures must be reported to the Department of Health where the data are analyzed on a yearly basis. In the most recent results released (1994) 2.5% of just over 18,000 patients undergoing coronary artery bypass grafting had a creatinine level of 2.5 mg/dl or higher and 0.9% were on dialysis preoperatively. These patients had mortality rates of 12.8 and 13.3%, respectively (2). This makes significant renal disease one of the biggest risk factors of all analyzed, edging out all but cardiogenic shock and the risk of reoperative bypass surgery. This is similar to results in other reported series (4).

With strict attention to patient selection, preparation and peri-operative management, the mortality over the last four years at Beth Israel Medical Center has been much lower. 54 patients with elevated serum creatinine (> 2.5 mg/dl) have undergone CABG with a mortality rate of only 3.7%, and 22 patients on dialysis had a mortality rate of only 4.5%. (These values approach but do not achieve statistical significance due to the small numbers of deaths.)

Acute renal failure developing after heart surgery carries a very bad prognosis. This dreaded problem occurred in 0.7% of patients in New York State and 59.7% of them died. Similarly, of 16 patients at our institution who developed renal failure requiring dialysis, 56.3% died. This makes postoperative renal failure second only to insertion of a Left Ventricular assist device (76.2% mortality) as a marker for death after CABG. It is worse than sepsis (49.3% mortality), respiratory failure (30.5% mortality), or needing an intra-aortic balloon pump postoperatively (25.7% mortality). It is little comfort, but this is similar to the mortality rate for renal failure following noncardiac surgery as well.

Clearly, postoperative renal failure is rarely an isolated event, but rather is most often a part of the multisystem organ failure that accompanies the low cardiac output syndrome. It is almost always preceded by some degree of respiratory insufficiency. However, it becomes a vicious cycle as it becomes almost impossible to dry out a pair of soaked lungs with dialysis in the setting of poor cardiac function.

The first step is to make the diagnosis. This seems obvious, but the surgeon is often incurably optimistic about the outcome of anyone he or she may have operated on and, therefore, could not possibly have a problem. When inappropriate oliguria is evident with no response to volume or to diuretics, the diagnosis must be entertained. Obviously, the cause must be sought and treated. Outcome is certainly a function of this underlying cause. Low Output Syndrome must be differentiated from the low resistance state of sepsis and appropriate volume replacement and inotropic support provided. Embolic etiology may be suspected if there are other signs of peripheral emoblization and, if found, may be a warning that other visceral vessels may have been compromised as well. Bedside renal blood flow scans or ultrasound may be useful as well as simpler, cheaper methods including urinary electrolyte measurements. Unfortunately, the diuretic therapy so often used before this is considered may alter the osmolality and sodium concentrations to the point where they can be misleading. The crucial thing is to accept the fact that the kidneys are not working and get on with treatment before the whole body is one big edematous lake. Every organ system is further compromised when this is allowed to occur. Dialzye the patient!

Goals of dialysis in acute renal failure are at least threefold. Troublesome fluid volume must be removed. Toxic solutes must be "excreted". Electrolyte imbalance, especially hyperkalemia, must be corrected. Unfortunately, these problems are ongoing in nature and most dialysis modalities are intermittent with access to only a limited fluid compartment.

Peritoneal dialysis is an alternative, but is often plagued by respiratory (diaphragmatic) compromise and poor solute clearance. Early, aggressive, and frequent hemodialysis should be pursued with judicious fluid removal and appropriate red cell replacement. A minimum of four and usually five or six hemodialysis treatments per week are needed to maintain adequate control of fluid and solute removal. Unfortunately, these sick patients do not tolerate the hemodynamic effects of taking out fluid too rapidly, so the need for vasopressor support often goes up dramatically as fluid is removed. This can aggravate the already sick renal situation with adverse vasoconstrictive effects.

Alternatively, we have used continuous hemofiltration in some of these very sick patients. Continuous veno-venous hemofiltration (CVVH) is one method but the current generation of equipment necessary to do this is cumbersome and requires specially trained personnel. Newer versions will soon be available to make this more user-friendly. We have chosen to use the simpler method of continuous arterio-venous hemofiltration with or without dialysis (CAVH, CAVHD).

Access is simple, usually involving a pair of femoral punctures. The fluid removal can be precisely controlled by the bedside ICU nurse and can be extremely efficient. Because it is not trying to do two days' worth of volume removal in a few hours, this is hemodynamically much easier for the unstable patient to tolerate than normal hemodialysis. Precise net fluid removal can be controlled on an hour-to-hour basis and solute clearance is impressively efficient. It can also be very discriminating in solute removal by varying the rinse solution run through the filtration device.

Obviously, this technique cannot be used for protracted periods, especially in the setting where sepsis is common and catheter changes are needed frequently. As soon as the patient has achieved sufficient hemodynamic stability to allow it, more durable venous access for standard hemodialysis should be the goal. Permanent access procedures are to be discouraged until several weeks into this kind of renal failure due to the high mortality on the one hand and the chance of renal recovery on the other. Fistulas and shunts are also apt to thrombose due to low flow states in the early phase.

Despite its high risk for mortality, renal failure after cardiac surgery can resolve. There is often a diuretic phase which requires careful attention to fluid replacement to avoid dehydrating the recovering kidney while continuing dialysis support for needed solute removal. The initial urine output may be adequate or even abundant, but the quality leaves a lot to be desired. Dialysis should continue until both volume and solute removal can be reliably trusted to the kidneys.

Summary

In summary, the patient with compromised renal function is at increased risk with an odds ratio of nearly 3.0 for death after coronary artery surgery, probably even more so after more complex cardiac operations. However, these patients can undergo operation with appropriate selection and careful preparation that optimizes the state of renal function before and during surgery. Hypotension must be rigorously avoided and agents such as dopamine and diuretics may play a protective role. Drugs cleared by the kidney must be used in adjusted doses and frequencies or alternatives sought. Dialysis should be done the day before and the day after surgery in the chronic dialysis patient. It should be considered early for any patient developing renal insufficiency even very early post-operatively and used aggressively but gently to prevent further multisystem organ damage. CAVHD is an effective tool for this purpose.

References

1. Ahmed WH, Krishenbaum JM (1994) Outcome of coronary artery angioplasty in hemodialysis patients. Seminars in Dialysis Vol 7 No 2: 96–97
2. Coronary artery bypass surgery in New York State 1992–1994 (1996): New York State Department of Health
3. Kahn JK, Rutherford BF, McConahay DR, Johnson WL, Giorgi LV, Hartzler GO (1990) Short- and long-term outcome of percutaneous transluminal coronary angioplasty in chronic dialysis patients. Am Heart J 119 (3 pt 1): 484–489
4. Rutsky EA, Rostand SG (1994) Coronary artery bypass graft surgery in end-stage renal disease: indications, contraindications, and uncertainties. Seminars in Dialysis Vol 7 No 2: 91–95

Author's address
Paul Stelzer, MD
Division of Cardiac Surgery
Beth Israel Medical Center
317 East 17th Street 11th Floor
New York, NY 10003 USA

Cardiac surgery in patients with liver disease

K. J. Oldhafer, M. Frerker

Klinik für Abdominal- und Transplantationschirurgie, Medizinische Hochschule Hannover, Germany

Introduction

Open heart surgery represents an invasive surgical procedure. Cardiac surgery is associated with a specific rate of morbidity and mortality even in patients without other cardiac diseases. The liver represents an important organ for lipid and glucose metabolism and protein synthesis. Thus, it is reasonable to assume that liver insufficiency has an influence on the outcome of patients undergoing open heart surgery.

There are several liver diseases which can be treated by cardiac surgery, e.g., the so-called Budd-Chiari syndrome by a hepato-atrial anastomosis (16, 24). Fig. 1 shows the interactions between cardiac surgery and liver diseases. Even complete acute liver failure has been observed after open heart surgery (7). Further, the liver has been injured by cardiac surgery (4).

This paper deals with the problem of cardiac surgery in patients with coexisting liver disease. But, there is not much data available in the literature about this topic. It is surprising because problems with patients suffering from liver disease, like alcoholism, are frequent. Many groups have their own definitions of contraindications based on various parameters like cholinesterase concentration in the serum. In this article a short review of what is found in the literature about cardiac surgery and liver disease and a few ideas for future investigations are given.

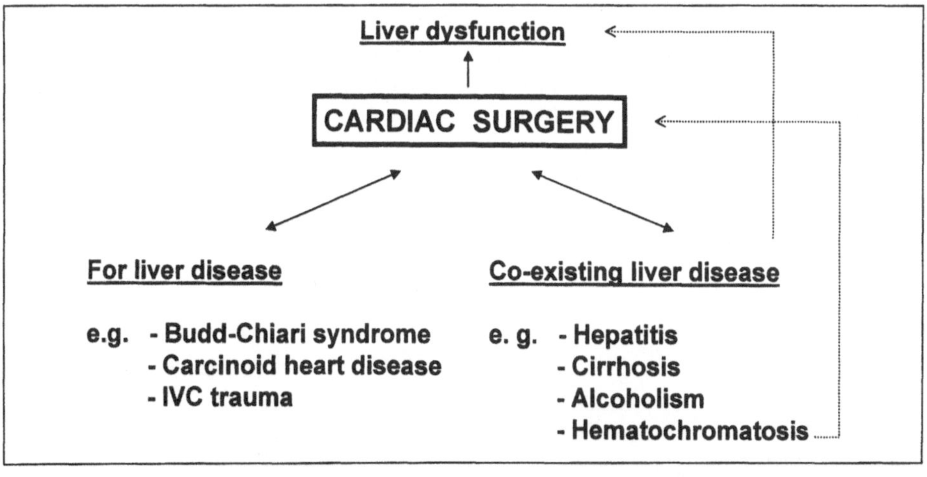

Fig. 1. Interactions between cardiac surgery and liver disease

Liver function tests

Several liver function tests are available. Besides special dynamic liver function tests, several daily routine parameters can be used for interpretation of liver function. Although clinical signs of liver disease must not be obvious, liver function can be reduced. Therefore, these tests and determinations, e.g., transaminase enzymes, are important in the preoperative work-up in every patient undergoing cardiac surgery. Hepatocytes contain large amounts of transaminase enzymes. Acute hepatocellular damage due to arterial hypoxemia, drugs, or viruses will cause an enzyme release into the systemic circulation. A problem is that other tissues as heart, lung, and skeletal muscle also contain transaminase enzymes. Thus, these determinations are not specific for liver damage. However, marked elevations of serum transaminase concentration (> four times) should suggest acute liver injury. In liver surgery, determination of clotting factors, serum cholinesterase, and albumin has shown to be useful for the estimation of the functional hepatic reserve. Bromsulfalein excretion tests and aminopyrine breath tests are applied since several years in many fields of medicine (6, 15). Recently, the arterial ketone body ratio (AKBR) was used to monitor the hepatic mitochondrial redox state in patients with cardiopulmonary bypass operations (11). The AKBR dropped to a critical level after the initiation of cardiopulmonary bypass and remained at a low level during the cardiopulmonary bypass, returning to the preoperative level on the second postoperative morning in a time dependent fashion. This data clearly showed that liver function is changed during or perhaps by open heart surgery. Thus, if patients preoperatively displayed partial hepatic insufficiencies, cardiac surgery could enhance liver injury.

Predictive scores

In order to assess the rate of postoperative morbidity and mortality various scores have been established in surgery. The basis of most of them were retrospective analyses of special patient populations. The Child-Pugh score was developed for cirrhotic patients undergoing decompressive shunt surgery (1). They are divided in three groups (Table 1). Meanwhile, the Child-Pugh score was used for many indications and could also be used for patients waiting for open heart surgery. A specific score for adult cardiac surgery was proposed by Parsonnet (12). This score consists of 18 different items, but no parameter of liver function is included. In 1997 a

Table 1. Child-pugh score

	1 Point	2 Points	3 Points
serum-bilirubin	< 2 mg/dl	2–3 mg/dl	< 3 mg/dl
serum-albumin	> 3.5 mg/dl	2.8–3.5 mg/dl	< 2.8 mg/dl
ascites	∅	+	++
encephalopathy	∅	+	++
Quick	> 50%	30–50%	< 30%

Child A. 5–6 Points
Child B: 7–9 Points
Child C: 10–15 Points

Table 2. Gastrointestinal complications after cardiac surgery

Author	No.	Total	Mortality	Cholecystitis	Pancreatitis	Liver Failure
Welling 1986	18	1596	12.0	3	–	?
Leitman 1987	60	6452	59.0	11	5	?
Krasnia 1988	25	1279	44.0	7	8	3
Yilmaz 1996	36	3158	13.9	3	2	2

modified Parsonnet's score was published by Gabrielle and co-workers (5). The number of items increased to 46, but also without any liver parameter. This might be due to the fact that no hepatic injury was mentioned on the list of postoperative events in their patient population (5).

Hepato-biliary complications

The patients who developed liver problems after cardiac surgery could be important for the analysis of the question what are risk factors or what are contraindications for cardiac surgery based on liver disease. Table 2 shows recent publications about gastrointestinal complications after cardiac surgery. Liver failure was observed in two out of four studies. Cholecystitis and pancreatitis were the leading clinical problems. The mortality was high with a range between 12.0 and 59.0%.

The problem of complete liver failure after cardiac surgery was described (18, 7). However, the underlying mechanisms remained unknown . A possible explanation could be the reduced liver perfusion during cardiac surgery under artificial perfusion conditions by the heart-lung machine. The major hemodynamic consequence of non-pulsatile cardiopulmonary bypass is the development of progressive, total systemic peripheral arterial vasoconstriction, leading to reduced perfusion of peripheral organs and increased left ventricular work. Several studies have shown the progressive increase in total peripheral vascular resistance from the onset of artificial circulation, extending into the early postoperative period. An increase of circulating levels of angiotensin II could be the explanation for this (21). Liver perfusion depends also on several other factors like sympathomimetics (13). Norepinephrine is routinely administered during cardiac surgery and during the early postoperative period. This substance causes vasoconstriction in gastrointestinal organs and can lead to a reduced liver blood flow.

The above mentioned acute cholecystitis represents a specific problem following open heart surgery. The cholecystitis is acalculous and occurs within the first postoperative week in the majority of cases (17, 14). Acute acalculous cholecystitis is a life-threatening condition especially in critically ill patients on the intensive care unit after cardiac surgery. Since gangrene and perforation were found, early cholecystectomy represents the therapy of choice. The underlying mechanisms remained unknown. Similar observations of acute cholecystitis were reported after regional chemotherapy in patients with non-resectable liver tumors due to regional ischemia to the gall bladder. Thus, a prophylactic cholecystectomy is routinely performed during the placement of port-catheters into the gastroduedenal artery. The acute acalculous cholecystitis may also be caused by temporary ischemia during the reduced perfusion conditions under non-pulsatile cardiopulmonary bypassing and its consequences.

Alcoholic liver disease

It is estimated that alcoholism afflicts about 10 million persons in the US and about 1.5 million in Germany. Critical dosages for the development of alcohol induced liver diseases are 60 – 80 g alcohol per day for males and 30 g alcohol for females. It is well-known that the postoperative morbidity is increased among alcohol misusers. Recently, Tonnesen and co-workers reported about a prospective study with symptom-free alcohol misusers undergoing colorectal surgery (19). The postoperative complication rate was higher in the alcohol-misuser group than in the control group. Alcohol misusers had longer bleeding times during the first postoperative week than control persons. An important finding is that there is an effect of alcoholism on cardiac muscle. Urbano-Marquez and co-workers reported that alcohol is toxic to striated muscle in a dose-dependent manner (20).

Cardiac surgery in liver transplanted patients

Patients after liver transplantation show a normal liver function in the majority of cases early after transplantation. However, recurrence of the underlying liver disease and chronically impaired graft function are problems in the long term post-transplant period. Furthermore, it can not be excluded that liver grafts display a reduced tolerance to invasive surgery like open heart surgery. In literature reports about five liver transplanted patients with open heart surgery were found (2, 3, 8). In the department of surgery at Hannover Medical School one liver graft recipient underwent combined valvular and coronary surgery (Dresler, personal communication). This patient received a mitral valve replacement and coronary artery bypass grafting 38 months after liver transplantation. Three weeks after cardiac surgery the patient was discharged in good condition and is now doing well more than 16 months after cardiac surgery.

Conclusions

Based on the literature search and discussions with many cardiac surgeons, it turns out that there is a need for clear definitions of contraindications for cardiac surgery in patients with coexistent liver disease. In patients with severe cirrhosis the decision is probably untroubled. However, in patients with unknown low-grade liver insufficiency, this can be complicated. Therefore, different dynamic liver function tests should be applied in patients undergoing cardiac surgery. But these tests are expensive and time consuming. Thus, the first step could be the retrospective analysis of liver function by routine parameters like cholinesterase, clotting factors, albumin and bleeding time in the huge patient population. These data should be available in many centers.

Fig. 2 shows a proposal of a possible treatment strategy in patients with apparent liver cirrhosis. The Child-Pugh classification is used. Child A patients with a lower mortality rate could be operated after specific preoperative therapy. In Child B and C patients liver transplantation should be considered in the treatment protocol.

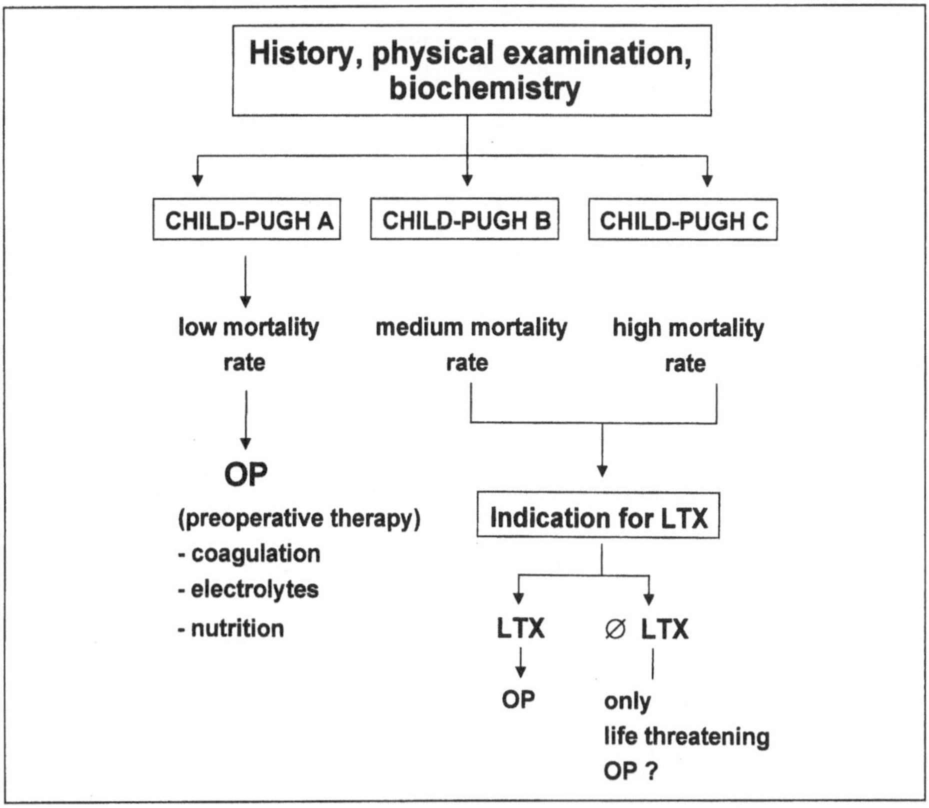

Fig. 2. Flow sheet for patients with cirrhosis and planned cardiac surgery (according to Levine JS (1992) Decision making in gastroenterology. Mosby, St. Louis, pp 414–415)

The liver blood flow during cardiopulmonary bypass represents in our hands an interesting target for further studies to analyze the influence of liver disease in open heart surgery. The reduced liver blood flow could be the explanation for early postoperative liver failure and also for the acute cholecystitis. Today, various methods of monitoring of the hepatic microcirculation are available and can be used in the clinic without problems. It is also possible that the disturbed liver microcirculation represents the target for treatment protocols in the future to avoid liver insufficiency after cardiac surgery or to allow open heart surgery in patients with coexisting liver disease.

References

1. Child CG, Turcotte JG (1964) Surgery in portal hypertension. In: Child CG (ed) Major problems in clinical surgery: The liver and portal hypertension. WB Saunders Philadelphia, pp 1–85
2. Dillow JR, Larrieu AJ, Fine RH (1995) Emergency coronary revascularization in a liver transplant recipient. Chest 108: 1763–1764
3. Dunton RF, Karlson KJ, Leonardi HK, Jenkins RL, Berger RL (1994) Coronary artery bypass grafting in patients with transplanted livers. Ann Thorac Surg 58: 1054–1058
4. Eugene J, Ott RA, Stemmer EA (1986) Hepatic trauma during cardiac surgery. J Cardiovasc Surg 27: 100–102

5. Gabrielle F, Roques F, Michel P, Bernard A, de Vicentis C, Roques X, Brenot R, Baudet E, David M (1997) Is the Parsonnet's score a good predictive score of mortality in adult cardiac surgery: assessment by a French multicentre study. Eur J of Cardiothorac Surg 11: 406–414
6. Gill RA, Goodman MW, Golfus GR, Onstad GR, Bubrick MP (1983) Aminopyrine breath test predicts surgical risk for patients with liver disease. Ann Surg 198: 701–704
7. Hill DM, Warren SE, Mitas II JA, Swerdlin AHR (1980) Hepatic coma after open heart surgery. South Med J 73: 906–911
8. Klima U, Wimmer-Greinecker G, Harringer W, Mair R, Groß C, Brücke P (1993) Homograft replacement of the aortic valve after liver transplantation. Transpl Int 6: 242–243
9. Krasna MJ, Flancbaum L, Trooskin SZ, Fitzpatrick JC, Scholz PM, Scott GE, Spotnitz AJ, Mackenzie JW (1988) Gastrointestinal complications after cardiac surgery. Surgery 104: 773–780
10. Leitman M, Paull DE, Barie PS, Isom OW, Shires GT (1987) Intra-abdominal complications of cardiopulmonary bypass operations. Surgery, Gynecology & Obstetrics 165: 251–254
11. Nomoto S, Shimahara Y, Kumada K, Okamoto Y, Ban T (1996) Influence of hepatic mitochondrial redox state on complement biosynthesis and activation during and after cardiopulmonary bypass operations. Eur J Cardiothorac Surg 10: 273–278
12. Parsonnet V, Dean D, Berstein AD (1989) A method of uniform stratification of risk for evaluating the results of surgery in acquired adult heart disease. Circulation 79: 3–12
13. Reilly PM, Bulkley GB (1993) Vasoactive mediators and splanchnic perfusion. Crit Care Med 21: S55–S68
14. Savino JA, Scalea TM, Del Guercio LRM (1985) Factors encouraging laparotomy in acalculous cholecystitis. Crit Care Med 13: 377–380
15. Schneider JF, Baker AL, Haines NW, Hatfield G, Boyer JL (1980) Aminopyrine N-demethylation: A prognostic test of liver function in patients with alcoholic liver disease. Gastroenterology 79: 1145–1150
16. Senning A (1983) Transcaval posterocranial resection of the liver as treatment of the Budd-Chiari syndrome. World J Surg 7: 632–640
17. Sessions SC, Scoma RS, Sheikh FA, Mcgeehin WH, Smink RD (1993) Acute acalculous cholecystitis following open heart surgery. Am Surg 59: 74–77
18. Strunin L, Davies JM (1995) Hepatic necrosis after cardiac surgery. Anaesthesia and Intensive Care 23: 755–756
19. Tonnesen H, Petersen KR, Hojgaard L, Stokholm KH, Nielsen HJ, Knigge U, Kehlet H (1992) Postoperative morbidity among symptom-free alcohol misusers. Lancet 340: 334–337
20. Urbano-Marquez A, Estruch R, Navarro-Lopez F, Grau JM, Mont L, Rubin E (1989) The effects of alcoholism on skeletal and cardiac muscle. N Engl J Med 320: 409–415
21. Watkins L, Lucas SK, Gardner TJ, Potter A, Walker WG, Gott VL (1979) Angiotensin II levels during cardiopulmonary bypass: A comparison of pulsatile and nonpulsatile flow. Surg Forum 30: 229–230
22. Welling RE, Rath R, Albers JE, Glaser RS (1986) Gastrointestinal complications after cardiac surgery. Arch Surg 121: 1178–1180
23. Yilmaz AT, Arslan M, Demirkilic U, Özal E, Kuralay E, Bingöl H, Öz BS, Tatar H, Öztürk ÖY (1996) Gastrointestinal complications after cardiac surgery. Eur J Cardiothorac Surg 10: 763–767
24. Zogno M, Danieli G, Pardini A, Fucci C, Ferrari M, Caradonna E, Vassalli M, Alfieri O (1990) Hepato-atrial anastomosis as emergency treatment for traumatic rupture of suprahepatic inferior vena cava and hepatic veins. Eur J Cardio-thorac Surg 4: 675–677

Author's address:
Karl J. Oldhafer
Medizinische Hochschule Hannover
Klinik für Abdominal- und Transplantationschirurgie
Carl-Neuberg-Straße 1
D-30625 Hannover, Germany

Cardiac surgery in patients with chronic renal failure

Ch. Fischer, O. Elert

University of Würzburg, Department for Cardiothoracic Surgery, Würzburg, Germany

Introduction

Recently, the prognosis for patients on chronic hemodialysis concerning their renal disease has improved so much that cardiovascular disease has become their leading cause of death and an increasing number of these patients is introduced to the cardiac surgeon. Chronic renal failure as a concomitant disease is itself accompanied by a number of concomitant diseases.

We reviewed the management and outcome of 44 dialysis dependent patients, who underwent cardiac surgery in our clinic.

Results

Patients

- 33 men and 9 women
- average age 57 years (36–72 years)
- mean period on dialysis prior to surgery 53 months (3 months to 12 years)

Causes of chronic renal failure

- glomerulonephritis 9 (20%)
- diabetes 6 (14%)
- nephrosclerosis 4 (9%)
- other (each in 1 case) 5 (11%)
- pyelonephritis 7 (16%)
- polycystic disease 6 (14%)
- lupus erythematodes 3 (7%)
- unknown 4 (9%)

Coexisting diseases

- secondary hyperparathyroidism 11 (25%) with osteopathy
- peripheral atherosclerosis II–III 9 (20%)
- duodenal ulcers 4 (9%)
- cerebral atherosclerosis 6 (14%)
- other 10 (23%)

Heart disease and operation

36 (82%) coronary artery bypass grafting with 3 grafts on average
- 10 (28%) patients suffered from unstable angina pectoris and urgent surgery was required
- 14 (39%) patients experienced myocardial infarctions
- 3 (8%) patients underwent CABG once before

8 (18%) valve replacement, of which
- 4 (50 %) were mitral and 4 (50%) were aortic valves
- 4 (50%) patients had emergency operation for acute endocarditis
- 2 (25%) aortic valve replacement plus each 1 coronary artery bypass

Special risk factors and considerations

Task force 1: Fluid balance

- All patients had their last dialysis on the day before surgery.
- Intraoperative ultrafiltration during CPB was done in all patients with a fluid extraction of 2765 ± 1605 ml (range: 100–5500 ml).
- Strict fluid restriction was kept postoperatively.
- In 43% a low dose of noradrenalin (Arterenol®) was used instead of volume to stabilize hemodynamics.
- Signs of hypervolemia were seen in 11% of the chest X-rays on the 1. p.o. day.
- Oxygenation was good in all patients and weaning from respirator was achieved after 4.8–31.5 h (mean 13 h).

Task force 2: Potassium balance

- Glucose/insulin infusion had to be administered in 50% to keep the potassium serum level below 6.0 mmol/l.
- The mean maximum serum potassium level was 5.98 ± 0.6 mmol/l.

Task force 3: Renal anemia

- The mean Hb at the beginning of serugery was 10.8 ± 1.8 g/dl and declined to 8.3 ± 1.2 g/dl at the end.
- The mean minimum Hb after surgery was 7.7 ± 1.1 g/dl.
- In 86% of the patients 3 units of blood on average (range: 1–13) were given.

Task force 4: Postoperative dialysis and bleeding

We tried to start dialysis as late as possible to prevent bleeding from heparin use.
- No patient had to be dialysed on the day of surgery.
- In 25% dialysis could be delayed until the second p.o. day.
- 80% of the patients were from the first postoperative dialysis onward back in their routine program with three times dialysis per week.

Under this policy:
- The mean loss of blood was 631 ml (range: 275–2375 ml).
- One patient required reoperation for bleeding on the 3rd p.o. day.
- One late hemorrhagic cardiac tamponade occured during dialysis on the 8th p.o. day.

Task force 5: Infections

Patients on maintenance dialysis are said to be prone to infections.

- Four (9%) leg wound infections occured. This is not half of the patients with severe peripheral atherosclerosis.
- One patient suffered from pneumonia.
- Two patients underwent reoperation for sternal dehiscence, both died from sepsis 6 weeks later.

Task force 6: Hyperparathyroidism

- No acute ionic alteration, neither hypocalcemia nor hypermagnesemia nor hyperphosphatemia occurred.
- Despite of 50% osteoporotic patients only two experienced sternal dehiscence.

Complications

- None in 21 patients (48%).
- Minor in 14 (32%), which are
  - non-persistent atrial fibrillation in 5 patients
  - inadequate state of mood with transient moderate confusion in 4
  - pericardial effusion without tamponade or intervention in 1
  - leg wound infection without systemic infection in 4
- Severe in 4 (9%), yet without prolonged hospital stay, which are
  - thrombosis of the arteriovenous shunt for hemodialysis in 2 patients
  - late hemorrhagic cardiac tamponade in 1
  - reoperation for bleeding in 1
- Lethal in 5 (11%), which are
  - pneumonia in 1 (patient died after 6 weeks)
  - sudden death on 5th p.o. day in 1
  - severe delirium → sternal dehiscence → sepsis in 2

Conclusion

Patients suffering from chronic renal failure carry a number of special risk factors, if they have to undergo cardiac surgery. Their altered fluid and potassium balance have to be considered carefully. Strict fluid restriction is as well essential as the adapting of drug dosage to their impaired excretory function. 80% of our patients were free of severe complications and the overall mortality was 11%. These results show that cardiac surgery can be performed in dialysis dependent patients at higher, yet still reasonable risk.

Author's address:
Charlotte Fischer, M.D.
Universitätsklinik für Herz- und Thoraxchirurgie
Josef-Schneider-Str. 6
97080 Würzburg, Germany

Cardiac surgery and pulmonary function: Does lung function testing predict pulmonary complications of cardiac surgery?

M. M. Borst and F. J. Meyer

Abteilung Innere Medizin III, Medizinische Klinik und Poliklinik, Ruprecht-Karls-Universität Heidelberg, Heidelberg, Germany

Introduction

Both cardiac surgeons and pulmonologists are aware of the interplay between pulmonary function and surgical interventions involving the heart. Cardiac surgery may induce dramatic changes in respiratory mechanics, in the pulmonary ventilation-perfusion ratio (9), and in pulmonary gas exchange. These effects can influence perioperative morbidity and mortality. On the other hand, pre-existing pulmonary disease may severely affect the postoperative course of patients undergoing cardiac surgery. Therefore, it is desirable to estimate the risk for pulmonary complications preoperatively and possibly to reduce it by adequate perioperative management (14). Focusing on patients with chronic obstructive lung disease (COPD), this review is intended to evaluate current approaches to the preoperative assessment of pulmonary problems during the postoperative period after open heart surgery. In particular, the impact of preoperative lung function testing for risk assessment will be discussed.

Effects of cardiac surgery on pulmonary function

Pulmonary function may be affected by cardiac surgery in many ways, especially in the early postoperative period. Incidence and mechanisms of surgery-induced disturbances have been reviewed extensively elsewhere (14, 17). A selection of possible interactions is given in Table 1. Among those, two types of problems are unique to cardiac surgery:

- specific changes in the lung induced by cardiopulmonary bypass (the "post pump syndrome") and
- pulmonary effects resulting from postoperative cardiac dysfunction.

During cardiopulmonary bypass, pulmonary vascular endothelium is damaged, leading to neutrophil sequestration and activation, platelet aggregation, and release of great amounts of vasoactive and inflammatory substances (2). These processes facilitate the permeation of plasma into the interstitial and possibly alveolar compartment, as indicated by a significant increase in pulmonary protein accumulation (13). Thus, cardiopulmonary bypass may result in a doubling of the alveolo-arterial difference in PO_2 and a significant drop in diffusion capacity (13). By this and other mechanisms, an increase in functional right-to-left shunt is induced by

Table 1. Types of Pulmonary Dysfunction Complicating Cardiac Surgery

Pulmonary Vascular Disease
• pulmonary arterial embolism
• irreversible elevation of PVR
• hypoxic vasoconstriction
• left ventricular failure
Restrictive Disease
• reduced respiratory drive
• reduced respiratory muscle function
• thoracic instability
• pleural effusion
• atelectasis
• pain
Obstructive Disease
• exacerbation of COPD or asthma
• tracheal stenosis
• mucous impaction
Alveolar Disease
• pulmonary edema
• alveolitis
• pulmonary hemorrhage
Infectious Disease
• tracheobronchitis, pneumonia
• pleural emphysema
• sepsis

cardiopulmonary bypass which is reversible within a few hours under normal circumstances (9). It remains to be clarified whether the incidence or severity of the "post pump syndrome" might be increased in the presence of pre-existing pulmonary disease such as COPD.

Respiratory complications from postoperative left ventricular failure are common in the presence of poor left ventricular function, such as in ischemic cardiomyopathy. Since the management of cardiogenic pulmonary edema is beyond the scope of this article, it will not be discussed further.

Respiratory complications in cardiac surgery

Among the specific pulmonary vascular problems listed in Table 1, pulmonary arterial embolism usually occurs unexpectedly and may have catastrophic consequences. In a series of 1033 patients undergoing cardiac surgery, pulmonary arterial embolism definitely diagnosed by angiogram, by ventilation/perfusion-scan, or by autopsy had an incidence of 3.2%, mostly in the first two weeks postoperatively (11). All cases of pulmonary embolism occurred in patients undergoing coronary bypass surgery with or without simultaneous valve replacement, but none in isolated valve replacement surgery. The overall perioperative mortality was 18.7% in patients suffering from pulmonary arterial embolism as opposed to 3.3% in the unaffected group (11). Thus, pulmonary arterial embolism is a serious complication of cardiac surgery which occurs not infrequently after coronary bypass grafting (CABG).

12. Morris AD, [illegible] (1997) [illegible]
13. National Diabetes Data Group: [illegible]
14. [illegible]
15. [illegible]
16. Royal College of Physicians of London [illegible]
17. [illegible]
18. [illegible]

Author's address:
[illegible]

Influence of blood cardiolegia or crystalloid cardioplegia on serum glucose in diabetic or non-diabetic patients

W. Kallweit, J. Braun, L. Eckel

Clinic for Thoracic and Cardiovascular Surgery, Klinikum Karlsburg, Germany

An increased serum glucose level during cardiopulmonary bypass is due to a decreased utility of glucose by postaggression metabolism, hypothermia, and cardiac depression. Nevertheless, some cardioplegic solutions contain glucose to nutriate the ischemic myocardium. Some entremely high serum glucose levels by diabetic and non-diabetic patients under cardiopulmonary bypass and blood cardioplegia prompted us to investigate different cardioplegic solutions.

In 37 patients undergoing open heart surgery in conventional extracorporal circulation (ECC), cardioplegic arrest, and mild hypothermia, we measured the serum glucose levels at different times (pre-ECC, while cardioplegia was installed, post-ECC, arrival in ICU and 3, 4, 6, 12, 14 hours postoperatively)

We formed two groups: Group I with 10 diabetic patients and group II with 27 non-diabetic patients. Each group was divided and given St Thomas cardioplegia

Table 1. Group I (10 diabetic patients) and group II (27 non-diabetic patients) results

group I

non-diabetic	pre ECC	cardio-plegia	post ECC	ICU	3 h
STC	106	103	133	147	184
BCP	118	175	190	185	176
p	> 0.05	< 0.05	< 0.05	> 0.05	> 0.05
	4 h	6 h	12 h	14 h	
STC	184	190	170	150	
BCP	188	171	163	150	
p	> 0.05	> 0.05	> 0.05	> 0.05	

group II

non-diabetic	pre ECC	cardio-plegia	post ECC	ICU	3 h
STC	106	103	133	147	184
BCP	118	175	190	185	176
p	> 0.05	< 0.05	< 0.05	> 0.05	> 0.05
	4 h	6 h	12 h	14 h	
STC	184	190	170	150	
BCP	188	171	163	150	
p	> 0.05	> 0.05	> 0.05	> 0.05	

44. Rathke V, Schmitt DV, Walther T, Mohr FW (1997) Fast-track-intensive care after cardiovascular operations. Thorac Cardiovasc Surgeon 45, Suppl 1: 182
45. Searle N, Sahab P (1993) Propofol in patients with cardiac disease. Can J Anaesth 40: 730–747
46. DeSouza G, deLisser EA, Turry P, Gold MI (1995) Comparison of propofol with isoflurane for maintenance of anesthesia in patients with chronic obstructive pulmonary disease: Use of pulmonary mechanics, peak flow rates and blood gases. J Cardiothorac Vasc Anesth 9: 24–28
47. Stoelting RK, Dierdorf SF (1993) Anesthesia and co-existing disease. Third Edition; Churchill Livingstone, New York, Edinburgh, London, Madrid, Melbourne, Milan, Tokyo
48. Taylor GJ, Mikell FL, Moses HW, Dove JT, Katholi RE, Malik SA, Markwell SJ, Korsmeyer C, Schneider JA, Wellons HA (1990) Determinants of hospital charges for coronary artery bypass surgery: the economic consequences of postoperative complications. Am J Cardiol 65: 309–313
49. Westaby S, Pillai R, Parry A, O'Regan D, Giannopoulos N, Grebenik K, Sinclair M, Fisher A (1993) Does modern cardiac surgery requir late intensive care? Eur J Cardiothorac Surg 7: 313–318

Author's address:
Matthias Angrés, MD
Department of Anesthesiology and Intensive Care
Cottbus Heart Center
Thiemstr. 111
03048 Cottbus
Germany

Indications and results of combined heart and lung surgery

A. Hoffmeier, M. Semik, B. Asfour, T. D. T. Tjan, H. H. Scheld

Department of Cardiothoracic Surgery, Westphalian Wilhelms-University, Münster, Germany

Background

Little data exists proving that simultaneous open heart and lung surgery can be performed at low risk [1–8].

Patients

From 1/93 to 6/97 we performed open heart procedures with cardiopulmonary bypass and simultaneously lung surgery on 17 patients (mean age 64, range from 56–74). Twelve patients suffered from coronary artery disease (CAD), 5 patients had aortic valve disease (AVD). Pulmonary surgery was indicated in 15 patients due to suspected lung cancer, and in 2 patients with emphysematous lung disease. Twelve patients received CABG (11 patients with use of LITA). Five patients had aortic valve replacement (3 xenografts including 1 stentless, 2 artificial). In 12 patients a lung wedge-resection and in 5 patients a lobectomy with lymphadenectomy were performed. All procedures but one were performed by median sternotomy. One patient with pulmonary hypertension and aortic valve disease had a 3 stage surgery (1st exploratory thoracotomy, 2nd MIC-AVR, 3rd extended pneumectomy).

The cases of combined heart and lung surgery were compared to those with "single" heart surgery (n = 746) during a 6 month period.

Results

The perioperative course was mostly uneventful in 13 patients (76%); 2 patients developed pneumothoraces, 2 respiratory insufficiency, which were treated successfully. One patient died on POD 8 from biventricular heart failure (30 day mortality 5.8%). The mean hospital stay on ICU was 2.6 days, overall hospital stay was 16.2 days (Fig. 1). Mean postoperative assisted ventilation was necessary for 18.6 hours. Amount of blood loss was comparable to single cardiac procedures, patients required 1.6 packed cell units (mean). The mean duration of chest tube drainage was 4 days.

Table 1. Data for the 17 patients receiving cardiopulmonary bypass and simultaneous lung surgery

ID	Initials	Sex	Age	Diagnosis	Operation
1	B. H.	m	56	Lung tumor left upper lobe, CAD, AVD	Wedge resection, CABG (ACVB → RCA) and AVR (Baxter Stentless Bioprothesis 25 mm)
2	B. F.	m	70	Lung tumor left lower lobe, AVD	Lobectomy, Lymphadenectomy, AVR (Carpentier Edwards Bioprothesis 23 mm)
3	G. P.	m	74	Lung tumor left lower lobe, AVD	Wedge resection, CABG (LITA → LAD; ACVB → RMI and RIP)
4	G. A.	m	60	Lung tumor left upper lobe, AVD	Lobectomy, Lymphadenecotomy, AVR (Carpentier Edwards Bioprothesis 27 mm)
5	H. W.	m	58	Lung tumor left lower lobe, CAD	Wedge resection, CABG (LITA → LAD; ACVB → RMI and RDI)
6	I. R.	m	66	Lung tumor left upper lobe, CAD	Lobectomy, Lymphadenectomy, CABD (LITA → LAD)
7	K. H.	m	60	Emphysematous lung disease, CAD	Wedge resection, CABG (LITA → LAD; ACVB → RMI)
8	K. A.	m	60	Emphysematous lung disease, CAD	Wedge resection, CABG (LITA → LAD; ACVB → RD and RIP)
9	M. B.	m	73	Lung tumor right lower lobe, CAD	Wedge resection, CABG (LITA → LAD; ACVB → RMI and RCA)
10	N. W.	m	67	Lung tumor right lower lobe, CAD	Wedge resection, CABG (LITA → LAD; ACVB → RMI)
11	S. B.	m	64	Lung tumor right lower lobe, Oropharyngeal Ca 1989, CAD	Wedge resection, CABG (LITA → LAD, ACVB → RIP)
12	S. I.	f	69	Lung tumor left upper lobe, CAD	Wedge resection, CABG (LITA → LAD, Possis-Graft → LAD and RMI)
13	S. F.	m	65	Lung tumor left lower lobe, CAD	Wedge resection, CABG (LITA → LAD, ACVB → RCX)
14	W. J.	m	56	Lung tumor left lower lobe, CAD	Wedge resection, CABG (ACVB → LAD, RMI and RMII)
15	W. K.-H.	m	67	Lung tumor right upper lobe, CAD	Wedge resection, CABG (LITA → LAD; RD, RM and RIP)
16	W. A.	m	60	Lung tumor left lower lobe, AVD	Lobectomy, Lymphadenectomy, AVR (Tekna 23 mm)
17	K. H.	m	63	Lung tumor left lower lobe, AVD	3 stage surgery: 1st exploratory thoracotomy, 2nd MIC-AVR (Tekna 21 mm) 3rd extended pneumectomy

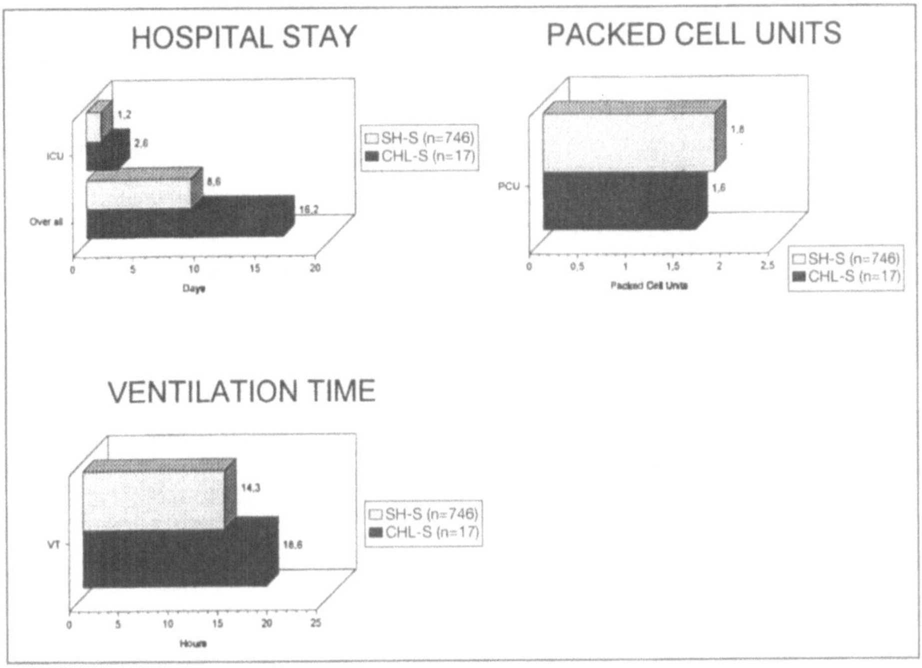

Fig. 1: The comparison between hospital stay, the use of packed cell units and ventilation time of combined heart and lung surgery (CHL-S) (n=17), and "single" heart surgery (SH-S) (n=746) are shown. The reason for longer hospital stay in combined surgery is our experience in special complications following lung surgery and, therefore, longer observation of these pts. compared to other departments of cardiology, who take care for postoperative follow-up and rehabilitation of our "single" cardiac pts.

Conclusion

In certain indications combined surgery for heart and lung diseases can be performed at low risk with acceptable perioperative morbidity and mortality. Combined cardiac and pulmonary surgery spares the patient the risk and cost of a second major surgical procedure.

References

1. Brutel de la Riviere A, Knaepen P, Van Swieten H, Venderschueren R, Ernst J, Van den Bosch J (1995) Concomitant open heart surgery and pulmonary resection for lung cancer. Eur J Cardiothorac Surg 9 (6): 310–13
2. Gillinov AM, Greene PS, Stuart RS, Heitmiller RF (1996) Cardiopulmonary bypass as an adjunct to pulmonary surgery. Chest 110 (2): 571–574
3. Irie T, Oonuki T, Kei J, Sone Y, Nitta S (1996) Peri- and postoperative courses in patients undergoing concomitant cardiac and pulmonary operations. Nippon Kyobu Geka Gakkai Zasshi 44 (6): 747–754

4. La Francesca S; Frazier OH, Radovancevic B, De Caro LF, Reul GJ, Cooley DA (1995) Concomitant cardiac and pulmonary operations for lung cancer: Tex Heart Inst J, 22 (4): 296–300.
5. Rao V, Todd TR, Weisel RD, Komeda M, Cohen G, Ikonomidis JS, Christakis GT (1996) Results of combined pulmonary resection and cardiac operation: Ann Thorac Surg 62 (2): 342–346
6. Terzi A, Furlan G, Magnanelli G, Conti F, Chiavacci P, Petrilli G, Ivic N (1994) Lung resections concomitant to coronary artery bypass grafting: Eur J Cardiothorac Surg, 8 (11): 580–584.
7. Ulicny KS Jr, Schmelzer V, Flege JB Jr, Todd JC, Mitts DL, Melvin DB, Wright CB (1992) Concomitant cardiac and pulmonary operation: the role of cardiopulmonary bypass: Ann Thorac Surg 54 (2): 289–295
8. Yokoyama T, Derrick MJ, Lee AW (1993) Cardiac operation with associated pulmonary resection: J Thorac Cardiovasc Surg, 105 (5): 912–916

Author's adress:
Andreas Hoffmeier, M.D.
Department of Cardiothoracic Surgery
Westphalian Wilhelms-University
Albert-Schweitzer-Str. 33
D-48149 Münster, Germany

Cardiac surgery and skeletal disorders

A. Schiessler and M. Angrés

Herzzentrum Cottbus, Cottbus, Germany

Introduction

Skeletal disorders in combination with cardiac lesions, requiring surgical correction, are quite a rare entity in surgical practice. There are a number of congenital systemic diseases which influence the developement of the skeleton as well as other tissues, resulting in increased problems if cardiac surgery is needed.

Chest wall malformations are the most important, especially in patients with disorders of the vertebral column and/or malformations of the sternum. These concomitant diseases can complicate the surgical treatment of cardiac lesions through a midsternal incision. There are also similiar problems with some aquired diseases which make it technically difficult to access the heart due to displacement of the heart, either in the left or right hemithorax.

The resulting problems render not only the surgical procedure but also anaesthesia and postoperative mobilization of the patient. Of course, in systemic diseases the difficulties may be increased by factors influencing the hemostatic system, the quality of the connecting tissue, and the wound healing.

In the following, experiences from literature research and from personal practice are presented.

Pathology of relevant concomitant diseases

The etiology of considerable malformations is in most cases due to *genetic systemic skeletal diseases.* They are predominantly inherited, whether connatal or with manifestation during the period of adolescent growth. The most important inheritable connective-tissue disorders are osteogenesis imperfecta and Marfan's Syndrome.

Osteogenesis imperfecta

Osteogenesis imperfecta is a heterogenous group of disorders of collagen biosynthesis characterized by osseus fragility and familial incidence. Osteogenesis imperfecta is divided into four categories. The severe form affects the fetus in utero or in early infancy and is associated with high early mortality. The "tarda"-types are compatible with long survival and even normal longevity. The major body systems affected are skeletal, ocular, auditory, integument, and teeth, and to a much lesser extent cardiovascular.

Cardiovascular manifestations in osteogenesis imperfecta are virtually similiar to those in Marfan's syndrome.

Cardiac operation in patients with osteogenesis imperfecta carries a high mortality rate. This is mainly due to bleeding, friability of the tissue, and impaired wound healing. There has been some speculation that patients with this disease may suffer from some platelet abnormalities, although there is no convincing evidence to this effect.

Marfan's syndrome

Marfan's syndrome is an autosomal dominant disorder of connective tissue associated with mutations in the fibrillin gene on chromosome 15 coding for fib 15-polypeptide. The fib 15 is the main element of the microfibrillar network of the extracellular matrix of connective tissue.

Cardiovascular, skeletal, and ocular abnormalities are linked with the fibrillin. Marfan's syndrome is characterized by large inter- and intrafamilial variation in clinical phenotypes. Cardiovascular complications account for 95% of the fatal complications in patients with the syndrome.

There are *aquired systemic disorders* like Rachitis, Osteomalacia, and Osteoporosis senilis or presenilis (M. Cushing) of interest in this context.

Rachitis and osteomalacia are similiar diseases. The developement of regular bone structure is not possible because of a lack of calciumapatite, which cannot be implanted in the osteoid. The main cause for that is seen in a D-avitaminosis, often in correlation with a malresorption of fat or protein-malnutrition. This results in an impaired resistance of the bone to stress. Often the patients present with scoliosis and kyphosis of the vertebral column.

Osteoporosis is clearly differentiated from these diseases, because there is a normal bone-tissue, but due to an imbalance in the metabolism it is becoming atrophic. The vertebrae are formed like a wedge due to the weight of the thoracal content, and a thoracal kyphosis results.

Inflammatory disorders

Ankylosing spondylarthritis (Bechterew's disease) is one form of rheumatic inflammation. The disease is characterized by ossification of the vertebral column. During the developement of the illness an increasing fixation of a kyphosis is observed. The patients often suffer from lung emphysema and cardiopulmonary insufficiency. Specific skeletal manifestations are listed below.

Malformation of the sternum

Pectus excavatum (Funnel chest, Trichterbrust)

This is a congenital deformity, most often sporadic, although familial incidence is common. This deformity tends to be progressive from birth. It is, in general, unassociated with other congenital lesions although it is one of the types of chest deformity that occurs in association with congenital cardiac deformities and is specifically associated with Marfan's disease.

There are two principal types, both affecting the costal cartilages. The second through eighth cartilages develop in a concave position, thus, forming a sternal depression which is maximal above the xyphoid appendix:

- a purely central defect with the manubrium in proper position, and the chest on each side well formed.
- a broader, more flatter deformity, which may even involve a depression of the manubrium. The cubic displacement of intrathoracic space is likely to be greater in this case and is in fact more significant physiologically.

The displacement of the heart is invariably to the left. The thoracic wall is the site of paradoxical movement. In most serious cases, compression of the right atrium or of the right ventricle by the sternum provokes disturbances in cardiopulmonary function.

Sternal fissure

There are three principal types of sternal fissure (14).

- In the superior sternal cleft skin covers the midline defect, and the pericardium, pleural envelopes, and diaphragm are intact. The heart is orthotopic.
- Complete clefts of the sternum are more complex defects. An associated anterior defect in the diaphragm and a wide diastasis recti are also present. This allows free communication between the pericardial and peritoneal cavities.
- The third type is a cleft in the distal sternum, which is part of Cantrell's pentalogy. This is a rare syndrome of omphalocele, deficiency of the anterior diaphragm, deficiency of the diaphragmatic portion of the pericardium with free communication between the pericardial and peritoneal cavities, and a congenital heart defect.

Malformation of the vertebral column

Scoliosis

There are multiple factors of etiology and pathogenesis resulting in a scoliosis. It is defined as a rotation and torsion of the vertebrae.The scoliosis is the result of primary or secondary asymmetric changes of the componing parts of the vertebral column, like the bones, the intervertebral disks, and the articulations.

In 90% of the patients with scoliosis an ideopathic genesis is assumed. The cause of its development is unknown. A specific pathogenesis is given in osteochondropathic, neuropathic, myopathic, and fibropathic forms of this disease.

Klippel-Feil-deformity is a congenital dysraphic disorder with scoliosis due to impaired coalescence of the mesenchymal vertebral construction.

Kyphosis

The bending of the vertebral column is in a dorsal convex curve. Connatal kyphosis is the result of maldevelopment (fission) of the vertebral bodies. Kyphosis is quite common in systemic diseases (chondrodystrophia, osteogenesis imperfecta) and can be acquired in rachitis, ankylosing spondylarthritis, and Scheuermann's disease. It is the most important affection of the juvenile spine (Scheuermann's disease), but very few patients have a symptomatic clinical course. It is probably a form of diskal disease with a constitutional predisposition. Kyphosis in ankylosing spondylarthritis (Bechterew's disease) is due to an inflammatory process in the small articulations of the vertebral bodies with final periarticular ossification. The patients present with severely impaired thoracic excursions.

Malformations of the chestwall

Thoracoplasty

Thoracoplasty is an iatrogenic malformation. In some elderly patients this obsolete procedure was undertaken for operative treatment of a pleural empyema in the early fifties. In these patients respiratory dysfunction is common. Dislocation of the mediastinum, heart, and great vessels is regular as well.

Special considerations in concomitant diseases

Anesthesiologic problems

If ever possible, a thorough assessment of the pulmonary function is recommended. In most of the thoracic deformations a restrictive element to ventilatory mechanics is detected. For this reason additional pulmonary problems should be ruled out.

Intubation is sometimes troublesome in patients with kyphosis and the head bent to the anterior chestwall. Personal experience in this case prooved the aid of a fiberoptic laryngoscope to be useful.

Postoperative the weaning from respirator is very delicate.

Various weaning techniques for those patients are used progressing through synchronized intermittent mandatory ventilation, continuous positive airway pressure ventilation, and nasal continuous positive airway pressure ventilation. The patient has to be fully awake and cooperative. Before extubation sufficient spontaneous breathing and mobilization of secretion is mandatory, because reintubation could be very difficult. Physiotherapy should be available at any time.

Central venous catheterization in patients with bent necks is very often impossible via the jugular veins. The approach of choise in these cases is via the subclavian vein.

Surgical problems

Before operating a patient with cardiac disease proper positioning of the patient's body on the operating table is problematic, if severe kyphosis is present. In this case the patient seems to be in a half-sitting position. Support of the spine with cushions and additional padding is necessary. The field of operation is reduced, since the head with the intratracheal tube is just above the manubrium. Special care has to be taken when performing a midline sternotomy. The cephalad extend of the incision should be sparing. Though division of the manubrium is possible in most cases.

In a few circumstances the approach to the heart is favorable through a lateral incision (3). Because the new minimally invasive techniques are rapidly becoming part of the cardiac surgical armamentarium, in selected cases indication for lateral thoracotomy may be preferred.

The institution of cardiopulmonary bypass using iliac vessel cannulation can avoid some difficulties in case of dislocation of the heart and great vessels.

In very rare instances, it may be necessary not only to perform cardiac surgery but also to correct the malformation in a combined approach (6, 8, 12, 13). This will not only help to improve the access to the heart, it will also avoid potential postoperative complications of cardiac compression (15, 21).

The underlying systemic diseases will influence decisions (11), since excessive bleeding, friability of the tissue, and problematic wound healing have to be appreciated.

Surgical management

The necessary cardiac correction and the dislocation of the heart are the keypoints in planning the interventional procedure.

Valvular operations, aortic surgery, or even heart- and heart-lung transplantations demand median sternotomy in general. Severe chest wall deformity is not a contraindication in heart-lung transplantation (16). Accomodation of the donor lung within the chest cavity occurs without difficulty so long as the donor total lung capacity is smaller than the predicted total lung capacity of the recipient.

In a patient with pectus excavatum coronary artery bypass grafting with the internal mammary artery is difficult or even impossible through a median sternotomy.

Coronary bypass procedures are facilitated through a left lateral thoracotomy when the heart is in the left hemithorax and the target vessels are anteroposterior because of the lesions not including the right coronary artery. Even harvesting of the internal thoracic artery is not a problem (3) like in minimally invasive procedures.

In our experience there are two patients with a chestwall deformity caused by thoracoplasty. One patient had a dislocation of the heart and great vessels to the right hemithorax. Cardiopulmonary bypass using standard aortic and atrial cannulation was not possible after median sternotomy. Also cannulation of the iliac vessels was impossible because of severe aorto-iliac occlusive disease. The displacement of the heart in the right hemithorax, provided an excellent exposure of the left ventricle. Bypass grafting with the use of the internal mammary artery was performed with the heart beating.

The other patient presented with dislocation of the heart in the left hemithorax after thoracoplasty. Despite of the displacement of the heart, exposure of the heart was satisfactory to perform "off pump"- bypass grafting with the use of the internal mammary artery. In this case severe impairment of renal function and a high Parsonnet (17) risk estimation score (>20) induced the decision to avoid cardiopulmonary bypass.

The Cottbus experience

Since June 1995, when the cardiac service in Cottbus, Germany, was opened, more than 2500 open heart operations have been performed. We report in this paper nine patients with severe concomitant skeletal disorders and where severe malformations of the chest made cardiac surgery and anesthesia more difficult.

Seven patients have been discharged with satisfactory clinical results. Two patients died on the third and fourth postoperative day. One patient (male, 74 years old) suffered from coronary heart disease and Bechterew's disease (Fig. 1). He died due to intractable pulmonary infection. Another patient with osteogenesis imperfecta (male, 35 years old) was operated under emergency circumstances because of acute infective mitral regurgitation and pulmonary edema (Fig. 2). In this case, a massive preoperative stroke due to septic embolism was the cause of death three days after surgery despite successful mitral valve replacement. At the time of surgery, the patient was deeply sedated and on respirator therapy. The patient had a history of bleeding complications in several orthopedic interventions (7, 9, 19, 20), but the use of cardiopulmonary bypass did not induce hemorrhagic complications.

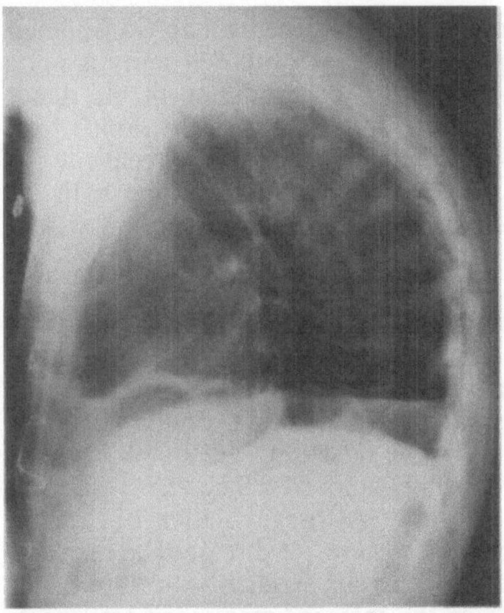

Fig 1. Preoperative chest roentgenogram of a 74 year old patient with Bechterew's disease and coronary lesions

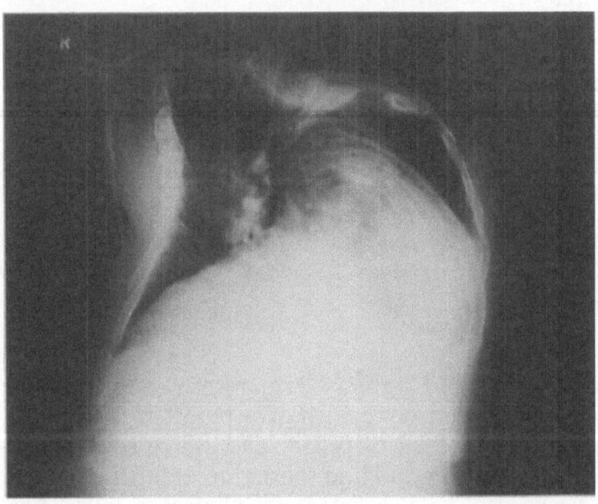

Fig. 2. Chest roentgenogram of a 35 year old patient with osteogenesis imperfecta and acute infective mitral insufficiency

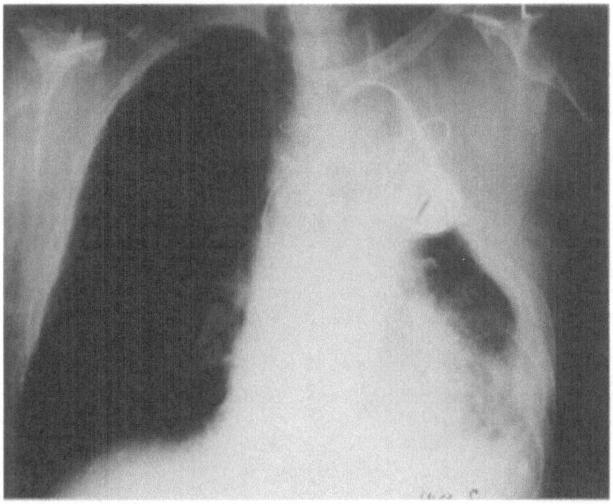

Fig. 3. Chest roentgenogram of a 71 year old patient with thoracoplasty on the left side

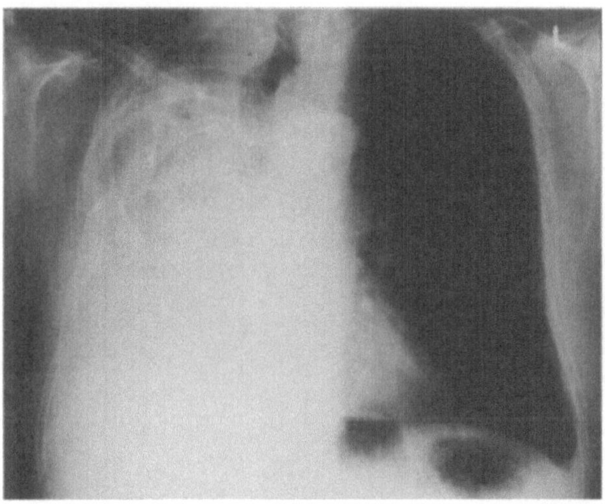

Fig. 4. Chest roentgenogram of a 73 year old patient with thoracoplasty on the right side

Two patients with dislocation of the heart due to thoracoplasty (Figs. 3 and 4) had coronary artery bypass procedures (beating heart without the aid of cardiopulmonary bypass). They have been weaned of the respirator and extubated early. In one of them a right-sided lobar pneumonia was diagnosed at the second postoperative day (Klebsiella pneumoniae). Antibiotic treatment was successful and the patient was discharged at postoperative day 20.

Three patients with severe kyphosis in Bechterew's disease had coronary bypass surgery with vein grafts and the use of the internal thoracic artery. The harvesting

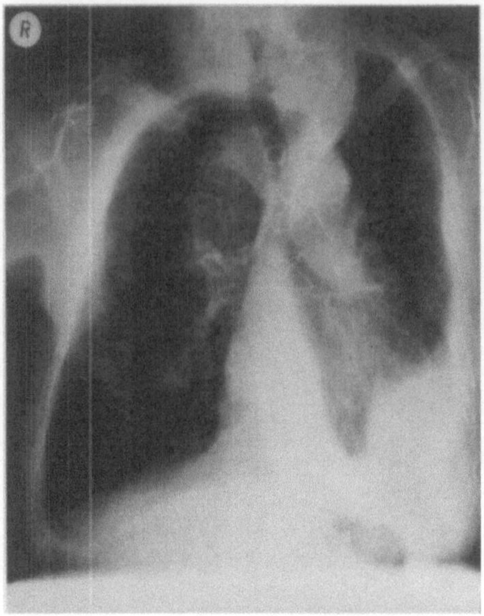

Fig. 5. Postoperative chest roentgenogram of a 67 year old patient with kyphoscoliosis

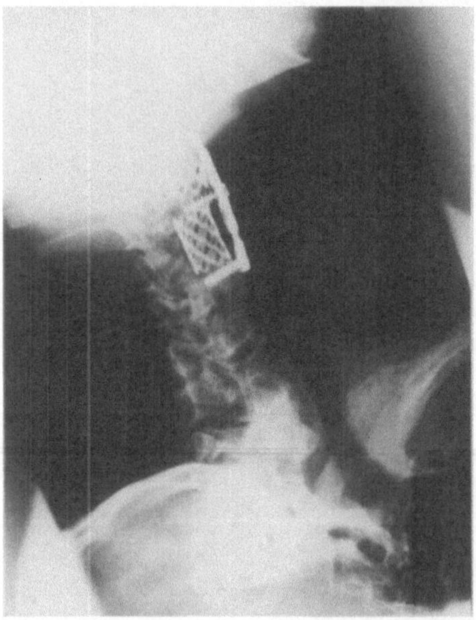

Fig. 6. Immobilization of the neck (spinal stenosis) in a 72 year old patient with aortic valve stenosis

of this vessel did not produce problems. The exposure of the mammary artery is impaired by the rigidity of the thorax. In these cases a Cleveland-IMA-retractor prooved to be very useful. One patient died in postoperative day 3. In this case, we experienced another but fatal septic complication of the respiratory system.

Two patients had coronary bypass surgery and aortic valve replacement. Kyphoscoliosis (Fig. 5) and immobilization of the neck due to spinal stenosis (Fig. 6) with operative stabilization did not negatively influence an uneventful postoperative recovery.

Conclusion

Concomitant skeletal malformations are a rare entity in cardiac surgery. In the literature most authors report on malformations in systemic disorders, like Marfan's disease (15). This is due to the well-known association of certain cardiovascular conditions with this connective tissue disease. The surgical treatment of cardiac diseases in osteogenesis imperfecta was not reported widely (10, 22). It is overshadowed by the bony, ocular, otologic, cutaneous, and dental manifestations of the disorder.

The scarcity of cases cited in the surgical literature may be attributed to the rarity of symptomatic cardiac manifestations in this heterogeneous patient population (1, 2, 4, 5, 18, 19, 22).

Surgical procedures performed in this group carry a higher risk of complications related to platelet dysfunction, friable tissue, impaired wound healing, and musculoskeletal weakness and deformity.

Surgery in all these patients suffering from concomitant diseases is technically more demanding, pre- and postoperative care affords a high adaptation to the patient's needs. Time and patience is required to allow an uneventful recovery.

Improved techniques in surgery, anesthesia, and intensive care give patients with cardiac and skeletal disorders a better chance to profit from surgical treatment.

References

1. Almassi GH, Hughes GR, Bartlett J (1995) Combined valve replacement and coronary bypass grafting in osteogenesis imperfecta. Ann Thorac Surg 60: 1395–1397
2. Ashraf SS, Shaukar N, Masood M, Lyons TJ, Keenan DJM (1993) Type I aortic dissection in a patient with osteogenesis imperfecta. Eur J Cardio-thorac Surg 7: 665–666
3. Choghari C, Heymans O, Geens M, Joris M (1996) Left thoracotomy for coronary bypass in a patient with pectus excavatum. Ann Thorac Surg 62: 1182–1183
4. Criscitiello MG, Ronan JAJ, Bestermann EMM, Schoenwetter W (1965) Cardiovaccular abnormalities in osteogenesis imperfecta. Circulation 31: 255–262
5. Cusimano RJ (1996) Repeat cardiac operation in a patient with osteogenesis imperfecta. Ann Thorac Surg 61 (4): 1294
6. DeLeon MM, Magliato KE, Roughneen PT, Graham L, Kudukis TM, DeLeon SY (1997) Simultaneuos repair of pectus excavatum and congenital heart disease. Ann Thorac Surg 64: 557–559
7. Estes JW (1968) Platelet size and function in the heritable disorders of connective tissue. Ann Intern Med 68: 1237–1249
8. Gould WL, Jett GK, Bostwick J, Jones EL, Mansour KA (1988) Simultaneous repair of severe pectus excavatum and aortic valve replacement following previous open-heart surgery. Ann Thorac Surg 45: 82–84
9. Hathaway WE, Solomons CC, Ott JE (1972) Platelet function and pyrophosphates in osteogenesis imperfecta. Blood 39: 500–509
10. Hortop J, Tsipouras P, Hanley JA, Maron BJ, Shapiro JR (1986) Cardiovascular involvement in osteogenesis imperfecta. Circulation 73: 54–61
11. Jones WG, Hoffman L, Devereux RB, Isom OW, Gold JP (1994) Staged approach to combined repair of pectus excavatum and lesions of the heart. Ann Thorac Surg 57: 212–214
12. Kalangos A, Delay D, Mutith N, Pretre R, Bruschweiler I, Faidutti B (1995) Correction of pectus excavatum combined with open heart surgery in a patient with Marfan's syndrome. Thorac cardiovasc Surgeon 43: 220–222
13. Laborde F, Redonnet M, Hubscher C, Touchot B, Greze M, Letac B, Soyer R (1979) Considerations about one stage surgical treatment of pectus excavatum, aortic dissection and aortic incompetence in a patient with Marfan's syndrome. Ann Chir 33: 183–187

14. Landolfo KP, Sabiston DC (1995) Disorders of the sternum and thoracic wall. In: S.F. Sabiston DC Jr (eds) Surgery of the Chest. Saunders Philadelphia, pp 494–515
15. Miller D, Pugh DM (1970) Repair of ascending aortic aneurysm and aortic regurgitation complicated by acute cardiac compression by pectus excavatum in Marfan's syndrome. J Thorac Cardiovasc Surg 59: 678–684
16. Parry AJ, O'Fiesh J, Wallwork J, Large SR (1994) Heart-lung transplantation in situs inversus and chest wall deformity. Ann Thorac Surg 58: 1174–1176
17. Parsonnet V, Dean D, Bernstein AD (1989) A method of uniform stratification of risk for evaluating the results of surgery in acquired adult heart disease. Circulation, 79 (suppl) (I-3-I-12)
18. Passmore JM, Walker WE, Fuentes F (1987) Successful aortocoronary bypass in osteogenesis imperfecta. J Am Coll Cardiol 9: 960–963
19. Reguillo F, De La Llana R, Castanon J, Alswies M, Trujillo J, Rodriguez G, Ramos W, O'Connor F (1996) Osteogenesis imperfecta and coronary artery surgery. A case report. J Cardiovasc Surg 37 (6): 621–622
20. Siegel BM, Friedman IA, Schwartz SO (1957) Hemorrhagic disease in osteogenesis imperfecta: study of platelet functional defect. Am J Med 22: 315–321
21. Tschirkov A, Natschev G, Mishev B, Savova A, Ovanessjan H (1989) An easy and safe approach for simultaneous repair of severe pectus excavatum and the underlying lesions of the heart and thoracic aorta. J Thorac Cardiovasc Surg 98: 305–307
22. Wong RS, Follis FM, Shively BK, Wernly JA (1995) Osteogenesis imperfecta and cardiovascular diseases. Ann Thorac Surg 60: 1439–1443

Author's address
Arnulf Schiessler MD, PhD
Leibnizstr. 44
10629 Berlin

Cardiac surgery and dental problems

A. Schmidt-Westhausen and P. A. Reichart

Dept. of Oral Surgery and Dental Radiology, Center for Dental Medicine, Charité Campus Virchow-Klinikum, Humboldt University Berlin, Germany

Introduction

The oral cavity is a significant site for ingress of microorganisms. About 10^7-10^8 microorganisms are harbored in one milliliter of saliva. The ratio between anaerobic and aerobic bacteria is approximately 30 : 1 (Table 1).

Concerning the complexity between cardiac surgery and oral problems, the number and severity of oral problems is increased due to immunosuppressive therapy in operations which are rarely performed (i.e., cardiac transplantations), whereas routinely performed surgical treatments such as coronary artery bypass grafts only lead to minor oral problems (nifedipin-induced gingival hyperplasia due to medication with antihypertensive agents).

There are several important aspects of dental and oral diseases; the two most common diseases to affect humans are dental caries and periodontal disease. It is not unusual for either disease to progress considerably before a patient experiences any symptoms.

Dental caries produced by the formation of acids and of proteolytic enzymes can lead to the destruction and necrosis of the dental pulp. Subsequently, an abscess or inflammatory foci within the alveolar bone and at the apex of a tooth can develop. Generally, such areas are not self-healing and remain chronic. Dental granulomas are frequently discovered during routine radiographic evaluations of the jaw. The dental granuloma may remain dormant for many years, but always retains the potential for developing into an acute abscess. These latent chronic infections may

Table 1. Microorganisms harbored in the oral cavity

aerobic	anaerobic	transient colonizers
Streptococci (mutans, salivarius, viridans), Lactobacteria, Neisseria, Haemophilus spp., Eikenella corodens, Micrococci, Staphylococci, Corynebacteria, Campylobacter sputorum	Bacteroides, Fusobacteria, Leptotrichia, Selenomonas, Treponema, Wolinella, Veillonella, Actinomyces, Arachnia, Bifidobacteria, Corynebacterium, Eubacterium, Lactobacillus, Propionibacterium, Rothia, Peptococcaceae	Candida spp., Enterobacteriaceae, nonpathogenic Protozoa

exacerbate during immunosuppressive therapy, and therefore it is most important that all such chronic infections be detected and treated before cardiac transplantation is performed. As a result of dental caries the dental pulp necrotizes and the tissue then produces the chronic bone-destroying inflammatory response seen at the apex of a tooth. This area of infection can either be treated by root canal therapy combined with root resection or by extraction of the tooth. The important fact to point out is that this inflammatory lesion is often discovered by chance during the course of a routine radiographic examination and the patient has no symptoms of dental disease.

Nearly every adult suffers from some form of periodontal disease. The periodontal ligament supporting a tooth is gradually destroyed and deep pockets develop, lined by chronically inflamed gingiva. These pockets may develop insidiously, without causing discomfort to the patient and yet they represent a significant foci of inflamed mucosa. This widespread periodontal disease may be a continuing source of chronic infection.

Groups at risk for infective endocarditis

In 1903 Glynn first suggested that "it is likely that microorganisms may gain an entrance into the circulation through the mouth when there is a gingivitis or stomatitis" (3). Until now the link between endocarditis and dental disease remains a serious concern. Antimicrobial prophylaxis has become a mainstay of prevention although optimum dental care and prudent treatment planning might also be potent factors of prevention. It is generally agreed that the dentist should try to identify those patients particularely susceptible to infective endocarditis. If there is any doubt, it makes sense to arrange a cardiology consultation and in the meantime carry out only urgent treatment with all precautions. The decision on prophylaxis and dental treatment planning should be arrived at following discussion involving all the parties concerned and not dedicated by one of them (6).

Patients at risk are mainly those with rheumatic carditis, congenital heart disease, and prosthetic cardiac valves. The Deutsche Gesellschaft für Kardiologie and the

Table 2. Antibiotic guidelines prior to dental treatment (Deutsche Gesellschaft für Kardiologie and the Paul-Ehrlich-Gesellschaft)

patients	antibiotics (1st choice)	antibiotics (2nd choice)
adults	penicillin 2 mio IU or Amoxicillin 2-3 mg 1 h prior to treatment	clindamycin 600 mg 1 h prior to treatment
children	penicillin 50.000 IU/ kg BW or amoxicillin 50 mg/kg BW 1 h prior to treatment	clindamycin 15 mg /kg BW 1 h prior to treatment

Paul-Ehrlich-Gesellschaft have recommended an antibiotic protocol which must be used prior to dental treatment in these patients (Table 2). Additionally, rinsing or irrigation with an antimicrobial agent containing chlorhexidine is also recommended to reduce the number of colony forming units directly before treating a patient.

Individuals with cardiac valves not only remain at risk but may develop a rapidly destructive and deadly form of endocarditis. Any dental treatment which may cause oral bleeding (tooth extraction, subgingival scaling, surgery involving the gingival margin) requires premedication. It is not possible to treat these patients with antibiotics continuously, so excellent oral hygiene and dental prophylaxis in these patients is mandatory. Patients with prosthetic valves are often therapeutically anticoagulated. When planning procedures likely to cause bleeding, the physician is requested to adjust the dosage necessary to keep the prothrombin time within the safety level. Adjustments may need to be initiated 2 to 3 days prior to the procedure.

Patients with pacemakers

Concerning pacemakers, modern bipolar devices present only few problems for dental treatment. However, patients with older pacemakers are at risk from interference if ultrasonic scalers for plaque and tartar removal are used. The European Pacemaker Patient Identification Card carried by the patient warns against exposure to ionizing radiation; however if the x-ray tube is correctly positioned the radiation dose from the dental sets is most unlikely to cause any problems.

Heart transplantation

Every prospective cardiac transplant patient should have an oral assessment as part of the standard evaluation protocol. One of the consultations required in the protocol is a dental evaluation.

The dentist should follow a standard protocol in order to be certain that there is no dental infection or any suggestion of possible future infections. This protocol includes

- Review of the patients record and medical history

It is most important that the examining dentist reviews the medical record before treatment. Particular attention must be paid to the cardiac status of the patient, as it might indicate a need for subacute bacterial endocarditis prophylaxis. In these cases consultation with the patient's medical advisor is necessary.

- Oral examination for identification of any soft tissue disease
- Radiographic examination

A panoramic film is recommended for it demonstrates many anatomic structures in addition to teeth (maxillary sinuses, translucencies and opacities in the alveolar bone)

- Dental status
  - Periodontal examination
  - Dental caries examination
- Prosthetic appliance examination

The long term prognosis of each appliance (bridges, crowns, dentures) must be considered. Dentures for instance can provide an ideal environment for bacterial and fungal growth. All transplant candidates should be given instruction in proper care and hygiene of their protheses.

Recommendations concerning the dental status and proposed treatment in patients with cardiac transplantation is divided into three categories (4). The first category includes active infections or situations that, if untreated, might be expected to result in an acute infection within the succeeding 6 months. All dental extractions and restorative work involving teeth with large carious cavities are classified in this category.

The second category includes all situations that if untreated might be expected to result in an acute infection in the succeeding 6 months to 1 year. Also included in this category are patients with active gingivitis or periodontitis.

The third category includes any dental condition not likely to reach an acute stage for at least 12 months as the construction of dentures and other elective procedures.

Concerning oral-surgical interventions in heart transplant patients a study by Schmelzeisen et al. (11) showed that only 2.5% complications after local treatment occurred in interventions which were performed prior to heart transplantation. In the group of patients where oral surgery was performed after organ transplantation, all 123 procedures were free from complications. Comparing these data with the complication rate of 3.2% in immunocompetent patients cited in the literature (7), these results indicate that post-oral surgery complications such as delayed wound healing are rare events in the management of patients prior to or after heart transplantation, and there appears to be no need for routine antibiotic prophylaxis during dental extractions in these patients.

In co-operation with Berlin transplant centers we have taken an approach to dental rehabilitation that is rather conservative, provided that the patient's oral hygiene is excellent. Completely impacted teeth are left in place. To avoid tooth extractions, root canal fillings and root resections are performed in selected patients prior to heart transplantation (14).

Oral manifestations in heart transplant patients

Immunosuppressed organ transplant recipients are more susceptible to oral infections, especially those of either fungal or viral origin (Table 3). Immunosuppressive

Table 3. Oral manifestations in heart transplant patients

1. Fungal infections
candidiasis, aspergillosis, mucormycosis, cryptococcosis
2. Viral infections
Herpes simplex Virus, Epstein Barr Virus, Cytomegalovirus, Human Papillomavirus
3. Malignancies
Lymphoproliferative disorders, Kaposi's sarcoma, squamous cell carcinoma
4. drug-induced lesions
azathioprine-induced ulcers, cyclosporin-induced gingival hyperplasia

agents may mask early manifestations of oral infection, or feature atypical presentations of common lesions such as recurrent oral herpes simplex, candidiasis or aspergillosis. Even unusual fungal infections such as cryptococcosis or mucormycosis, which lead to severe disseminated disease may occur. Viral infections are also common, mainly with human cytomegalovirus, herpes simplex virus, Epstein-Barr virus, and human papillomaviruses. An evaluation by cytological examination, culture, and/or biopsy is mandatory.

Candidiasis remains the most frequent fungal infection in these patients. The incidence seems to be dependent upon the patient's immunosuppressive regimen. Those medicated with a combination of azathioprine, cyclosporin, and prednisolone have significant higher incidence of candidiasis than those on either azathioprine and prednisolone or cyclosporin and prednisolone (5). A variant of candidiasis other than the pseudomembranous type (trush) is the erythematous type which may be overlooked during superficial oral examination (Fig. 1). The median rhomboid glossitis also represents a variant of erythematous candidiasis. It is located on the dorsal tongue and the lesion is associated with the loss of filiform papillae (Fig. 2). The erythematous type of oral candidiasis usually presents without disturbing symptoms.

Patients suffering from oral candidiasis are treated with topical antifungal agents, for instance nystatin pastilles or miconazole oral gel. For recurrent infections and those that appear resistant to topical antifungals, systemic fluconazole is the drug of choice. In patients treated with fluconazole and cyclosporine, the plasma cyclosporine concentration has to be monitored because there is an increased risk of nephrotoxicity. Early detection of Candida spp. and the early treatment of candidiasis is recommended. This can be facilitated by regular oral screening of heart transplant patients.

Hairy leukoplakia was first described in 1984 and appeared to be associated with HIV infection. Subsequently, case reports and reviews have now confirmed that the lesion occurs in organ transplant or other chronically immunosuppressed patients. Hairy leukoplakia is associated with the presence of the Epstein-Barr-Virus. In 1990, the first case of hairy leukoplakia in a heart transplant recipient

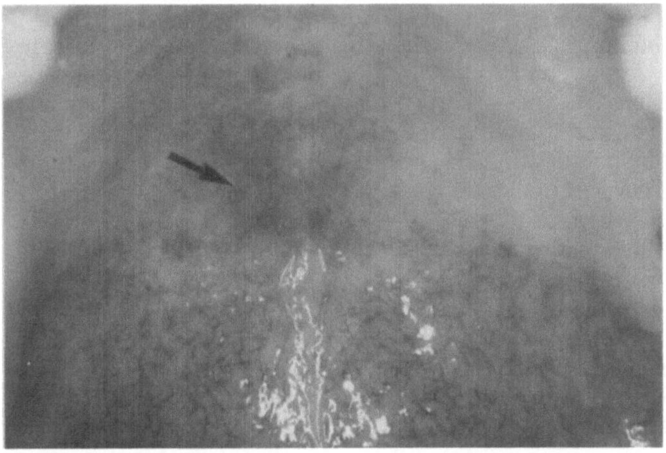

Fig. 1. Erythematous candidiasis on the palate of a patient treated with a combination of azathioprine, cyclosporin, and prednisolone

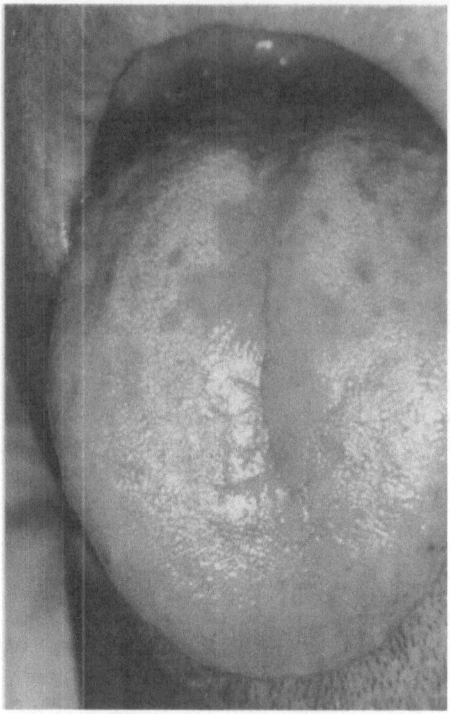

Fig. 2. Rhomboid glossitis due to infection with Candida albicans. This variant of erythematous candidiasis is associated with the loss of filiform papillae

was described (13). Immunohistochemically, EBV capsid antigen was detected. The lesion is symptom-free or can go into "remission". In another study fifty heart transplant patients treated at the Deutsche Herzzentrum Berlin were orally examined, 4% showed clinical signs of hairy leukoplakia, while EBV could be recovered by electron microscopy in 20% of the scrape material from the lateral border of the tongue (12).

Infections related to the herpes simplex virus (HSV) are also common in transplant patients. Clinically primary and recurrent HSV infections of the oral mucosa are characterized by clustered vesicles on an erythematous background. Typically, the vesicles on mucosal surfaces rapidly erode and leave an ulcerated area. HSV lesions can present as white plaques that closely resemble chronic pseudomembranous candidiasis. This emphazises the importance of biopsy of such lesions in order to ascertain the diagnosis. Mucosal ulceration is sometimes associated with Cytomegalovirus. The gastro-intestinal tract is a common site for such ulcerations, but the oral cavity can also be involved.

It is well recognized that immunosuppressed organ transplant patients are more susceptible to malignant neoplasms with the mouth and associated structures being an important "target area". Longitudinal studies have shown an increased incidence of lymphomas, skin and lip cancer, and Kaposi's sarcoma (1, 9, 10) This emphasizes the need for regular screening of all transplant patients by appropriately trained personnel.

Immunosuppressive drugs such as azathioprine may cause painful erosive oral lesions. However, they may present as oral manifestations of acute or chronic graft versus host disease (Fig. 3).

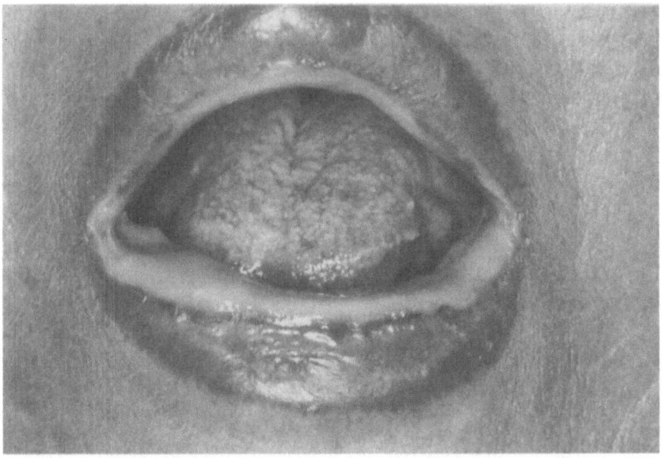

Fig. 3. Painful, erosive oral lesions on the lips of a female heart transplant patient. The tentative diagnosis was graft vs host disease

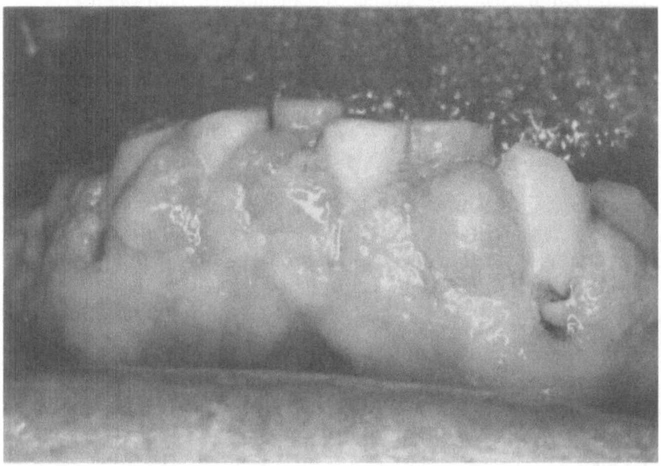

Fig. 4. Cyclosporin-induced gingival hyperplasia on the labial side of the mucosa (lower jaw)

Long-term administration of both cyclosporin and calcium channel blockers is associated with gingival hyperplasia (Fig. 4). Up to 70% of dentate patients medicated with cyclosporin experience mild gingival hyperplasia. Thus, it is quite likely that transplant patients with gingival symptoms will be seen by dentist. Hyperplasia occurs within 3 months of treatment and the labial mucosa appears to be a predilection side (15). Age is also an important determinant since children are more susceptible than adults. Approximately 30% of cyclosporin-treated patients are likely to develop significant gingival overgrowth that requires surgical correction. Approximately half of these will undergo repeated gingival surgery because of recurrence of hyperplasia (2).

Another complication associated with the use of cyclosporin and other immunosuppressants is an increased incidence of malignancies. Long-term use of cyclosporine also is associated with a spectrum of hyperproliferative disorders ranging from reactive lymphoid hyperplasia to aggressive malignant lymphomas. Cyclosporin-related lymphoproliferative disorders have been widely reported and even a case of an oral presentation as the first manifestation of this disease was recently described (8). Posttransplant lymphoproliferative disorders may occur months or even years after organ transplantation, so it may be seen first in institutions that are not involved in transplantation. It is essential that the lymphoproliferative syndrome be recognized early and treated, as many cases can be cured, without accurate diagnosis and prompt treatment it is rapidly fatal.

References

1. Birkeland SA (1983) Cancers in transplanted patients- the Scandia-transplant material. Transplant Proc 15: 1071
2. Daley TD, Wysocki GP, May C (1986) Clinical and pharmacological correlations in cyclosporin-induced gingival hyperplasia. Oral Surg Oral Med Oral Pathol 62: 417–21
3. Glynn TR (1903) Infective endocarditis mainly in its clinical aspects. Lancet 1: 1007–10
4. Golder GT, Drinnan AJ (1993) Dental aspects of cardiac transplantation. Transplant Proc 25: 2377–80
5. Gupta KL, Ghosh AK, Kochmar R et al. (1994) Esophagal candidiasis after renal transplantation: comparative study on different immunosuppressive protocols. Am J Gastroenterology 89: 1062–5
6. McGowan D (1995) Infective endocarditis. In: Porter SR, Scully C (eds) Oral Health Care for those with HIV Infection and Other Special Needs. Science Reviews Lonsdale Press Limited, London, pp 117–125
7. MacGregor AJ (1968) Aetiology of dry socket: A clinical investigation. Br J Oral Surg 6: 49-52
8. Oda D, Persson GR, Haigh WG, Sabath DE, Penn I, Aziz S (1996) Oral presentation of posttransplantation lymphoproliferative disordes. Transplantation 61: 435–40
9. Penn I (1987) Cancers following cyclosporin therapy. Transplantation 43: 32–5
10. Qunibi WY, Akmtar M, Ginn E, Smith P (1988) Kaposi's sarcoma in cyclosporin-induced gingival hyperplasia. Am J Kidney Dis 11: 349–52
11. Schmelzeisen R, Eckhardt A, Knoll M, Girod S (1991) Zahnärztlich-chirurgische Besonderheiten bei Patienten mit Organtransplantationen. Dtsch Z Mund Kiefer Gesichts Chir 15, 431–4
12. Schmidt-Westhausen A, Gelderblom HR, Hetzer R, Reichart PA (1991) Demonstration of Epstein-Barr virus in scrape material of lateral border of tongue in heart transplant patients by negative staining electron microscopy J Oral Pathol Med 20: 215
13. Schmidt-Westhausen A, Gelderblom HR, Reichart PA (1990) Oral hairy leukoplakia in an HIV-seronegative heart transplant patient J Oral Pathol Med 19: 192
14. Sonner S, Neuhaus R, Schräder S, Becker J, Reichart PA (1996) Zahnärztlich-chirurgische Sanierung von 320 Lebertransplantatpatienten. Dtsch Zahnärztl Z 51: 794–796
15. Thomason JM, Kelly PJ, Seymour RA (1996) The distribution of gingival overgrowth in organ transplant patients. J Clin Periodontol 23: 367–71

Author's adress:
A. Schmidt-Westhausen
Dept. for Oral Surgery and Dental Radiology
Center of Dental Medicine, Charité Campus Virchow-Klinikum
Humboldt University Berlin
Föhrer Str. 15
13353 Berlin, Germany

Dental problems in cardiac surgery

A. Böning[1], A. Bremerich[2], N. C. Gellrich[2], A. M. Laczkovics[1], E. Machtens[2]

Ruhr-Universität Bochum, [1]Klinik für Herz- und Thoraxchirurgie, Bergmannsheil Bochum, Universitätsklinik, [2]Klinik für Mund-, Kiefer- und Gesichtschirurgie, Knappschaftskrankenhaus Bochum, Universitätsklinik, Bochum, Germany

Abstract

To investigate the frequency of dental problems before cardiac operations, 102 patients admitted for valve replacement or aortocoronary bypass graft (CABG) procedures were preoperatively examined at the Department of Oral and Maxillo-Facial Surgery at the Ruhr-University Bochum. Only in 21% of the patients was the dental status good. Examples of dental pathology, such as parodontitis, cysts, and caries were found in 61% of the patients; in 18%, evidence of superficial parodontitis or mild forms of caries were seen.

These results show, that a search for dental foci before cardiac surgery is not considered as necessary by general practitioners.

Despite this trend, we conclude that – especially in valve replacement patients – a preoperative evaluation and subsequent therapy of dental diseases should be carried out because of the high risk and mortality of prosthetic valve endocarditis and because of problems concerning the necessity of postoperative anticoagulation.

Introduction

The spectrum of adult cardiac surgery in Germany in 1996 included CABG procedures (70%), valve procedures (25%), transplantations (1%), and other procedures (4%).

Preoperative evaluation for dental problems as a potential infectious focus is routine before heart transplantation. At the beginning of this investigation we asked the question: should patients undergoing other cardiac procedures be evaluated for dental pathology as a potential source of infection?

We divided this question into two parts:

- What is the frequency of dental problems in our cardiac patients?
- What is the role of preoperative therapy in such patients?

Material and methods

To investigate the frequency of dental problems before cardiac operations, 102 patients admitted for valve replacement or aortocoronary bypass graft procedures

Table 1. Dental diseases in cardiac patients

Patients (%)	Dental Pathology	Infectious focus	
22	None	no	
15	Superficial parodontitis		no
2	slightly carietic teeth	no	
26	Parodontitis Marginalis profunda	yes	yes
16	Parodontits Apicalis		
12	Cysts, root rests		yes
7	Destroyed carietic teeth		yes

were preoperatively examined at the department of Oral and Maxillo-Facial Surgery at the Ruhr-University Bochum.

Results

For cardiac surgeons surprisingly, we found that many patients with potential dental infectious foci were admitted to the hospital for cardiac surgery.

Discussion

The incidence of infectious endocarditis in the USA is 1/100,000 per year (2) and in Great Britain is 23–25/1,000,000 per year (5). The mortality of endocarditis of a native heart valve is 10–20% (5).

Dental pathology as a source for infectious endocarditis was found in 24% (3) or 25% (5) of patients undergoing valve replacement. Even more serious is the natural history of endocarditis after heart valve procedures (prosthetic endocarditis): the incidence of endocarditis after heart valve replacement is between 1.8 and 5.7%, and the mortality is 32 to 53% (1, 4). In addition to the high risk of prosthetic endocarditis, patients with mechanical heart valve prostheses are in need of long-term postoperative anticoagulation therapy. The danger of thromboembolic complications in addition to perioperative bleeding after stopping warfarin therapy for dental surgery adds additional risks to the patient.

IN CABG patients, there is no higher risk for endocarditis and no need for a postoperative warfarin – therapy.

Conclusions

We draw the following conclusions:

- The preoperative dental evaluation before valve surgery makes sense, because 61% of the cardiac patients suffer from dental diseases.

- The preoperative dental evaluation of patients undergoing prosthetic valve procedures is necessary to decrease the incidence of prosthetic endocarditis and postoperative complications from anticoagulation therapy.

References

1. Calderwood SB, Swinski LA, Waternaux CM, Karchmer AW, Buckley MJ (1985) Risk factors for the development of prosthetic valve endocarditis. Circulation 72: 31–37
2. Greenman RL, Bisno AL (1992) Prevention of bacterial endocarditis. In: Kaye D. (ed) Infective Endocarditis, 2nd ed. Raven Press, New York pp 171–175
3. Janatuinen MJ, Vänttinen EA, Rantakokko V, Nikoskelainen J, Inberg MV (1990) Prosthetic valve endocarditis. Scand J Cardiovasc Surg 25: 127–132
4. Sett SS, Hudon MPJ, Jamieson WRE, Chow AW (1993) Prosthetic valve endocarditis. J Thorac Cardiovasc Surg 105: 428–434
5. Skehan JD, Murray M, Mills PG (1988) Infective endocarditis: incidence and mortality in the North East Thames Region. Br Heart J 59: 62–68

Author's address:
Andreas Böning, M.D.
Klinik für Thorax- Herz- und Gefäßchirurgie
Med. Hochschule Hannover
30623 Hannover, Germany

Cardiac surgery and hematological disease

M. Barthels

Division of Hematology and Oncology Medical School Hannover, Germany

Introduction

It is not frequently observed that a patient with a hematological disease is in need of cardiac surgery in as far as hematological diseases are understood as disorders of the blood cells and the bone marrow. More often cardiac surgery is combined with a disorder of the coagulation system either already present or due to cardiac surgery and cardiopulmonary bypass.

Blood cell disorders

Most times the blood cell disorders will be malignant diseases:
- myeloproliferative syndromes, e.g., leucemias, polycythemia vera, essential thrombocythemia
- monoclonal gammopathies.

But also congenital defects may induce special problems like
- the mediterranean hemoglobinopathies,
- siccle cell anemia, and
- paroxysmal nocturnal hemoglobinuria.

These hematological diseases may influence cardiac diseases by reducing the blood flow, e.g., the hyperviscosity syndrome in monoclonal gammopathies or the high red cell volume in polcythemia vera leading to microcirculatory disturbances. Hematological diseases may complicate the outcome of any cardiac disease or cardiopulmonary bypass by the additional reduced immune status frequently observed. Last but not least, many of these diseases, like promyelocytic leucemia, thrombocythemia or siccle cell anemias, are often combined with chronic DIC or a higher incidence of thrombohemorrhagic complications, which could be an additional risk factor in cardiopulmonary bypass situations (9).

Coagulation disorders

Most patients with a coagulation disorder, who may undergo cardiac surgery, are those with an imbalance on the thrombophilic side of the coagulation system either due to a genetic defect or due to acquired thrombophilia. Congenital or acquired bleeding disorders are less frequent.

Thrombophilia

Thrombophilia research is a rather young branch of the medical sciences. Thrombophilia can be defined as a disposition which leads to a higher risk of mainly venous thromboembolic complications with the risk factor to be found in the coagulation or fibrinolytic system (12).

Congenital Thrombophilia

Today we know that in about 60–80% of all patients with a thromboembolic event before age 40 a genetic defect can be found which may contribute to venous thromboembolism (for reviews see 10, 11). Acknowledged risk factors for congenital thrombophilia are listed in Table 1. The most frequent genetic defect in the coagulation system leading to thrombophilia is a point mutation in clotting factor V (G1691A), called factor V Leiden. The altered clotting factor V in its activated form is no longer recognized by activated protein C (APC resistance) and is therefore not inactivated. Factor V Leiden occurs in the heterozygous form in 3–7% of the normal western population. These data show that the factor V mutation alone is a rather weak risk factor. But combined with other risk factors, e.g., oral contraceptives or surgery the risk for thromboembolic complications increases (4). Another rather low risk factor is the point mutation, factor II Leiden (G20210A) which is found in 1–2% of the general population (15). A risk factor not belonging to the coaguloation system is the homozygous C 677 T mutation of the MTHFR gene (methylenetetra-hydrofolate reductase). This mutation is extremely common in the general population (12% homozygous and about 40% heterozygous). It leads to impaired methionine synthesis, sometimes decreased plasma folate, and hyperhomocysteinemia. Hyperhomocysteinemia has been reported to be mainly associated with cardiovascular diseases and less with venous thromboembolism (14). In contrast to these three genetic defects, the well known congenital deficiencies or dysproteinemias of the physiological coagulation inhibitors: antithrombin, protein C or protein S occur very seldom. While the heterozygous form of factor V Leiden, factor II Leiden in both forms, protein S-deficiency and subnormal protein C-deficiency are rather low risk factors for thromboembolic complications, homozygous factor V Leiden, antithrombin deficiency and especially combined genetic defects like factor V Leiden combined with protein S deficiency are high risk factors. On the whole it seems that statistically every 10th patient undergoing cardiac surgery is supposed to have an imbalance of the clotting mechanism toward higher clottability. Whatever this means, either a higher risk for thromboembolism or a lesser danger for bleeding problems the hemostatic situation in cardiopulmonary bypass calls for a new evaluation. It is generally agreed that before surgery a routine diagnostic screening of each patient is not thought necessary. A careful case history may reveal former thromboembolic events in the patient or his family. Thromboembolic events occuring at an early age or at unusual sites, e.g., mesenteric vein thrombosis will point to higher risks. A special treatment or prophylaxis for these higher risk patients is not possible at this time as special clotting factor concentrates are not available except in the rare cases of congenital antithrombin deficiency. Some patients may need an anticoagulant prophylaxis especially adapted, e.g., to body weight and dosage if possible in higher concentrations than usual, and controlled by coagulation tests. In special cases there could be an indication for the use of the recently introduced recombinant thrombin inhibitor hirudin.

Table 1. Congenital thrombophilias

defect in:	Form	thromboembolic risk	prevalence in general population	prevalence in pat. with ven. thromboembolism
Antithrombin	deficiency (typ I) dysform (typ II):	homozygot: not compatible with life, heterozygot: higher risk than protein C- or S deficiency, especially in pregnancy	0.02-0.17%	1%
Protein C	deficiency (Typ I) dysform (Typ II)	homozygot: purpura fulminans and thromboembolism in the newborn heterozygot: fam. Protein C deficiency 8-10 fold risk, general pop: prot. C def. in 0.5-0.8 without thromboembolic complications!	0.5–0.8%	2–3%
Protein S	deficiency (typ I) total and free protein S and protein S activity reduced dysform (typ II): total Prot. S normal, but activity and free protein S reduced	homozygot: like protein C deficiency heterozygot: like protein C deficiency	?	2%
activated protein C resistance (APCR)	in 80–90% due to G1691A mutation of the factor V gen (factor V Leiden)	homozygot: 100-fold risk for thromboembolic complication heterozygote: 10-fold risk for TE compared to general population	3–7%	20–30%
Factor II Leiden	due to mutation G20210A of the factor II gen, often combined with elevated factor II levels	lower risk for thromboembolic complications than in APCR for heterozygotes (3fold) and probably also for homozygotes	1–2%	20%
Hyperhomocysteinemia	homozygous defect of MTHFR or homozygous defect of cystathionin-ß synthetase	higher risk for cardiovascular diseases, but also for venous thromboembolism	0–11%	5.7–25%

Table 2. Coagulation disorders in various diseases

Diseases	Coagulation and platelet disorders
Impaired liver function	mostly impaired synthesis of coagulation factors and inhibitors antithrombin, protein C, platelet dysfunction besides thrombocytopenia, hyperfibrinolysis, DIC, various inhibitors of coagulation
sepsis	thrombocytopenia, antithrombin deficiency, but also protein C and/or S deficiency, DIC
massive blood loss	low levels of all coagulation factors, inhibitors and platelets due to dilution
hematologic disorders:	
acute promyelocytic leucemia	→ (DIC, bleeding, and thrombotic events
polycythemia vera	→ thromboembolic and bleeding events
essential thrombocythemia	→ thromboembolic and bleeding events, acquired von Willebrand disease
paroxysmal nocturnal hemoglobinuria	→ thromboembolic events
lymphoproliferative diseases (monoclonal gammopathies)	→ acquired von Willebrand disease
malignancies (especially tumors of the pancreas, lower gastrointestinal tract), but also nearly all other tumors	increased incidence of thromboembolic events, DIC but also inhibitors like LA
autoimmune diseases	thromboembolic events, especially in the presence of lupus anticoagulants (LA), seldom: bleeding due to inhibitors to clotting factors
uremia	platelet dysfunction
nephrotic syndrome	antithrombin deficiency

Acquired thrombophilia

Acquired thrombophilia is also rather frequent, especially in the elderly and in patients with multivariate and severe diseases (Table 2). During the next years the need of cardiac surgery could increase. As already pointed out the latent DIC will be the main problem.

Heparin induced thrombocytopenia

The most actual problem in cardiac surgery is a special acquired thrombophilia, the heparin induced thrombocytopenia (HIT) (for review see 16) which is an immunological disease accompanied by life and limb threatening thromboembolic complications. The immunoglobulin, mostly IgG, becomes detectable five or more days after the first exposure to heparin. It is directed against a complex of unfractionated heparin or any other highly sulfated oligosaccharide complexed with platelet factor 4 (antiheparin factor) on the platelet surface. In the presence of heparin and the immunoglobulin platelets become activated. The platelet count begins to fall continuously 5–8 days sometimes up to three weeks after the first application of heparin to a median low about 50 000/µl frequently accompanied by a new thromboembolic event. Deep vein thrombosis of the lower limbs and pulmonary embolism are mostly observed. Arterial thrombosis presents in most cases as acute limb ischemia or stroke. Injured or diseased vessels are at increased risk. In contrast to other drug induced thrombocytopenias purpura and bleeding are seldom observed.

HIT is diagnosed by functional assays where normal platelets aggregate in the presence of the patient's serum and low heparin concentrations and not when high heparin concentrations are used. Cross – reactivity exists for low molecular weight heparins and in about 10% even to other glycosaminoglycans like danaparoid sodium. Immunological assays are also available. The concordance to these two test systems unfortunately is only 80–90%. Because of the dangerous situation one cannot wait for the laboratory results but must suspect a HIT if the platelet count drops by 50% or more and especially if it is accompanied by a new thromboembolic event. Other causes of thrombocytopenia, like the frequently occuring sepsis or DIC, must be excluded. The combination of sepsis with HIT has been described and DIC may be a complication of HIT.

The therapeutic approach consists in stopping the heparin therapy immediately and in using for prophylaxis or therapy either danaparoid sodium or recombinant hirudin (Refludan®). For dosage see Table 3. A special problem is cardiac surgery when the presence of HIT is already known. First promising results with recombinant hirudin during and after cardiopulmonary bypass have been published by Riess et al. (13).

Table 3. Prophylaxis or treatment of thrombosis in patients with heparininduced thrombocytopenia (from (16))

Prophylaxis: Danaparoid sodium: 750 anti-Xa units two or three times daily by subcutaneous injection.

Treatment of thrombosis:
Danaparoid sodium: *loading dose:* 2,250 U i.v. bolus*, followed by 400 U / hour x 4 hours, then 300 U / hour x 4 hours; then *maintenance:* 150-200 U / hour, with subsequentdosis adjustments made using anti-Xa levels (target range 0.5-0.8 anti-Xa U/ml) if assay available**.
Or
recombinant hirudin: *loading dose:* 0.4 mg / kg bw bolus, followed by
maintenance: 0.15 mg/kg bw per hour infusion, with dose adjustments to maintain APTT 1.5-3.0 times the mean of the normal laboratory APTT range.

Other indications:
for danaparoid sodium see "compassionate use" of the producer,
for hirudin, see for example (13).

The authors do not recommend starting oral anticoagulants (e.g., warfarin, phenprocoumon) until several days after stopping heparin (generally not until the thrombocytopenia has resolved or unless the patient is satisfactorily anticoagulated with danaparoid sodium or hirudin). If the patient is already fully anticoagulated with oral anticoagulants (OA) when the HIT is recognized, the authors recommend continuing with the OAs

* Adjust bolus for body weight: < 60 kg: 1,500 U; 60-75 kg: 2,250 U, 75-90 kg: 3,000 U, > 90 kg: 3,750 U. The recommendations are based on the 750 ampoule availability; for 1,250 ampoules, the loading dose would be 2 500 U etc.

** the calibration curve for anti-Xa testing must be derived using danaparoid rather than low-molecular weight heparin.

Bleeding disorders

Acquired bleeding disorders are one of the major problems of cardiac surgery. Compared to them congenital bleeding disorders are of less importance.

Congenital bleeding disorders

The general opinion is that congenital bleeding disorders are extremely rare and when they occur they are obvious. This is true for the classical severe hemophilias A or B and similar severe clotting factor deficiencies. It is less known about the congenital von Willebrand disease in its mild form type 1 that occurs rather frequently. Subnormal concentrations of von Willebrand factor in the peripheral blood in the range of 40–50% are present in 1–2% of the normal population (2). Furthermore, during the last years the von Willebrand factor as an adhesive protein and as an endothelial factor has gained importance. Von Willebrand factor (VWF) is a large multimeric and multifunctional protein synthezised in the endothelial cell. It binds the platelets to the subendothelium and with each other and protects factor VIII against premature fibrinolytic degradation. In type 1 von Willebrand disease, the VWF is still measurable and its activity is accordingly reduced. Type 2 is characterized by various defects of the von Willebrand molecule, mainly with a lack of the large multimers, and type 3 by the complete lack of VWF.

Severe congenital bleeding disorders are easily recognized with clinical symptoms like abnormal skin bruises, abnormal bleeding even after minor surgery and the danger of deformed joints due to hemophilic arthropathy, and distinctly abnormal coagulation tests. But mild bleeding disorders are most times inobtrusive without provocation and blood coagulation tests can give intermittently normal results (1). Here the careful case history will give clues which point to a haemostatic imbalance. Leading symptoms are prolonged or even life threatening bleeding after tonsillectomy or adenotomy in early childhood or after tooth extraction, frequent severe nose bleeding especially in childhood, and in women unexplained menorrhagia. Less informative is the postoperative course after such surgery as for example appendectomy or herniotomy.

Today cardiac surgery presents no major problem and has been performed in severe congenital coagulopathies as highly purified and virus inactivated factor concentrates are available. Using the formula that 1 IU clotting factor / kg bw will increase plasma factor levels about 1–2%, one can keep the coagulation factor within the normal range of 80–120% until wound healing is completed. This is also due for mild bleeding disorders. Here, too, the factor level must be kept within the normal range. Subnormal levels of VWF about 40–50% and without a history of bleeding as mentioned above should present no problem as von Willebrand factor (normal range 50–150%) is an acute phase reactant like factor VIII and will rise during and after surgery at least threefold. Furthermore, von Willebrand factor-concentration is elevated in inflammatory processes, liver diseases, tumors, all stress situations, and in the elderly. Still in some cases postoperative abnormal bleeding may occur and should be treated with a von Willebrand factor concentrate.

A severe problem is the rare case of severe congenital M. Glanzmann. These patients lack certain glycoprotein receptors on the surface of their platelets and will easily produce special inhibitors against transfused normal platelets. These inhibitors are easily recognized as the bleeding time does not shorten to normal after platelet transfusion. To prevent abnormal bleeding in spite of substitution therapy, one should ascertain before surgery that normalization has been obtained in the coagulation and platelet function tests.

Acquired bleeding disorders

Acquired bleeding disorders in cardiac surgery have been recently surveyed by Dapper in 1997 (5). According to this report, postsurgical bleeding occurs in 10–20% of the patients and the need to rethoracotomy in about 3–5%. As the hemostatic system reacts mostly to the various disorders quite a number of diseases are not only combined with thrombophilia but also with an acquired bleeding diathesis (Table 2). Either due to these disorders or to cardiopulmonary bypass, there are three compartments where hemostasis could be impaired:

- deficiency of coagulation factors or inhibition of coagulation,
- platelet dysfunction due to thrombocytopenia and/or platelet dysfunction,
- highened fibrinolysis.

The hemostatic situation during and after cardiopulmonary bypass in regard to the danger of abnormal bleeding can be summarized as follows:

1. The abnormal bleeding is most times not provoked by the intermittendly low levels of fibrinogen and coagulation factors during cardiopulmonary bypass as already shown in the early 1970s and recently (7). The routine use of fresh frozen plasma in operations with cardiopulmonary bypass is not justified (3).

2. Thrombopathy which is more extensive than assumed by the drop in platelets and can be demonstrated by a prolonged bleeding time. Platelet function tests are generally not available. The new platelet function analyzer might prove valuable here (8). The therapy consists in transfusion of platelet concentrates.

3. The intraoperative application of the proteinase inhibitor aprotinin has reduced the blood loss markedly (survey see (6)). The reason for it is still not clear. Aprotinin is a plasmin inhibitor and, therefore, inhibits fibrinolysis which is activated by cardiopulmonary bypass. But several investigators could show that the protective effect of aprotinin on platelet adhesive function might be the main cause.

4. A rebound effect of heparin must be excluded.

5. In the early 1970s patients routinely received factor VIII concentrates after CPB which contained not only factor VIII but also von Willebrand factor. After it was shown that factor VIII levels were such that substitution therapy was not necessary, the therapy was dropped. But there may be some cases with bleeding problems because of low levels of von Willebrand factor either due to congenital or to acquired von Willebrand disease. So in cases with unexplained bleeding complications the infusion of a von Willebrand factor concentrate might prove useful.

References

1. Barthels M, Poliwoda H (1997) Gerinnungsanalysen. Georg Thieme Verlag Stuttgart – New York, p 191
2. Budde U, Drewke E, Schneppenheim R (1996) Hämostaseologische und molekularbiologische Diagnostik des von Willebrand Syndroms. DG klinische Chemie Mitt 27: 41–54
3. Consten CJ, Henny ChP, Eijsman L, Dongelmans DA, van Oers MHJ (1996) The routine use of fresh frozen plasma in operations with cardiopulmonary bypass is not justified. J Thorac-Cardiovasc-Surg 112: 162–167
4. Dahlbäck B (1995) The protein C anticoagulant system. Thromb Res 77:1–44
5. Dapper F (1997) Blutungskomplikationen in der Kardiochirurgie. In: Blutgerinnung und Blutungskomplikation: Wirkung von Hämostasefaktoren ausserhalb des Gerinnungssystems. XXXIX. Hamburger Symposion über Blutgerinnung. V. Tilsner u. F. R. Matthias. F. K. Schattauer (eds) Verlag Stuttgart p 47–70
6. Dietrich W, Barankay A, Hähnel Ch, Richter JA (1992) High dose aprotinin incardiac surgery: three years's experiencein 1,784 patients. J Cardiothorac Vasc Anesth 6: 324–327

7. Gelb AB, Roth RI, Levin J (1996) Changes in blood coagulation during and following cardiopulmonary bypass: lack of correlation with clinical bleeding. Am J Clin Pathol 106: 87–99
8. Kolde HJ, de Haan J (1998) Eine neue Methode zurBestimmung der Plättchenhämostasekapazität. Hämostaseologie 18: 41–48
9. Landolfi R, Marchioli R, Patrono C (1997) Mechanisms of bleeding and thrombosis in myeloproliferative disorders. Thrombos Haemost 78: 617–621
10. Lane DA, Mannucci PM, Bauer KA, Bertina RM, Bochkov NP, Boulyenkov V, Mammen C, Dahlbäck B, Ginter EK, Miletich JP, Rosendaal FR, Seligson U (1996) Inherited thrombophilia: part 1. Thrombos Haemost 76: 651–662
11. Lane DA, Mannucci PM, Bauer KA, Bertina RM, Bochkov NP, Boulyenkov V, Mammen C, Dahlbäck B, Ginter EK, Miletich JP, Rosendaal FR, Seligson U (1996) Inherited thrombophilia: part 2. Thrombos Haemost 76: 824–834
12. Lechner K (1983) Gesichertes und Ungesichertes in der Diagnostik der Thrombophilie. Med Welt 34: 103–106
13. Riess FC, Poetzsch B, Müller-Berghaus G (1997) Recombinant hirudin as an anticoagulant during cardiac surgery. In: New anticoagulants for the cardiovascular patient. Pifarré R (ed.) Hanley and Belfus Inc. Philadelphia, p 197–219
14. Selhub J, D'Angelo A (1997) Hyperhomocysteinemia and thrombosis: acquired conditions. Thromb Haemost 78: 527–531
15. Swibertus R, Rosendaal F, Reitsma PH, Bertina RM (1996) A common genetic variation in the 3'-untranslated region of the prothrombin gene is associated with elevated plasma prothrombin levels and an increase in venous thrombosis. Blood 88: 3698–3703
16. Warkentin TE, Chong BH, Greinacher A (1998) Heparin-induced thrombocytopenia: towards consensus. Thromb Haemost 79: 1–7

Author's address:
Prof. Dr. med. M. Barthels
Division of Hematology and Oncology
Medical School Hannover 1
Carl-Neuberg-Straße 1
30625 Hannover, Germany

Practical use of recombinant R-Hirundin in cardiac surgery for prevention of perioperative thrombosis

R. Kaiser, H. Schwarz, Th. Wenzel, H.-G. Wollert, L. Eckel

Dept. of Thoracic and Cardiovascular Surgery Klinikum Karlsburg, Karlsburg, Germany

Introduction

The most serios complications of peri- and postoperative use of heparin are bleeding and heparin-induced thrombocytopenia (HIT) (4). HIT is classified into type 1, which is characterized by a temporary decrease of platelets without the presence of mediating antibodies. Despite the ongoing use of heparin, platelets will increase again, whereas type 2 is medicated by platelet activating antibodies that are directed against heparin/PF4 complexes. Impaired coagulation is referred in 0.5–5% to HIT type 2 with a complication rate of 20%, mostly vascular obstruction by thromboembolism (3).

In 2 out of 978 following patients a history of HIT type 2 was found preoperatively. Diagnosis was confirmed routinely by HIPA-Test (heparin induced platelet aggregation), and alternative drugs (orgaran and r-hirudin) were tested for perioperative anticoagulation.

Two cases are presented, which were treated with r-hirudin perioperatively. The regimen is described and the course is discussed.

The patients were enrolled in a clinical study conducted by the Behringwerke, Marburg, Germany, in which r-hirudin was used instead of heparin.

Methods

For both patients (patient 1: female, 68 y, 166 cm, 78 kg, coronary artery bypass grafting; patient 2: male, 63 y, 172 cm, 86 kg, aortic valve replacement) a bolus regime was used intraoperatively and a continuous regime was chosen postoperatively in order to avoid irregular dosage.

Shortly before start of cardiopulmonary bypass (CPB) a bolus of 0.2 mg/kg body weight (BW) r-hirudin was given and 0.25 mg/kg BW was added to priming solution. During CPB the anticoagulatory effect was monitored by the ecarin clotting time (ECT) in 10 min intervals. Additional boluses of 5 mg r-hirudin were administered when r-hirudin plasma levels fell below 2.5 μg/ml. Postoperatively r-hirudin was given intravenously by continous infusion of 0.1 mg/kg BW/h for four days. The activated partial thromboplastin time (aPTT) was monitored in at least four hour intervals. We tried to keep the aPTT between 2–3 times of the reference aPTT. If a PTT fell 20% below this range, the infusion raste of r-hirudin was increased by 20%. If risen above that range, the infusion was stopped for two hours.

Table 1. Intra- and postoperative characteristics of the patients

	Patient 1	Patient 2
HB (mmol/L Preop.	6.9	6.4
Dosage of r-hirudin (mg/ml)	4.6–9.2	1.8–4.6
aPTT-range (s)	51–92	49–84
duration of r-hirudin administration (days)	4	4
total dosage of r-hirudin (mg/kg BW)	3.8	2.0
platelets (10^9/L) postop.	125–252	247–275
perfusion time (min)	105	115
transfusion of blood (ml) intra-/postop.	750/0	2500/1750
transfusion of fresh frozen plasma (ml) postop.	0	1600
blood loss via thoracic drain (ml) postop.	680	4280

Results

The intra- and postoperative characteristics of the patients are shown in Tab.e 1

Discussion

For monitoring anticoagulation with r-hirudin postoperatively we used the aPTT. Although the aPTT values do not always correlate with the plasma r-hirudin level (1), it is reported to be sufficient to screen the anticoagulatory effectivity of r-hirudin (2, 4).

Despite a BW-dependent continous regimen of r-hirudin prolonged bleeding of patient 2 postoperatively could be triggered by a different individual response to the specific thrombin inhibitor r-hirudin. The postoperative aPTT values were not associated with the bleeding amounts. As r-hirudin cannot be neutralized (like heparin with protamine) bleeding complications may be more likely to persist if commenced.

References

1. Pötsch B et al. (1997) Monitoring of r-Hirudin Anticoagulation during Cardiopulmonary By-pass-Assessment of the Whole Blood Ecarin Clotting Time. Thrombosis and Haemostasis 77 (5): 920–925
2. Riess F-C et al. (1997) Rekombinantes Hirudin als Antikoagulans für kardiopulmonalen Bypass in der Herzchirurgie: Klinische Erfahrungen. Z Herz- Thorax- Gefäßchir 11: 79–87

3. Shorten GD et al. (1996) Heparin-Induced Thrombocytopenia. J Cardiothor Vasc Anesth 10 (4): 521–530
4. Westphal K et al. (1997) Heparin-induzierte Thrombozytopenie Typ II als Komplikation der Heparingabe nach einem Eingriff bei Aorta ascendens Dissektion.

Author's address:
Rolf Kaiser, M.D.
Department of Thoracic and Cardiovascular Surgery
Klinikum Karlsburg
Greifswalder Straße 11A
17495 Karlsburg, Germany

Progeria adultorum (Werner's syndrome) in a young patient undergoing double valve replacement due to massive calcification of the aortic and mitral valve

H. Grubitzsch, S. Beholz, H.-G. Wollert, L. Eckel

Department of Thoracic and Cardiovascular Surgery, Klinikum Karlsburg, Karlsburg, Germany

Abstract

We report on an aortic and mitral valve replacement due to heavy endocardial calcification in an 18 year old girl suffering from Werner's syndrome (progeria adultorum). Prominent features in this case were progressive dyspnoe (NYHA III) in accordance with rapid deterioration of aortic as well as mitral valve stenosis and prolonged postoperative recovery resulting from the difficulty of the operation and the syndrome itself.

Results

Werner's syndrome (WS; McKusick catalogue No. 27770) is are autosomal recessive disorder, which was first described in 1904 (3). It is characterized by the appearance of premature aging in young adults and reduced life time expectance (2). The limiting cardiovascular finding is early occurrence of ateriosclerosis (2). However, the most striking cardiac lesions are severe calcifications of the aortic and/or mitral valve leaflets and rings (1, 2).

We describe the perioperative course of an 18 year old girl (152 cm; 37.5 kg) presenting prominent features of WS as a bird-like face, a squeaky voice, growth arrest at puberty, hypogonadism, diabetes, scleroderma-like skin changes, premature graying, and thinning of hair, who underwent aortic and mitral valve replacement due to massive calcification of these valves. Clinical diagnosis of WS was established in 1993. At that time echocardiography revealed calcification of aortic valve leaflets and mitral anulus with mild aortic stenosis and reduced deflection of mitral valve opening. However, deterioration of these findings in accordance with progressive dyspnoe (NYHA III) occurred until 1997. Now a severe aortic stenosis, a severe mitral stenosis, and pulmonary hypertension were evident. No arteriosclerotic plaques of the coronary arteries were found. Because of clinical worsening and progressive valve dysfunction, a double valve replacement was indicated.

The operation was carried out in mild hypothermia with cardiac arrest induced by cold crystalloid cardioplegia. Intraoperatively the following pathological findings were seen: an enormous hypertrophy of the left and right heart with congestin of both atria, a hypoplastic aorta demonstrating about half the diameter of the pulmonary artery and widespread calcification of both the leaflets and the anulus of the aortic as well as the mitral valve proceeding into the left atrium. After removement of the calcific deposits at the mitral anulus and the inner atrial tissue, a prosthetic mitral valve (St. Jude, 25 mm) was implanted. Due to the small aortic root, aortic valve replacement was conducted with a 17 mm mechanical prosthesis (St. Jude). Considering the body surface area there was no need for root enlargement. Careful removement of calcific deposits resulted in a total ischemic time of 221 minutes. High dosages of catecholamines were necessary for weaning of cardiopulmonary bypass. Finally the chest had to be left open avoiding compromised cardiac performance.

After cardiopulmonary stabilization during the 6 following days, the chest was definitely closed. The patient made a prolonged recovery. During the postoperative course the following problems occurred: respiratory insufficiency with need of controlled and supported ventilation for 23 days, oliguria with need of temporary hemofiltration for 6 days, transient right hemiparesis, nosocomial pneumonia by coagulase-negative staphyloccocus, enteroccocus, and E. coli followed by klebsiella with a systemic inflammatory response syndrome at 49th day. Because of an acute gall bladder hydrops due to cholecystolithiasis conventional cholecystectomie had to be performed. Finally, almost complete regression of hemiparesis and mobilization at normal level could be reached by consequent physiotherapeutic training. The patient was discharged after 73 days and echocardiographic examination at that time demonstrated normal function of the aortic and mitral valve prosthesis, almost normal ejection of the hypertrophied left ventricle, and a reduction of the pulmonary hypertension.

Conclusions

We conclude that detailed cardiovascular examination as well as scheduled follow-up should be performed in young patients with WS to determine the optimal time for surgical intervention. Aggressive surgical procedures are proper treatment in this very special subset of patients although there is a risk for developing postoperative problems resulting from the syndrome itself.

References

1. Cohen JI, Arnett EN, Kolodny AL, Roberts WC (1987) Cardiovascular Features of the Werner Syndrome. Am J Cardiol 59: 493–495
2. Epstein CJ, Martin GM, Schultz AL, Motulsky AG (1966) Werner's syndrome: a review of its symptomatology, natural history, pathologic features, genetics and relationship to the natural aging process. Medicine 45: 177–221
3. Werner O: Ueber Katarakt in Verbindung mit Sklerodermie (Inaugural-Dissertation). Kiel: Schmidt & Klaunig, 1904

Author's address:
Herko Grubitzsch, M.D.
Department of Thoracic and Cardiovascular Surgery
Klinikum Karlsburg
Greifswalder Str. 11A
17495 Karlsburg, Germany

Cardiac surgery and pregnancy

A. J. Parry[1], S. Westaby[2]

[1]University of California, San Francisco, California, USA; [2]Oxford Heart Centre, Oxford, England

Introduction

Unlike the other topics in this symposium cardiac surgery during pregnancy is different for a number of reasons. First, pregnancy is a physiological state rather than a pathological condition; second, obviously there are 2 lives at stake rather than one; and third, the increased risk from the surgery is not sustained by the individual with the pathology. Indeed, if one were to ask what is the impact of cardiac surgery on the pregnant woman, the answer nowadays is nothing. The real problem is that the other individual involved is at significant risk; although we understand the physiology of the mother and the effects of cardiopulmonary bypass on this physiology, we know very little about the effects of maternal bypass on the physiology of the fetus.

In developed countries the virtual eradication of rheumatic fever has reduced the incidence of maternal heart disease during pregnancy from 3.6 % to 1.5 % over the last 25 years, though rheumatic valve disease still accounts for 60–75 % of this (11). Nevertheless, cardiac disease remains the principle cause for maternal death during pregnancy. However, in developing countries, as expected, rheumatic valve disease still contributes significantly to maternal and fetal mortality.

Determining the best management for the pregnant patient who requires intervention for cardiac disease is difficult as the literature is biased by reporters only documenting their successes. Therefore, what we interpret from these reports must be treated with some caution.

Pathologies usually encountered during pregnancy

Cardiac pathology requiring intervention during pregnancy may either be preexisting or acquired. If it is preexisting this implies that it is well tolerated in the unstressed state, but there is no reserve to cope with the dramatic hemodynamic challenge of pregnancy. Most commonly this is due to post-rheumatic mitral or aortic stenosis which 'fix' the cardiac output so that the mother cannot meet the increased demands of a hyperdynamic circulation. Increasingly, complications related to previous cardiac valve replacement occur; a hypercoagulable state exists in pregnancy which may result in thrombosis of a mechanical valve, or prosthetic valve endocarditis may occur due to the relatively, immunocompromised state of pregnancy. Acquired cardiac pathology is primarily due to hypertension and the hyperdynamic circulation which accompany pregnancy. Spontaneous dissection of the aorta or coronary arteries very rarely occurs in young women without evidence of other cardiovascular disease but when it does it almost always occurs during pregnancy and usually has catastrophic results.

Relevant physiologic changes occurring with pregnancy

The maternal physiological hemodynamic adaptions which occur with pregnancy start by the 5th week of gestation and place a significantly increased demand on the cardiovascular system (6). The crucial consideration in successfully managing cardiac surgery in pregnant women is to provide adequate perfusion of the uterus and thereby adequate perfusion of the fetus. For this reason, understanding the physiologic changes which occur with pregnancy will aid both in appreciating why cardiac decompensation occurs in otherwise well adapted patients and also in managing the patient correctly during surgery.

The earliest change is an increase in cardiac output, initially due to an increase in heart rate and left ventricular performance associated with a fall in peripheral vascular resistance by up to 40 % (7). This appears to be due to an insensitivity to vasoconstrictors induced by elevations in plasma estrogen levels which are found early in pregnancy. Later an increase in stroke volume contributes to the increase in cardiac output and peaks at 20 weeks gestation 33 % above pre-pregnancy levels. All these changes result in a cardiac output 20 % above non-pregnant levels by the 8th week of gestation, 30–60 % by the 32nd week of gestation, and peaks at 80 % above non-pregnant levels during the second stage of labor. Accompanying these changes, left ventricular remodeling starts early in the second trimester with increased left ventricular end systolic and end diastolic volumes, and an increase in left ventricular wall mass and thickness due to myocyte hypertrophy. In addition, there is an increase in pulmonary, mitral, and aortic valve area (9). Mean red cell mass increases, but this is outweighed by the increase in blood volume which increases by 30 % and hematocrit, therefore, falls. Heart rate correspondingly increases and oxygen consumption is elevated to 15–18% above non-pregnant levels. Finally, there is an alteration in the levels of various plasma coagulation proteins which induces a hypercoagulable state. This leads to problems with the management of anticoagulant regimens, and prosthetic valve thrombosis is not uncommon during pregnancy. This problem is exacerbated by the fact that warfarin has in the past been considered to be a teratogen, and it has been recommended that it should be discontinued with the substitution of heparin during early pregnancy. The period of conversion between these two is particularly risky.

Drug administration

A discussion of the impact of various drugs on the mother and fetus during pregnancy is beyond the scope of this chapter. However, some general principals apply and are critically important for the correct management of these patients. All drugs should be considered to be teratogenic during pregnancy and therefore used cautiously. Also, due to an increased glomerular filtration rate drug levels will be lower than normal by 10–15 %. Antibiotic prophylaxis is routine in all cardiac operations and these drugs are generally considered to be about the safest drugs prescribable during pregnancy. Tetracycline should be avoided due to the risk of fetal tooth enamel staining, and aminoglycosides due to a risk of fetal ototoxicity. However the more widely used penicillins are considered safe.

Fetal age and the timing of surgery

Though there is no proven relationship between the gestational age of the fetus at the time of intervention and mortality, congenital malformatins occur more commonly when cardiopulmonary bypass is performed during the first trimester due to drug administration and possibly cardiopulmonary bypass. However, this does not imply a universally unfavorable outcome and 6 successful pregnancies have been reported when cardiopulmonary bypass was carried out early in the first trimester before the patients were aware they were pregnant. After this period, open cardiac surgery is significantly safer and there are many reports of fetal survival to term after operations performed in the second or third trimesters. However, recent advances in neonatal care have improved survival of premature infants to such an extent that, while for neonates less than 26 weeks gestation there is still a very high mortality (90%) and for survivors a 20% risk of neurological damage, for those greater than 26–30 weeks survival is 80%, and for infants greater than 30 weeks, 99%.

For this reason we and others have reported successful cesarean section immediately prior to commencing cardiopulmonary bypass and suggest that this may be the most appropriate approach during the third trimester (13, 14). This philosophy is particularly relevant when there are indications of reduced placental reserve such as intrauterine growth retardation and pre-eclampsia (10). In these circumstances there is a very high incidence of fetal loss if maternal cardiac surgery with continuation of the pregnancy is attempted. When the approach of cesarean section immediately prior to cardiac surgery is adopted, the abdominal wall is best left open to allow ready access to the uterus to ensure that undue hemorrhage does not occur.

Prior to the third trimester, if cardiac intervention is essential and the pregnancy is to continue, it is essential to obtain full informed consent from the parent(s). Bypass should be conducted as discussed below, but it is essential that care be concentrated on the mother and that this care is not compromised in an attempt to reduce the risk to the fetus. As yet the best management for the fetus is not known, and 'experimenting' on the mother cannot be justified.

Closed surgical procedures

At any stage of pregnancy avoiding bypass is best, and closed mitral valvotomy has historically held an important position in the management of women with mitral stenosis during pregnancy since it produces adequate palliation yet avoids the insult to both mother and fetus of cardiopulmonary bypass (1). In countries where rheumatic mitral stenosis remains prevalent, large numbers of closed mitral valvotomies are performed each year with approximately 1% of the caseload made up of pregnant women. With this population the results are excellent; the maternal mortality is the same as for non-pregnant women undergoing the same procedure. Indeed, all the mortalities in reported series occurred prior to 1965. Likewise, the overall reported fetal mortality is low at 7.7%. Over recent years the fetal mortality has gradually decreased but it has remained appreciable at 5.3% since 1980. Although advocates claim no teratogenic effects from the procedure and that it is safe at any stage of pregnancy, the later the intervention occurs the better since there is the option of cesarean section prior to the cardiac procedure if the mother can be carried to the third trimester as discussed above.

However, closed mitral valvotomy is not without risk, and in one series 2.8% of patients required emergency mitral valve replacement for torn mitral leaflets. In addition, the indications are somewhat restrictive; there must be isolated mitral stenosis with reasonably well preserved valvar and subvalvar apparatus, and no evidence of left atrial thrombus. A significantly calcified valve is a relative contra-indication.

More recently the role of closed mitral valvotomy has been challenged by balloon valvuloplasty as the radiation dose required for this procedure is 0.002 Gy, well below the 0.005 Gy threshold accepted (8, 12). The reported complication rate is low, but the procedure is still limited in scope by the same contra-indications as for closed mitral valvotomy. However, where interventional cardiology is unavailable, closed surgery will continue to be used in a large number of cases.

Most recently, coronary artery bypass grafting without using cardiopulmonary bypass has allowed us to palliate coronary artery disease without the risks of bypass. We may assume that the risk to the fetus is also reduced with this technique but this has not yet been proven. In some units percutaneous coronary angioplasty has been performed in pregnant patients to palliate them through the pregnancy, and although the experience is small, the results have been very encouraging (2). Finally, for patients with cyanotic congenital heart disease, systemic-pulmonary artery shunts may allow adequate palliation for the duration of the pregnancy without the risk of cardiopulmonary bypass.

Open cardiac surgery

Cardiopulmonary bypass is bad for the fetus. Coagulation abnormalities, leukocyte degranulation, complement activation, air and particulate embolization, and cellular changes have all been implicated. The risk to the mother has dramatically decreased with improvements in bypass techniques and while maternal mortality over the entire history of cardiac surgery during pregnancy is 3.2%, there has not been a maternal death during open heart surgery reported in the literature during the last 22 years despite far more complex operations being undertaken during pregnancy (3, 4, 14). Inevitably there is an element of reporting bias in these results but the trend appears to be true. However, though fetal mortality has also fallen, now being 18.8% overall and 11.1% over the last 6 years, there still remains a significant risk to the child.

When open surgery is inevitable during pregnancy the philosophy regarding the management of the operation must be based on the following considerations:

1) how to maintain the physiology as normal as possible,

and 2) how best to maintain placental/fetal perfusion.

The first decision concerns the nature of the prime solution. These data are very poorly documented in the literature, and hence no firm conclusions can be drawn. There are no reports of significant uterine or fetal reactions to a non-sanguineous prime except for a mild fetal bradycardia at the start of bypass, and although this appears to conflict with our stated aims, it should be considered that we do not know where the correct balance lies between viscosity and oxygen carrying capacity on bypass. With this uncertainty, our practise has been pragmatically to add blood to the prime to maintain a hematocrit of around 25%.

The temperature should be maintained at 35 °C or above. Hypothermia adversely affects placental gas-exchange and increases uterine vascular resistance producing a fall in placental perfusion. With a hypothermic prime there is a significant fetal bradycardia associated with the commencement of bypass. Review of the literature to date reveals that fetal mortality is higher in those cases in which hypothermia was used during the conduct of the operation than those in whom normothermia was maintained (8% versus 0%). Recently, there have been reports of operations for aortic dissection using profound hypothermic circulatory arrest with good outcome for both mother and fetus (5). However, it is clear from these articles that more unsuccesful cases had been performed prior to the succesful reported one, and the problem of reporting bias is again evident. What is certain, however, is that success may be achieved with most approaches, and although it is possible to suggest what is the most ideal approach to adopt, when circumstances necessitate a less ideal approach it may still be possible to obtain a satisfactory outcome.

Bypass flows should be kept high, above 2.5 l/min/m^2. There is no direct evidence to support this recommendation but the fetal bradycardia which often accompanies the start of bypass, or occasionally occurs during bypass, is reversible in almost all cases by increasing the flow. Some authors have actually claimed that fetal heart rate is directly related to the flow rate. In addition, venous return should always be considered, and after 20 weeks gestation, the right flank of the mother should be elevated to ensure unimpeded venous return.

Flow is not the whole issue and adequate blood pressure is also essential. In the relaxed state, uterine perfusion is dependent on a mean blood pressure of more than 70 mmHg as the uteroplacental bed is maximally dilated and unable to autoregulate. Hypotension always occurs at the start of bypass due to a fall in the systemic vascular resistance, and this must be anticipated and proactively treated. However, when uterine contractions occur the required perfusion pressure is much higher and during them fetal bradycardia is common. Preventing them is therefore of the utmost importance, and cardiotocography is an absolutely essential part of cardiac surgery in pregnant women. Uterine contractions are usually treatable by any of the available techniques, intravenous β_2 agonists, magnesium, or nitrates, but they must be aggressively treated both peri- and post-operatively. Close maternal and fetal monitoring must therefore continue well into the post-operative period and aggressive management of developing problems must be undertaken. In particular, the fetus should be closely monitored so that, should fetal death occur, immediate treatment may be instituted to prevent the significant hemorrhage which often accompanies this eventuality particularly during the post-bypass period when maternal coagulation remains derranged.

A pressure of more than 70 mmHg is however potentially dangerous for the mother, and a compromise must therefore be found. If pressures are less than 50 mmHg, there is a 20% risk of both fetal mortality and significant morbidity, while the risks are 11% and 5.5%, respectively, if the pressure is greater than 50 mmHg. For this reason, we have adopted 60 mmHg as an acceptable compromise.

There is no evidence that pulsatile perfusion is better, though rationally it would seem likely that it would perfuse the uterus better during periods of uterine contraction. Indeed, the only case reported in the literature in which pulsatile flow was used during pregnancy resulted in fetal death. Aprotonin should be avoided, but above all the duration of bypass should be kept as short as possible.

Fetal monitoring

Fetal heart rate monitoring is essential. Bradycardia often accompanies maternal cardiopulmonary bypass and indicates diminished fetal perfusion. Early identification may allow manipulation of bypass which can reverse the problem but severe bradycardia is irreversible. Treatment must therefore be early and aggressive and should continue into the post-operative period as fetal mortality is significant during this period also.

Preterm labor

Despite a successful operation, preterm labor remains a significant risk. It is often precipitated by hypovolemia and hypoxia, and both of these must therefore be treated aggressively. It is more common during the third trimester due to the maturation of receptors in the uterine smooth muscle and the contractile elements of the muscle cells. There is some evidence that a fall in plasma progesterone levels associated with the bypass prime can induce preterm labor as progesterone stabilizes the smooth muscle cells, but there is as yet no evidence that prophylactic progesterone supplementation in the pump prime is beneficial.

Most tocolytics have shown some success in treating preterm labor but the most favored at present are progesterone during the first half of pregnancy and terbutaline during the later part. There is increasing evidence that non-steroidal anti-inflammatory drugs can prevent pre-term labor though anxiety over their impact on ductal closure has limited their use. Most recently drugs with selective action against one cyclooxygenase subtype, responsible for fetal membrane prostaglandin synthesis and thereby probably induction of labor, have been developed. The results are awaited with interest.

Reducing the likelihood of maternal cardiac surgery during pregnancy

Correct management of women with cardiac disease starts well before pregnancy. Diagnosis of maternal disease must be accomplished early in life well before the risk of pregnancy. As soon as the woman has been diagnosed, a full and open discussion must be undertaken during which the risks and benefits of early intervention are discussed and, most importantly, the woman is educated so that she knows the risks of pregnancy with her heart disease and the risks she may incur with pregnancy even after the cardiac defect has been corrected. An example of this is the risk of mechanical prosthetic valve thrombosis due to the hypercoagulable state which accompanies pregnancy and the potentially teratognic effects of warfarin.

Second, corrective/palliative surgery should be scheduled before the risk of pregnancy so that women with known heart disease do not have an unnecessary risk during pregnancy.

Third, the use of allografts, or even better the 'Ross' procedure, for young women of childbearing age is to be strongly encouraged. There is a significant risk of prosthetic valve thrombosis or endocarditis in pregnancy after prosthetic valve replacement, and this may be significantly reduced if a living tissue prosthesis is used instead.

Finally, there must be meticulous medical management of women with borderline lesions so that adequate therapy may be given to maintain homeostasis during pregnancy. Later, if symptoms worsen, this will also allow prompt treatment of a decompensating cardiovascular system by medical or surgical means before the physiologic state of the mother has deteriorated to risk the fetus even prior to operation. Meticulous anticoagulant management of women with mechanical protheses should be included in this management approach for the previously mentioned reasons.

Conclusion

From our current understanding the following recommendations may be made.

1. Open heart surgery should be avoided, if at all possible, during the first trimester. If this is not feasible, precautions as for the later stages of pregnancy should be taken.
2. When the fetus is more than 28 weeks gestation, it is a safe option to deliver the child by cesarean section immediately before, and at the same operation as, the cardiac surgery.
3. The duration of cardiopulmonary bypass should be kept to a minimum.
4. High-flow (greater than 2.5 $l/min/m^2$), high-pressure (maternal blood pressure around 60 mmHg), normothermic bypass offers the least risk to the fetus.
5. Fetal heart and uterine monitoring should be used both during and after the operation to allow adjustments to the flow and pharmacological manipulations to ensure adequate placental perfusion.
6. Fetal bradycardia must be recognized early, recognized for what it is (a sign of fetal compromise), and aggressively treated by increasing bypass flow, increasing maternal blood pressure (if feasible), and treating uterine contractions.
7. Uterine contractions should be aggressively treated using one of the proven pharmacological agents.

References

1. Abid A, Abid F, Zargouni N, Khayati A (1990) Closed mitral valvotomy in pregnancy – a study of seven cases. International Journal of Cardiology 26: 319–321
2. Ascarelli MH, Grider JH, Hsu HW (1996) Acute myocardial infarction during pregnancy managed with immediate percutaneous coronary angioplasty. Obsterics and Gynecology 88(4): 655–657
3. Becker RM (1983) Intracardiac surgery in pregnant women. Annals of Thoracic Surgery 36(4): 453–458
4. Bernal JM, Miralles P (1986) Cardiac surgery with cardiopulmonary bypass during pregnancy. Obstetrical and Gynecological Survey 41(1): 1–6.
5. Buffolo E, Palma JH, Gomes WJ, Vega H, Born D, Moron AF, Carvalho AC (1994) Successful use of deep hypothermic circulatory arrest in pregnancy. Annals of Thoracic Surgery 58: 1532–1534

6. Crapo RO (1996) Normal cardiopulmonary physiology during pregnancy. Clinical Obstetrics and Gynecology 39(1): 3–16
7. Duvekot JJ, Cheriex EC (1996) Pieters FAA, Menheere PPCA, Peeters LLH Early pregnancy changes in hemodynamics and volume homeostasis are consecutive adjustments triggered by a primary fall in systemic vascular tone. American Journal of Obstetrics and Gynecology 169(6): 1382–1392
8. Farhat MB, Maatouk F, Betbout F, Ayari M, Brahim H, Souissi M, Sghairi K, Gamra H (1992) Percutaneous balloon mitral valvuloplasty in eight pregnant women with severe mitral stenosis. European Heart Journal 13: 1658–1664
9. Geva TG, Mauer MB, Striker L, Kirshon B, Pivarnik JM (1997) Effects of physiologic load of pregnancy on left ventricular contractility and remodeling. American heart Journal 133(1): 53–59
10. Izquierdo LA, Kushnir O, Knieriem K, Wernley JA, Curet LB (1990) Effect of mitral valve prosthetic surgery on the outcome of a growth-retarded fetus. American Journal of Obstetrics and Gynecology 163(2): 584–586
11. Kahler R (1975) Cardiac Disease. In: Burrow G, Ferris T (eds.) Medical complications during pregnancy. Philadelphia: WB Saunders; p. 105
12. Patel JJ, Mitha AS, Hassen F, Patel N, Naidu R, Chetty S, Pillay R (1993) Percutaneous balloon mitral valvotomy in pregnant patients with tight pliable mitral stenosis. American Heart Journal 125(4): 1106–1109
13. Shah AM, Kulatilake ENP, Pearson JF, Hall RJC (1992) Emergency mitral valve replacement immediately following Caesarean section. European Heart Journal 13: 847–849
14. Westaby S, Parry AJ, Forfar JC (1992) Reoperation for prosthetic valve endocarditis in the third trimester of pregnancy. Annals of Thoracic Surgery 53: 263–265

Author's address:
Andrew Parry, Assistant Professor
Box 0118
University of California, San Francisco
505 Parnassus Ave.
San Francisco, CA 94143-0118 USA

The impact of gender on cardiac surgical outcome

I. C. Ennker

Herzzentrum, Lahr/Baden

Introduction

The most frequent cause of death for a woman in Germany today is myocardial infarction. Annually about 120,000 women suffer from myocardial infarction and 2/3 of them die (6). This cause of death is prior to all causes of death due to cancer. However, there is a rare incidence of myocardial infarction before menopause. Causes of death due to myocardial infarction have increased during the last 50 years enormously.

Discussion

In autopsies done at the University of Minnesota Medical School from 1910–1938, there were 50 out of 1000 cases of death in male and only 20 cases out of 1000 in female patients related to coronary artery disease (5). Nowadays, the annual mortality due to coronary artery disease in the United States is the same in male and female patients (3), and in Germany it is slightly higher for females. If we look at the numbers of the Statistisches Bundesamt Wiesbaden from 1986 in comparison to the numbers of 1996, we see an increase in the total number of deaths related to cardiac disease for women from 15.8 to 16.3%, and over the same time period we see a decrease in the total numbers of deaths related to cardiac disease for men from 14.1 to 12.5% (Table 1).

At the age of 75 and older, women exceed men in the frequency of heart attacks. For female patients there is a dramatic increase in coronary heart disease after menopause, which is about the age of 50 to 55. And there is a steady increase in angina after menopause. In male patients there is a plateau at the age of about 45 years and the peak of angina in males is at the age of 52 to 55 (6).

Table 1. Gender dependent mortality, Statistisches Bundesamt Wiesbaden

	1986			1996		
	male	female	n	male	female	n
acute myocardial infarction	58%	42%	80240	56%	44%	84951
ischemic heart disease	44%	56%	55331	40%	60%	95584
heart failure and other cardiac compliactions	36%	64%	62719	32%	68%	62240

The prevalence of coronary artery disease in the United States for females in the age group from 45 to 64 is 1 : 7 and for female patients older than 65 it is about 1 : 3 (3). The percentage of female patients confronted with CABG below 55 years of age in our own hospital is about 8.6%.

There are some differences concerning coronary artery disease in males and females:

- onset of CAD,
- the protective effect of hormones pre-menopausal, and
- the difference in type of arteriosclerotic lesions.

In male patients there is a more dense fibrous tissue and in females a more cellular fibrous tissue (3).

Even at the time of 1953 it was known that there were some differences. Wüst postulated it as early as 1953. "At the present time there are two main schools of though concerning the explanation for differences in degree of coronary arteriosclerosis in men as compared to women. One, which employs the anatomic differences in the heart and coronary arteries of men and women and the other, which postulates an ovarian hormonal factor responsible for delaying the development of arteriosclerosis in women over men." (17)

One may consider, that coronary heart disease manifest 10 to 20 years later in women. Women are less likely to experience typical angina as the presenting symptom. Standard exercise tests to diagnose coronary artery disease in women lack specifity and sensitivity. Women are less frequently referred for angiography and, when they are, they receive CABG less often. Even thrombolysis is performed less often (14).

The most typical symptoms of myocardial infarction in female patients are

- emesis,
- queasiness,
- epigastric abdominal pain, and
- pyrosis.

A male patient shows a more typical symptoms, as pain in the left arm and shoulder and more the typical pain.

Owen experiences and results

The analysis of the consecutively effected operations within the period of time from Jan. 1, 1995 until May 30, 1997 has been done retrospectively by interpretation of the combined surgical and anesthological data banks by means of SPSS. The comparision between men and women is based on the comparison of average data (age, EF, body mass index, operation times, number of grafts) by t-test for independent spot checks or on non-parametric tests (Mann-Whithney U) for ordinated data. Nominal data (IABP, hypertonia, etc.) were compared by means of the Chi-Square test.

In 1996 the total number of coronary angiographies at our institution was 1,643, 460 in female patients (28%) and 1,183 in male patients (72%).

Coronary angiographies were performed in 30.3% of female and 69.7% of male patients. PTCA was performed in 25.1% of female and 74.9% of male patients. Stenting was done in 28% in female and 71.4% in male patients (Table 2).

In the time period from January 1, 1995 to May 30, 1997 in the Heart Institute Lahr/Baden, 3342 patients were operated for coronary artery disease. The percentage of female patients was 24% (Fig. 1).

Table 2. Invasive diagnostic and treatments in relation to gender (total number of coronary angiogrpahies in 1996 = 1643)

	n = 460 (28%) female	n = 1183 (72%) male
coronary angiographies	30.3%	69.7%
PTCA	25.1%	74.9%
Stents	28.6%	71.4%

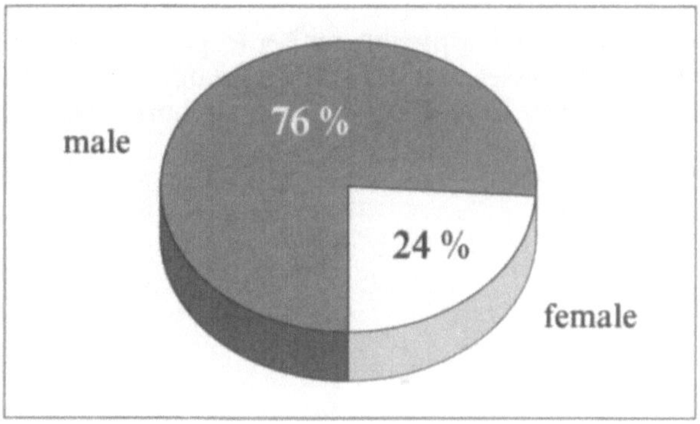

Fig. 1. Patients operated for coronary artery disease; sitribution by gender

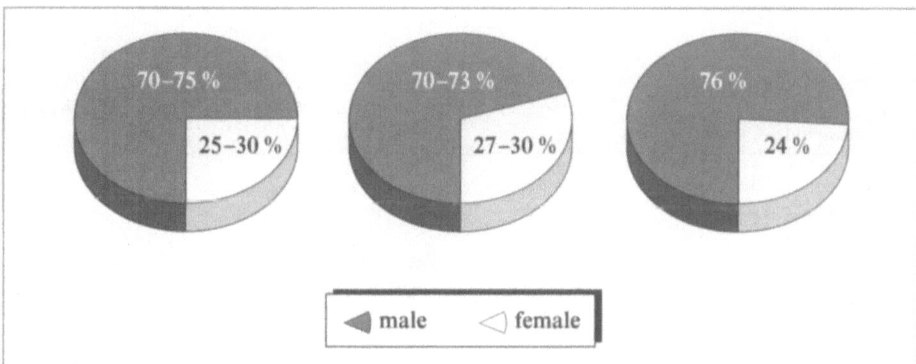

Fig. 2. Coronary artery bypass grafting, male/female ratio for the U.S., Germany, and our institute, respectively

The comparison of the percentage concerning the male/female ratio between the United States, Germany, and our own institute are basically the same (Fig. 2).

There is an enormous increase in the total number of open heart procedures. In 1985 there were about 33 departments performing open heart surgery, whereas in 1996 there were 77 and two planned departments. The total number of operations increased from 21,705 in 1985 up to nearly 90,000 in 1996.

Interestingly, the male/female ratio was first established as an individual statistical parameter by the German Society of Thoracic Cardiovascular Surgery as early as 1994. So we do not have exact data whether the male/female ratio changed during the last 10 years (10).

The clinical data are shown in Table 3; there were 810 women and 2,532 men. The women differed from the men in the following ways. Women were older and more likely to have associated diabetes, hypertension, and hyperlipoproteinaemia. Not surprisingly, the women were smaller in body surface area, height, and weight than men, but similar proportions of female and male patients wer obese with a BMI in both groups of 27.3. Women needed more emergency operations, and they were more symptomatic than their male counterparts. The number of unstable anginas was significantly higher in female patients (1).

In our experience, women and men were comparable with a respect to injection fraction, operation data as number of bypasses, arterial grafting, clamp time, perfusion time, and their need for postoperative intra-aortic balloon support. The total

Table 3. Clinical data, medical history

	femalse	males	total	p value
n	810	2532	3342	
age	68.1	63.5	64.6	$p < 0.001$
emergency op.	8.0%	6.2%	6.6%	$p < 0.05$
unstable a.p.	21.6%	16.0%	17.3%	$p < 0.01$
Ef	56%	54%	55%	$p < 0.001$

b

n	810	2532	3342	
hypertonia	76.5%	63.2%	66.4%	$p < 0.01$
diabetes mellitus	33.3%	23.3%	25.7%	$p < 0.001$
HLP	66.3%	58.5%	60.4%	$p < 0.001$
body mass index	27.3	27.3	27.3	n.s.

Table 4. Operation data

	females	males	total	p value
n	810	2532	3342	
number of bypasses	3.0	3.0	3.0	n.s.
arterial grafts	94%	94%	94%	n.s.
clamp time	50 min	51 min	50 min	n.s.
perfusion time	207 min	209 min	209 min	n.s.
bypasses valves	11%	7%	7.9%	$p < 0.001$

Table 5. Postoperative course data

	femalse	males	total	p value
n	810	2532	3342	
delayed mobilization	24%	18%	19%	$p < 0.01$
perioperative myocardial infarction	2.9%	2.9%	2.9%	n.s.
in hospital mortality	2.2%	2.1%	2.0%	n.s.

number of combinations of myocardial revascularization and valve repair were significantly higher in women.

Concerning the postoperative course, both groups were comparable in relation to intensive care stay perioparative myocardial infarction and the in-hospital mortality.

Only a delayed mobilization for female patients could be noticed, as shown in Tables 4 and 5.

The literature review shows a gender difference in recovery. Women experience more shortness of breath, engage in less physical activity, and the number of physical symptoms as chest pain and discomfort are significantly higher. There was also a trend for an increasing percentage of more cardiac dysfunction a longer stay in intensive care units, and a higher in-hospital mortality (1).

Mortality and morbidity in early recovery after treatment of coronary artery disease with angioplasty are higher in women. Women have been shown to have more adverse outcomes after a CABG than men including lower physical and social functioning, higher incidence of morbidity and death (1, 4). But there are also reports showing that there are no differences with regard to survival after CABG. This is be supported by our own experiences (8, 11, 13).

It could be shown that there is an imbalance concerning the total number of causes of death due to cardiac diseases and the total number of performed open heart operations or interventional treatment between females and their male counterparts. What might be the reasons for this situation, and what might be the causes of less favourable outcome in women after CABG?

Females have a higher incidence of concomitant disease as diabetes, hypertension, unstable angina, and a higher incidence of hyperlipoproteinaemia. Their body size is smaller and not surprisingly their coronary arteries are smaller. This may result in a reduced graft patency as some surgeons state, but it should not be too difficult for a trained surgeon to operate on a coronary artery with a diameter of 1.0 to 1.5 mm (1).

Some special psycho-social risk factors of women, who develop coronary heart disease, could be worked-out:

- low social class,
- low educational achievement,
- extra commitments to work and family,
- chronic troubling emotions, and
- lack of social support (4).

With regard to the knowledge that there is a rare incidence of myocardial infarction before menopause and the small number of open heart surgery for coronary artery disease in younger females, circumstances should be taken into consideration to prevent myocardial infarction (3). Angiographic studies in postmenopausal women indicate that estrogen replacement therapy reduces the risk of angiographically significant coronary artery disease. These results can be supported by several authors (3, 9, 15). The effect of estrogen deficit is decreased HDL, increased LDL, increased cholesterol and increased weight and blood pressure (3, 6, 16).

In the Framingham heart study, the lipid research clinics program could show that the HDL is a very sensitive and primary predictor of heart disease in women (3, 6). To prevent coronary artery disease and myocardial infarction in females, hormonal replacement therapy is requested (3, 6, 9, 16).

Many women are afraid of hormonal replacement therapy because they think this might increase the risk of breast cancer. Statistically there is a 20% risk of myocardial infarction for a female at the age of 70 but only a 5% risk of getting breast carcinoma (6). With this background a decreased desire for hormonal replacement therapy is unfounded as far as no severe contra-indications occur.

The indications for an estrogen replacement therapy are high risk patients, hypertonia, arterial hypertension, and hyperlipoproteinemia. Contraindications are metro carcinoma, mamma carcinoma, and severe hypertrigliceridemia (2, 12).

It could be shown that there are a number of gender differences concerning coronary artery disease, but concerning myocardial infarction studies, the rate of female patients involved in such studies is only 20% (6). Due to the differences, there should be a higher portion of females in myocardial infarction studies. It is not a men's disease anymore. For female patients as well as for male patients, myocardial infarction is the most frequent cause of death. But there is an imbalance concerning diagnostics, therapy, and outcome. It is to hoped or better postulated to equalize this imbalance, and the same quality of treatment for both gender should be possible.

References

1. Artinian NT, Hillebrand Duggan C (1996) Sex differences in patients recovery patterns after coronary artery bypass surgery. Heart Lung 24 (6) 483–494
2. Breckwoldt M, Hesch D., Kuhl H., Runnebaum B., Ziegler R (1996) Sonderdruck Endokrinologie, Inf. 20
3. Bush TL (1996) Evidence for primary and secondary prevention of coronary artery disease in women taking oestrogen replacement therapy. Eur. Heart J 17, (Supplement D): 9–14
4. Brezinka V, Kittel F (1995) Psychosocial factors of coronary heart disease in women: a review. Soc Sci Med 42 (10): 1351–1365
5. Clawson B (1941) Am Heart J 22: 607–624
6. Deutsche Liga zur Bekämpfung des hohen Blutdrucks (1995) Kardiovaskuläre Erkrankungen der Frau in der Postmenopause, Jahrestagung 1995, Potsdam
7. Douglas PS, Ginsburg Geoffrey S (1996) The evaluation of chest pain in women. The New England Journal of Medicine 334 (20): 1311–1315
8. Eakler ED, Kronmal A., Kennedy JW, Davis K (1989) Am Heart J 117 (1): 71–81
9. Holdright DR, Sullivan AK, Wirght CA, Sparrow JL, Cunningham D., Fox KM (1995), Eur Heart J 16: 1566–1570
10. Kalmar P, Irrgang E (1997) The impact of gender on cardiac surgical outcome, Thoracic Cardiovasc Surg 45: 134
11. King KM, Ross Kerr J (1992) The women's health agenda: Evolution of hormon replacement therapy as treatment and prophylaxis for coronary artery disease. Jorunal of Advanced Nursing 23: 984–991
12. Kuhl H, Runnebaum HP, Schneider G (1995) Langfristige Hormonsubstitution und Mammakarzinomrisiko: Aktuelle Bestandsaufnahme, Zentralbl. Gynäkol. 117: 549–553
13. Mickleborough LL, Takagi Y, Maruyama H, Sun Z, Mohamed S (1995) Is sex a factor in determining operative risk for aortocoronary bypass graft surgery? Circulation 92 (9) (Supp II): 80–84
14. Moore SM (1995) A comparison of women's symtpoms during home recovery after coronary artery bypass surgery. Heart Lung 24 (6): 495–501
15. Mosca L, Manson JE, Sutherland SE, Langer RD, Manolio T, Barret-Connor E (1997) Cardiovascular disease in women – a statement for healthcare professionals from the American Heart Association. Circulation 96: 2468–2482
16. Windler E (1996) Prävention kardiovaskulärer Erkrankungen durch Hormonsubstitution in der Postmenopause. Zentralbl Gynäkol 118: 184–194
17. Wuest JH, Dry TJ, Edwards JE (1953) The degree of coronary atherosclerosis in bilaterally oophorectomized women. Circulation 7: 801–808

Authors' address:
Dr. med. I. C. Ennker
Herz-, Thorax- und Gefäßchirurgie
Herzzentrum Lahr/Baden
Hohbergweg 2
77933 Lahr

Consequences of preexisting neurological disease in cardiac surgery – Literature survey and own experience

J. Ennker, A. Albert

Heartinstitute Lahr/Baden, Germany

Preoperatively existing neurological disease

Patients with preexisting neurological disease are quite common among cardiac surgical patients. As the rate of elderly people being operated on has been steadily increasing, we find besides various other concomitant diseases (Table 1) also more and more age-correlating neurological diseases, like neuropsychiatric syndromes, vertigo, tremor, neuropathy, Parkinson's syndrome, and cerebrovascular disease. The incidence of cerebrovascular diseases is disproportionally high, which is not only a consequence of cardio- and cerebrovascular arteriosclerosis but also of the cardiac disease itself. Especially patients with coronary artery disease in the state of acute myocardial infarction, patients with cardiomyopathy, mitral disease and enlarged atrium – with or without atrial fibrillation – develop intracardiac thrombi with the risk of cerebral embolism. Thus, patients awaiting cardiac surgery often have suffered from transient ischemic attacks (TIA), prolonged reversible ischemic neurological deficit (PRIND) or a completed stroke.

Especially high-grade asymptomatic carotid stenoses (17) and symptomatic carotid stenoses (25, 30, 43) have been identified to be an important risk factor regarding perioperative mortality and morbidity in cardiac surgical patients. This is also the case in preceding anamnestical ischemic incidents with perioperative stroke (59).

The incidence of non-cerebrovascular neurological diseases is not well known.

As the diagnosis of preexisting neurological diseases is of major importance for the evaluation of perioperative risk and for the distinction between preexisting syndromes and perioperative complications, the Heart Institute Lahr/Baden, FRG reguested a neurologist to evaluate the incidence of neurological diseases in cardiac

Table 1. General risk factors of the patients operated at the Heart Institute Lahr/Baden, FRG

risk factor	%
female gender	28.0
age > 70 years	34.0
diabetes mellitus	2.5
renal insufficiency, compensate	18.0
renal insufficiency, terminal	0.8
obstructive pulmonary disease	3.2
restrictive pulmonary disease	7.5
auto-immun disease	13.0
liver disease	1.3

Table 2. Preexisting neurological diseases in the patients operated at the Heart Institute Lahr/Baden, FRG (****see Table 3)

neurological disease	n	%
ischemic stroke****	154	3.80
diseases of the peripheral nervous system****	72	1.80
carotid artery stenosis	184	4.50
vertigo	4	0.10
cerebral trauma	20	0.50
seizures	24	0.60
essential tremor	20	0.10
neuropsychiatric disorders****	2	0.50
myasthenia gravis	2	0.05
multiple sclerosis	2	0.05
Parkinson's syndrome		0.05

Table 3. Specification of 'ischemic stroke', 'diseases of the peripheral nervous system' and 'neuropsychatric disorders' in the patients operated in the Heart Institute Lahr/Baden, FRG

neurological disease	specification	n	%
ischemic stroke****	with residuum	82	53.0
	without residuum	72	47.0
diseases of the peripheral nervous systems****	diabetic neuropathy	32	56.0
	nerve plexus damage	2	3.5
	peroneal paralysis	5	8.8
	intervertebral disc disorders	17	31.0
	unclear neuropathy	1	1.8
neuropsychiatric disorders****	vascular encephalopathy	4	20.0
	Alzheimer disease	2	10.0
	organic syndrome	10	5.0
	episodic amnesia	1	0.5
	disturbed consciousness	3	1.5

surgery. The results for the time span from 01. March 1995 to 30. May 1997 are demonstrated in Tables 2 and 3.

Perioperative neurological diseases

As stated above, neurological diseases may be present in cardiac surgical patients. However, all complicated operations bear the risk of negative effects on neurological functions. Anesthesia may cause hypotonia with hemodynamically induced insults or prolonged postoperative organic syndromes. Perioperative bleeding or thrombopathy may also result in neurological complications. The positioning during operation may cause peripheral paralyses.

Preexisting neurological diseases, such as, neuropsychological symptomes, Parkinson's syndrome, myasthenia gravis, may be aggravated by general anesthesia.

Various central and peripheral neurological disorders, for example, critical illness polyneuropathy, may result from postoperative complications with a prolonged stay in the intensive care unit or sepsis.

In cardiac surgery, there is a high perioperative occurrence of neurological symptomes, especially focal ischemic deficits or global neuropsychological deficits.

As a specific feature in cardiac surgery, the use of the heart-lung machine has been found to be responsible for a variety of complications due to enhanced coagulation in the tube system or oxygenator and infiltration of thrombogenic material (16, 26, 57), nonphysiological how (33, 69, 70), embolisation from the ascending aorta (3), gas embolism (31) or global hypoperfusion (29). In addition, preexisting thrombi can be detached (28) and, especially in valvular surgery, redissected material can enter the arterial circulation (13, 42).

It is often not easy to determine neurological complications in postoperative patients, especially focal ischemic deficits in intensive care patients are difficult to diagnose (27). In addition, focal ischemic deficits like TIA, PRIND or completed stroke can not be easily distinguished from global hypoxic and metabolic disturbances, which may also lead to neuropsychological changes. As a consequence, some focal neurological deficits are missed, or they are misdiagnosed as an organic syndrome. The data on neurological complications in our patients are summarized in Table 4. The organic syndrome was defined as an evident disturbance of time, local, and/or personal orientation. Mild cognitive deficits may have been missed in our group of patients, as longer lasting cognitive or psychic disturbances related to surgery were not recorded, as they would require complicated neuropsychological tests.

Table 4. Neurological complications in cardiac surgery patients determined from 4058 operations with the heart-lung-machine performed at the Heart Institute Lahr/Baden, FRG

neurological complications	incidence	%
ischemic stroke	48	1.2
organic syndrome	200	4.9
intracranial bleeding	0	0.0
paralysis of peroneal or ulnar nerve	15	0.4
seizures	4	0.2

Table 5. Incidence of Perioperative Stroke in the Literature

author	clinical course	n	%
Lytle et al. (37)	completed stroke	1689 AVR	1.7
Bojar et al. (6)	PRIND, stroke	3206	1.0
Shaw et al. (61)	completed stroke	1985	4.8
Bruer et al. (7)	completed stroke	421	5.2
Sotaniemi (65)	completed stroke	100 AVR	7.0
Lee (35)	completed stroke	943	0.7
Martin and Hashimoto (40)	completed stroke	253	3.7
Cernaianu et al. (11)	TIA, PRIND, completed stroke	2455	1.8
Rao et al. (54)	completed stroke	3910	1.4
McKhann et al. (41)	completed stroke	456	5.7
Heart Institute Lahr/Baden, FRG 1998	TIA, PRIND, completed stroke	4058	1.2

AVR = including aortic valve replacement

Perioperative focal ischemic deficits

In cardiac surgery, stroke is a serious complication and the most important non cardiac cause of perioperative morbidity and mortality. Earlier studies (8, 20, 29) reported a perioperative incidence of persisting neurological deficits of about 15%, whereas later studies (6, 7, 12, 23, 35, 61, 62) reported an incidence of 0.7–5.2%. While there has been a distinct decrease of cardiac mortality in recent years, the percentage of neurological fatalities has risen. According to the data of the Cleveland Clinic, USA, less than 10% of deaths in the seventies were primarily due to neurological complications compared to 20% in the eighties (14). These studies included strokes or major neurological deficits (see Table 5). Our own results correspond with those of Lee et al. (35). In general, prospective studies show a higher incidence of stroke than retrospective, especially in those, where all operated patients are seen by a neurologist (66). In our study, patients with obviously abnormal neurological functions were examined by a neurologist pre- and postoperatively. Thus, it is possible that some focal ischemias were not detected.

Perioperative focal ischemic deficits: Own experience

Among the 4058 operations performed in the Heart Institute Lahr/Baden, FRG, from the 1. March 1995–31. May 1997 there was an incidence of 48 ischemic strokes (1.2%), including 33 completed strokes (69%) , 10 PRINDs (21 %), and 5 TIAs (10 %) (see Table 1).

CT diagnosis

In 31 patients ischemia was confirmed by CT screening. Ischemia was located in the middle (18 patients, 58%), posterior (7 patients, 23%) and anterior cerebral artery territory (3 patients, 10%). Three patients (10%) exhibited a border zone infarction.

Clinical manifestations

Apart from 2 patients with hemianopsia, the main syndrome was hemiparesis (96%). An additional 25 patients (54 %) showed a distinct aphasia and in 13 patients (28 %) other distinct neuropsychological deficits such as neglect and speech apraxia were detected. A high number of patients (37 patients, 80%) showed a disturbance of consciousness. Out of these patients 9 (20 %) were comatose, 7 (15 %) stuporous, and 13 (28 %) somnolent. Eight (17 %) of the patients died as a direct consequence of the insult.

The results of our investigation with respect to the distribution of TIA, PRIND and completed stroke in cardiac surgical patients are shown in Table 6. The main symptoms and the affected territories are summarized in Tables 7 and 8.

Table 6. Distribution of principal stroke patterns according to the clinical course

completed stroke	33	69%
PRIND	10	21
TIA	5	10

Table 7. Symptoms of TIA, PRIND, and completed stroke

strokes	46	%
hemiparesis left side	25	52.1
hemiparesis right side	17	35.0
aphasia	26	54.0
hemianopsia	2	4.2
neuropsychiatric deficits	13	27.1
coma	9	18.6
stupor	7	14.6
death	8	16.6

Table 8. Differentition according to the affected artery territories

arterial territories	n	%
middle cerebral artery	22	45
anterior cerebral artery	4	8
posterior cerebral artery	7	15
unclear cerebral artery	12	25
border zone infarction	3	6

Etiologies of perioperative stroke: Use of the heart-lung machine

Ever since its use, the cardiopulmonary bypass has been related to cerebral damage (2, 48). In this context the following pathogenetical mechanisms can be of importance.

Atheroembolism of the ascending aorta

In most cases, the heart-lung machine is connected to the ascending aorta. Some authors observed an accumulation of strokes with increasing age, a high incidence of peripheral artery disease in stroke patients, and there was also evidence of systemic atheroembolism. This leads to the conclusion that atheroembolism originating from a sclerotic ascending aorta is the result of the cannulation or the 'sand blasting' effect where atheromatous material is detached from the aortic wall by the jet of the arterial cannula. This seems to be an important factor leading to perioperative strokes (3). As a consequence, transesophageal sonography has been used to determine the extent of atherosclerosis of the ascending aorta (38) in order to affect cannulation or insertion of the proximal anastomoses at less sclerotic regions or to apply the so-called 'no-touch technique' (15).

Gas embolism, Platelet aggregates

During temporary bypass with the heart-lung machine, diffuse embolisation of gas occurs, which has been repeatedly shown by retinal angiography and transcranial sonography (5, 45, 51). It has been shown that the extent of embolisation has a direct effect on the outcome of the operation in a way that patients who exhibited more symptoms of embolisation suffered more often from neuropsychological dysfunction (53, 68). Also histological changes of the cerebral microvascular system were observed as a consequence of air embolism (9). However, there was no evidence of a relationship between air embolism and stroke. Besides, gas emboli other microemboli can reach the cerebral vascular territories through temporary bypass with the heart-lung machine (4). Platelet fibrin aggregates can play an important role in this regard. Although the plasma coagulation system is controlled by heparinization, the function of the platelets is not, which can lead to activation and formation of platelet aggregates during operation and postoperative lack of platelets (2, 26).

Hyperthermia

A temporary hyperthermia may occur with warming up during the operation and in relation with the varying perfusion through the heart-lung machine or the gas embolism and may provoke postoperative neuropsychological dysfunction. In addition, hyperthermia could also cause a reduced ischemic in focal ischemic lesions (46). For better myocardial protection, it has been lately recommended to perform uncomplicated cardiac surgery in normothermia instead of hyperthermia as no differences concerning the stroke risk were determined (71). But some authors found a clearly higher stroke rate in normothermal perfusion vs. hypothermic perfusion: 3.1 % vs. 1.0 % (39). Our own results do not show any correlation between the incidence of a TIA, PRIND or complete stroke and the lowest rectal temperature (independent t-test, $p > 0.05$).

Hypoperfusion or non-pulsatile perfusion

It is still unclear whether hypoperfusion contributes to postoperative cerebral morbidity. According to a recently published study (22), the stroke rate (and mortality) could be significantly lowered by maintaining a high perfusion pressure of 80–100 mmHg, whereas most of the other authors report perfusion pressures of 50 mmHg to be sufficient. The primary of perfusion pressure over flow rates should be considered (60). An increased perfusion may theoretically lead to a higher load of microemboli from the heart-lung machine. This is underlined by the fact that a cerebral luxus perfusion provoked by the 'ph stat method' leads postoperatively to more disturbance of the cognitive functions than by the 'alpha-stat method' (74). The effect of the used either pulsatile or nonpulsatile flow patterns on cerebral function is still unclear (32, 69, 70).

Table 9. Possible etiologies of the perioperative insult at the Heart Institute Lahr/Baden, FRG

etiology (pressumption)	n	%
unclear atrial fibrillation	14	29
postoperative atrial fibrillation with conversion	8	17
anterior wall aneurysm or trial fibrillation	6	13
unclear	6	8
hemodynamical	4	8
symptomatic carotid stenosis	4	6
carotid endarteriectomy	3	4
lacunar insult	2	2
thromboembolism in dilatative cardiomyopathy	1	1

Table 10. Time interval between the end of surgery and the occurence of focal ischemia

interval after surgery	n	%
< 12 h	13	27
12–48 h	15	31
> 48 h	20	42

Table 11. Incidence of late stroke after surgery

study	interval: OP-stroke
New Jersey (11)	32% > 48 h
Buffalo (56)	59% > 24 h
Lahr	42% > 48 h

Etiologies of stroke: Evaluation in the Heart Institute Lahr/Baden, FRG

We tried to establish possible and probable etiologies of stroke in our patients, considering CT diagnosis, risk factors, and abnormalities of the clinical course. The results are listed in Table 9. In 2 patients with low output syndrome and border zone infarction in CT, we presume hemodynamic strokes. Two other patients with low output syndrome and intraaortic ballon pump had territory infarction in CT. Other possible causes are listed in Table 9. In 4 cases with an early appearence of stroke, a possible etiology could not be found. Atrial fibrillation is an established etiological factor in the development of stroke. The incidence of atrial fibrillation is known to increase greatly during the postoperative period. Thus, atrial fibrillation with conversion should be considered as an etiological factor of perioperative stroke. This is underlined by the fact that the distribution of stroke in our patients shows a distinct dependence on the postoperative time interval. A total of 27 % of strokes occured immediately after surgery and 42 % that occured in a noticeable interval after surgery (Table 10). The increased incidence of stroke in a late postoperative period was also observed by other authors (Table 11).

Effect of preexisting neurological diseases on the incidence of perioperative neurological diseases

Preexisting neurological diseases were found to correlate with neurological complications, postoperative morbidity, and mortality. The result from multiple studies are summarized in Table 12. A 7-fold increase in the stroke rate was determined in relation to a prior stroke (44) and a 9-fold increase connection with a carotid stenosis (56). Mortality rate even increase up to the 21-fold (11).

In our study, the risk of a perioperative stroke rose from 1.2 % to 2.6 % (2.4-fold) for patients who suffered from a perioperative prior stroke (Table 13). These

Table 12. Dependence of the postoperative stroke rate and mortality on the prior stroke and internal carotid artery stenosis

risk factors				prior stroke	prior stroke	ACI-stenosis
authors	n	postop. stroke rate	mortality rate	postop. stroke rate	mortality rate	postop. stroke rate
Cernaianu et al. (11)	2455	1.8		2.3	38.6	
McKhann et al. (41)	456	5.7	4.2	6.6	19.2	17.0
Mickleborough et al. (44)	1631	1.2	1.3	8.2	26.0	3.2
Newman et al. (49)	2417	3.2				11.0
Rao et al. (54)	3910	1.4	2.2	8.0	22.2	
Ricotta et al. (56)	1779	1.6	3.7	4.6	17.0	14.7

Table 13. Preexisting neurological disease and neurological complications I

		stroke	stenosis	syndrome	
complications	4058	154	184	20	24
ischemic stroke	1.2%	2.6%	5.4%		
organic syndrome	4.9%	12%	8%	95%	
subarachnoid-, intracerebral bleeding	0%				
paralysis of the peroneal or ulnar nerve	0.40%				
epilepsia	0.10%				8.30%
death	2.40%	6.50%			
intensive care stay	2.9 days	3.7 days		4.7 days	

Table 14. Preexisting neurological disease and neurological complications II

preexisting neurological disease	n	complications
peripheral nerve paralysis	72	differentiation to perioperative defects
cerebral trauma	20	none
vertigo	4	none
essential tremor	4	none
myasthenia gravis	2	prolonged intensive care
multiple sclerosis	2	prolonged intensive care
Parkinson's syndrome	2	prolonged intensive care

patients did stay significantly longer in the intensive care unit (3.7 d), the incidence of postoperative severe disorientation rose up to 12 %, and especially the mortality rate was raised to 6.5 % (2.7-fold). Besides the stroke in history, the high-grade carotid stenosis also raised the stroke incidence (to 5.4 %). The postoperative stay at the intensive care unit was significantly prolonged (4.7%) in patients with a preexisting organic syndrome due to an aggravation of neuropsychiatric disorders. All other preexisting neurological diseases were accompanied only by minimal postoperative problems (Table 14). Patients with myasthenia gravis, multiple sclerosis, and Parkinson's syndrome required a prolonged stay in the intensive care unit, due to retarded mobilization.

Table 15. Variables correlating with the perioperative stroke

risk factors	first author
age	Rao et al. (54), McKhann et al. (41),
	Mickleborough et al. (44), Newmann et al. (66)
calcification of the ascending aorta	Gardner et al. (20), Lynn et al. (36),
	Mickleborough et al. (44), Cernaianu et al. (11)
carotid bruit	Mc Khann et al. (41), Newmann et al. (49)
carotid stenosis > 50%	Ricotta et al. (56)
diabetes	Rao et al. (54), Lynn et al. (36),
	McKhann et al. (41)
hyperlipidemia	Ricotta et al. (56)
hypertension	Mc Khann et al. (41), Cernaianu et al. (36)
left ventricular thrombus	Lynn et al. (36)
peripheral vascular disease	Rao et al. (54), Mickleborough et al. (44)
prior stroke	Rao et al. (54), Gardner et al. (18), McKhann et al.
reduced ejection fraction	(41)
reoperation	Mickleborough et al. (44), Newmann et al. (49)
three vessel disease	Ricotta et al. (56)
valve replacement	Rao et al. (54)
	Ricotta et al. (56)

Table 16. Comparison of selected preoperative anamnestic parameters between patients with or without stroke

	stroke	no stroke	p-value
n	48	4112	
age	66	65	n.s.
female gender	1121	12	n.s.
β-blocker	15	1858	< 0.05
aneurysmectomy	4	41	< 0.0001
antiarrhythmic agent	4	84	< 0.01
aortic valve disease	13	709	< 0.05
carotid artery stenosis	10	174	< 0.0001
catecholamine	2	39	< 0.05
digitalis	14	670	< 0.05
diuretics	19	1042	< 0.01
ejection fraction	49%	71%	< 0.0001
preoperative stroke	38	3729	< 0.0001
ventricular aneurysm	8	625	< 0.0001

Risk factor analysis and prediction of stroke: Own experience

Focal ischemias: TIA, PRIND or completed stroke are the most important neurological complications in cardiac surgery. Therefore, it would be beneficial if the risk of such complications could be preoperatively predicted for each patient. In order to develop a pattern for the risk prediction, the following steps can be followed:

1. Exact detection of strokes to determine a statistical value.
2. Extensive study of anamnestical data as variable.
3. Identification of variables that are statistically related to the incidence of strokes.
4. Input of identified data in a statistical pattern of prediction (e.g., multiple regression analysis).
5. Evaluation of the prediction results by use of prospective tests.

However, the published results are often contradictory; especially such factors as high age, diabetes, hyperlipidemia, and valvular surgery could not be confirmed by all authors (Table 15). Moreover, in most cases only insufficient preoperative data were available. Finally, there was a preselection of data with respect to the typical atherosclerotic risk factors.

In our study, a total of 69 anamnestical parameters were evaluated from 4058 surgical patients. Analysis by univariate statistics shows that 11 of the parameters significantly ($p < 0.01$) correlated with the occurence of stroke (Table 16).

Risk factor analysis and prediction of stroke: Literature survey

According to these results patients with high age, diabetes, obesity, hypertonia, peripheral arterial disease, prior valvular surgery, repeated coronary surgery, 3 vessel disease did not show a higher risk of perioperative stroke. This is especially remarkable as far as age is concerned. Tuman et al. (80) observed a distinct age-dependency of perioperative stroke, the stroke, risk in his study was < 1 % for patients under 65 and about 5 % for patients over 65. This fact was observed by other authors too (see Table 15), whereas Cernaianu et al. (11) and Ricotta et al. (56) could not confirm these results. They found no correlation between age and perioperative stroke. In contrast to the results of Slogoff et al. (63) and Wong et

Table 17. Preexisting factors related to the occurence of a perioperative stroke

preoperative factor	score
aneurysmectomy	8
disturbance of the consciousness	8
ventricular aneurysm	3
carotid stenosis (> 50%)	3
administration of antiarrhythmic agents	3
prior stroke	2
administration of diuretics	1

al. (24), open-heart surgery (valvular surgery) did not represent a higher risk in our patients compared to coronary surgery.

The results of regression analysis are given in Table 17. There are 7 factors correlating with stroke. The weights in the regression analysis are presented as score points.

The prediction power of this analysis was rather low (predicted value 14 %). Intraoperative events, which were not registered during our extensive preoperativedata collection, play an important role in the etiology of the stroke. For example, the temporary bypass time with the heart-lung machine is a highly significant factor regarding the incidence of an insult (t-test, $p < 0.001$). This was also observed by other authors, e.g., McKhann et al. (41).

However, there remains a great discrepancy between our results and those of McKhann et al. (41). He calculated a perioperative stroke risk of 74 % for patients over 75 years of age with prior stroke, carotid stenosis, hypertonia, and diabetes mellitus. The above mentioned atherosclerotic risk factors are the only preoperative predictive factors that turned out to be relevant for the prediction pattern. Factors like chronic atrial fibrillation or ventricular aneurysm have not been considered, which is very astonishing if one looks at the high plausibility of these risk factors. In our group of patients, hypertonia, diabetes mellitus, and age did not correlate with the incidence of stroke.

Risk factor profiles

The discrepancy in the risik factor analysis (see Table 18) are related not only to the selection of the preoperative data, but also to the statistical problems as well. We could demonstrate this by 'semantic computing'. This statistical method enables the formation of groups of patients according to the risk factors (1). By this we could show that the group of patients with severe atherosclerosis, as described by McKhann et al. (41), form only one of these groups. Another risk group is formed by patients with preoperative antiarrhythmical therapy, probably because of their tendency to atrial fibrillation with the risk of intraatrial thrombi development. Another risk group are the patients with dilatative cardiomyopathy. In conventional statistics, the old patients in the group with severe atherosclerosis are mixed together with the young patients suffering from dilatative cardiomyopathy. Thus, the age of whole group becomes normal, and in statistical analysis a significant difference between the patients with and without stroke can not be found. In this way we could explain the differences concerning the stroke risk factors found in the literature (Table 18).

Intraoperative prophylaxis of a perioperative stroke

Table 19 shows a selection of intraoperative measures for the prevention of a perioperative stroke. However, some of the following points are not accepted by all authors (e.g., hypothermia).

Table 18. Discrepancy between the results of different studies concerning perioperative stroke

	Roach et al. (55)	McKhann et al. (41)	Cernaianu et al. (11)	mixed studies	Lahr 98	Lahr 98
method	multivariat analysis	multivariat analysis	univariat analysis	diverse	multivariat analysis	semantic computing
3 vessel disease	n.i.	n.s.	n.i.	****		****
age	****	****	n.s.		n.s.	****
aorta ascendens sclerosis	****	n.i.	n.i.		n.i.	n.i.
aortic valve disease	n.s.	n.i.	n.u.	****	****	****
aortic valve replacement	n.i.	n.i.	n.s.			n.s.
atrial fibrillation	n.i.	n.i.	n.i.		****	****
carotid stenosis	n.s.	****	n.s.		****	****
COPD	****	n.i.	n.i.		n.s.	****
diabetes	****	****	n.s.		n.s.	****
disturbence of the conciousness		n.i.	n.i.		****	
hyperlipidemia	n.s.	n.s.	n.s.			****
hypertonia	****	****	****		n.s.	****
instable angina	****	n.s.	n.i.			n.s.
LV-aneurysm		n.i.	n.i.		****	****
prior stroke	****	****	****		****	****
red. ejection fraction		n.i.	n.i.	****		****
reoperation		n.i.	n.i.	****		****

n.s. – non significant; n.i. – preoperative data not included in the study; **** – risk factors confirmed by the study group above

Table 19. Selected intraoperative measures for stroke prophylaxis

1.	Careful ventilation prior to the opening of the aortic clamp (34, 50, 52, 58)
2.	Head-down position at the beginning of cardiac output
3.	Use of isoflurane and theopental for protection against cerebral ischemia (75)
4.	Hypothermia during operation
5.	Maintenance of adequate blood flow and pressure
6.	Adequate anticoagulation during temporary bypass with heart-lung machine
7.	Alpha-stat instead of ph-stat (47)
8.	Maintenance of normoglycemia
9.	Aortic scanning for the selection of optimal cannulation site
10.	EEG monitoring
11.	Use of membrane oxygenators instead of bubble oxygenators (5, 31, 51)
12.	Use of arterial filter (19, 51)
13.	Insertion of proximal anastomoses intruncus brachiocephalicus in case of porcelain aorta

Postoperative prophylaxis of focal ischemic deficits

So far the issue of the postoperative stroke prophylaxis has been confronted in only a few publications. Our observations and those of the authors listed in Table 11 show that 30–60 % of perioperative strokes occur after a time interval of > 24 h after surgery. In view of this long postoperative time span, there must be other precipitating factors, other than direct manipulation on the heart or aorta with its risk of embolisation or infiltration of the thrombogenic material through the heart-lung machine. This accumulation of postoperative strokes asks for explanation. The following etiologies are to be considered:

1. The high incidence of atrial fibrillation (up to 70 %) lasting often several hours or even days, bearing the risk of formation of atrial thrombi with subsequent embolisation especially with the background of insufficient anticoagulation.
2. Exsiccosis mainly from insufficient fluid intake and/or enhanced fluid elimination in elderly patients with reduced cardiac function.
3. Rebound of heparin after extracorporal circulation, resistance to heparin or insufficient dosage. Latest studies show that an abrupt discontinuation of heparin, effect antagonization of heparin, result in hypercoaguability that manifests itself by increased thrombin activity and activation of protein C (24) and clinically by an accumulation of thrombotic events (21, 72). An immediate postoperative heparin administration is almost impossible after cardiac surgery due to the high bleeding risk. Therefore, hypercoagubility is always present and could be one of the reasons for the perioperative accumulation of strokes. The individual bleeding risk and the risk of thrombosis should be considered. In this context, the identification of patients with a higher risk of thrombosis, for example by means of a score or risk division as in Table 18, would be beneficial.

Treatment of focal ischemic deficits

The treatment of a postoperative stroke should be started right after the diagnosis or already when it is suspected, and it should comply with the general directions of the stroke therapy or the measures recommended by Hacke et al. (27) (see Table 20).

Table 20. Recommended treatment of perioperative stroke

1.	Neurologic examination by a neurologist/CT scanning
2.	80 mmHg < arterial blood pressure < 120 mmHg
3.	30% elevation of the trunk
4.	body temeprature < 37.5 °C if necessary by administration of antipyretic drugs or cooling
5.	100 mg/dl < blood glucose < 200 mg/dl
6.	Arterial blood gases: PCO_2 < 50 mmHg, early mechanical ventilation
7.	Hyperosmolar therapy
8.	Early transfer to the neurology department, if necessary trepanation

Neuropsychological dysfunctions

The identification of cognitive or neurological dysfunctions is difficult. A comparison of the pre- und postoperative condition by neuropsychological tests can lead to mistakes due to the influence of typical preoperative moods like fear. Repeated postoperative tests may be be of limited value due to adaptation by learning. The Rey test in relation with a control group, however, has turned out to be effective (10). However, there is an increasing evidence of disturbed cerebral function due to cardiac surgery. In 50–60% of the patients, neuropsychological disturbances have been found after bypass surgery (47, 64, 74).

In most cases, the disturbances resolve completely, although according to some studies neurological or psychical defects could still be detected years after surgery. Murkin et al. (47), for example, found disturbances of the cognitive function in 22 % of patients three years after bypass surgery, and in 18 % they found neurological symptoms in comparison to the preoperative state. According to Sotaniemi et al. (67) some patients suffered from cognitive disturbances even 5 years after surgery.

The same pathogenetic mechanisms that provoke TIA, PRIND, and completed stroke have to be considered. Further, diffuse cerebral damage caused by microembolisms, different perfusion due to temporary bypass or hyperthermia may play a role. It was shown that the use of arterial filters (53) have an impact on the neuropsychological outcome of the patients.

These studies are all based on the evaluation of elective bypass surgeries and patients without neurological symptoms. Therefore, little is known about the incidence of preoperative and postoperative neuropsychological disturbances in patients with nonelective cardiac surgery and those with prior neurological or neuropsychatrical symptoms.

Appendix

Spectrum of operations and data acquisition in the Heart Institute Lahr/Baden, FRG

Patients and operations

All patients that underwent cardiac surgery with the heart-lung machine since April 1995 were included in the study, except for aortic surgery, atrial septum defect- and ventricular septum defect-suture. In all, 4058 patients with the average of 65 years were included. Women represented 29% of the patients. The operation spectrum comprised: 75 % coronary surgery with an additional 4 % of re-surgery, 8 % aortic valve replacement, 3 % mitral valve replacement, 1.5 % aortic surgery, 5 % combined operations and 1 % double-valve replacement. Normally anesthesia was induced with Hypnomidate and continued with Midazolam and Sufentanyl occasionally Isofluran was added. The patients were paralyzed by i.v. Pancuronium. After median sternotomy and heparinization, cardiopulmonary bypass was initiated by cannulation of the atrium and the ascending aorta, or in exceptional cases with strong aortic calcifications, of the truncus brachiocephalicus. Jostra HL 20 heart-lung machines were used with the capillary oxygenerators Jostra Quadrox or Biocor

200 or GOBE Optima. An atrial filter with a pore size of 40 µm was connected. The aspired value of cardiac output was 120 % of the calculated value, where the body surface area was multiplied by 2.5. The mean blood pressures were to be about 60 mmHg; in patients with carotid stenoses higher. The flow profile was not pulsatile and the temperature was 34 (in short-term surgery, in most of the cases 30–32°, and in special surgery lower. Hematocrit was between 26 and 30 %.

Neurology

All patients received a preoperative ultrasound of the extracranial vessels. Patients with neurological diseases or incidences underwent a preoperative examination by a neurological specialist. Postoperatively, all patients with focal neurological deficits occurring 5–7 days after surgery underwent an examination by a specialist. With the exception of 6 patients with TIA, all other patients received a CT of the brain. Patients suffering exclusively from organic syndrome or discret neurological symptoms or patients with resuscitation defects were not considered. Immediately after a stroke was diagnosed, neuroprotective therapy was initiated by regulation of the blood pressure in the upper standard range, elevation of the trunk, hypothermia, CO_2 control – at signs of high intracranial pressure mannitol and glycerin were administered or trepanation was performed (2 cases).

Data acquisition

In order to obtain a common data bank, the data from the Data Pec System of our anesthesiological department (about 100 preoperative parameters) were combined with the data of the quality assurance system of our surgical department (about 40 preoperative parameters). The 'strokes' were recorded prospectively.

Statistical analysis

The dependence of the stroke recurrence in the preoperative variables was determined by statistical analysis using contiguity tables for category data and t-test or Mann-Whitney-U-Test for continuous data. The variables reaching a P-value < 0.1 entered the multiple logistic and hierarchic regression analysis which determined a small group of independent and significant variables. Semantic computing was performed with the software of ASOC AG, Offenburg/Baden, FRG (1).

References

1. Bernhard M, Borrelli P, Weineck J (1977) Semantic computing. Eine neue Lösung für wissensverarbeitende Systeme. ASOC AG
2. Blauth CL (1997) The role of cardiopulmonary bypass technique in cerebral protection. In: Ennker J, Coselli JS, Treasure T (eds) Cerebral Protection in Cerebrovascular and Aortic Surgery. Darmstadt, Steinkopff, pp 177–84
3. Blauth CL, Cosgrove DM, Webb BW et al. (1992) Atheroembolism from the ascending aorta. J Thorac Cardiovasc Surg 103:1104–12
4. Blauth CI (1995) Macroembolie and microembolie during cardiopulmonary bypass. Ann Thorac Surg 59:1300–3

5. Blauth CL, Smith PL, Arnold JV et al. (1990) Influence of oxygenator type on the prevalence and extent of microembolic retinal ischemia during cardiopulmonary bypass. Assessment by digital image analysis. J Thorac Cardiovasc Surg 99:61–9
6. Bojar RM, Najafi H, Delaria GA et al. (1983) Neurological complications of coronary revascularisation. Ann Thorac Surg 36:427–32
7. Breuer AC, Furlan AJ, Hanson MR et al. (1983) Central nervous system complications of coronary artery bypass graft surgery. BMJ 14:682–87
8. Brierley JB (1967) Brain damage complicating open heart surgery: A neuropathological study of 46 patients. Proc R Soc Med 858–9
9. Brown WR, Moody DM, Stump DA et al. (1995) Dog model for cerebrovascular studies of proximal-to-distal distribution of sequentialy injected emboli. Ann Thorac Surg 59:1304–7
10. Bruggemans EF, van Dijk JG, Huysmans HA (1995) Residual cognitive dysfunctioning at 6 months following coronary artery bypass graft surgery. Eur J Cardiothorac Surg 9:636–643
11. Cernaianu AC, Teimouraz V, Flum D et al. (1995) Predictors of stroke after cardiac surgery 10:334–339
12. Coffey CE, Massey W, Roberts KB et al. (1983) Natural history of cerebral complications of coronary artery bypass graft surgery. Neurology 33:1416–21
13. Coselli JS, Crawford ES (1986) Aortic valve replacement in the patient with extensive calcification of the ascending aorta (the porcelain aorta). J Thorac Cardiovasc Surg 91:184–7
14. Cosgrove DM, Loop FD, Lyttle BW et al. (1988) Primary myocardial revascularisation trends in surgical mortality. J Thorac Cardiovasc Surg 673–84
15. Culliford AT, Stephen BC, Rohrer K et al. (1986) The atherosclerotic ascending aorta and transverse arch: a new technique to prevent cerebral injury during bypass: Experience with 13 patients. Ann Thorac Surg 41:27–35
16. Evans EA, Wellington JS (1994) Emboli associated with cardiopulmonary bypass. J Thorac Surg 48:323–30
17. Furlan AJ, Craciun AR (1985) Risk of stroke during coronary artery bypass graft surgery in patients with internal carotid artery disease documented by angiography. Stroke 16:797–9
18. Gardner TJ, Horneffer PJ, Manolio Ta et al (1985) Stroke following coronary artery bypass grafting: a ten-year study. An Thorac Surg 40:574–81
19. Garvey JW, Wilner A, Wolpowitz A et al. (1983) The effect of arterial filtration during open heart surgery. Circulation 68 (Suppl II): 125–8
20. Gilman S (1965) Cerebral disorders after open-heart operations. N Engl J Med 272:489–94
21. Gold HK, Torres F, Garabedian H et al. (1993) Evidence for a rebound coagulation phenomenon after cessation of a 4-hour infusion of a specific thrombin inhibitor in patients with unstable angina pectoris. J Am Coll Cardiol 21:1039–47
22. Gold JP, Charlson ME, Williams-Russo P et al. (1995) Improvement of outcomes after coronary artery bypass. A randomized trial comparing intraoperative high versus low mean arterial pressure. J Thorac Cardiovasc Surg 110:1302–14
23. Gonzales-Scarano F, Hurtig H (1981) Neurologic complications of coronary artery bypass grafting:case-control study. Neurology 31:1032–5
24. Granger CB, Miller J, Bovill EG et al. (1995) Rebound increase in thrombin generation and activity after cessation of intravenous heparin in patients with acute coronary syndromes. Circulation 91:1929–35
25. Gravlee GP, Cordell AR, Graham JE et al. (1985) Coronary revascularization in patients with bilateral internal carotid occlusion. J Thorac Cardiovasc Surg 90:921–5
26. Guidoin RG, Awald JA, Laperche Y et al. (1975) Nature of deposits in atubular membrane oxygenotors after prolonged extracorporeal circulation. A scanning electron microscope study. J Thorac Cardiovasc Surg 69:479–91
27. Hacke W, Schwab S, de Georgia (1997) Intensive care of acute ischemic stroke. In: Ennker J, Coselli JS, Treasure T (eds) Cerebral Protection in Cerebrovascular and Aortic Surgery. Darmstadt, Steinkopff, pp 37–47
28. Hartman RB, Harrison EE, Pupello DF et al (1983) Characteristics of left ventricular thrombus resulting in perioperative embolism. A complication of bypass grafting. J Thorac Cardiovasc Surg 86:706–709
29. Javid H, Tufo HM, Najafi H et al. (1969) Neurological abnormalities following open-heart surgery. J Thorac Cardiovasc Surg 58:502–9
30. Jones EC, Craver JU, Michalik RS et al. (1984) Combined carotid and coronary operations: are they necessary? J Thorac Cardiovasc Surg 87:7–10

31. Kessler J, Patterson RH (1970) The production of microemboli by various blood oxygenators. Ann Thorac Surg 9:221–8
32. Kirklin JW, Barrat-Boyes BG (1993) Cardiac Surgery, 2nd edition, Churchill Livingston, New York pp 89–91
33. Kritikou PE, Branthwaite MA (1977) Significance of changes in cerebral electrical activity at onset of cardiopulmonary bypass. Thorax 2:534–8
34. Lawrence GH, McKay HA, Sherensky RT (1971) Effective measures in the prevention of intraoperative aeroembolus. J Thorac Cardiovasc Surg 62:731–5
35. Lee MC, Geiger J, Nicoloff D et al. (1997) Cerebrovascular complications associated with coronary artery bypass (CAB) procedures. Stroke 10:107
36. Lynn GM, Stefanko K, Reed JJ et al. (1992) Risk factors for stroke after coronary artery bypass. J Thorac Cardiovasc Surg. 104:1518–1523
37. Lytle BW, Cosgrove DM, Taylor PC et al. (1989) Primary isolated aortic valve replacement. J Thorac Cardiovasc Surg 97:675–94
38. Marschall K, Kanchuger M, Kessler K et al. (1994) Superiority of transesophageal echocardiography in detecting aortic arch disease: Identification of patients at increased risk of stroke during cardiac surgery. J Cardiothorac Vasc Surg 8:5–13
39. Martin TD, Craver JM, Gott JP et al. (1994) Prospective, randomized trial of retrograde warm blood cardioplegia: myocardial benefit and neurologic threat. Ann Thorac Surg 57:298–304
40. Martin WRW, Hashimoto SA (1982) Stroke in coronary bypass surgery: Can J Neurol Sci 9:21–6
41. McKhann GM, Goldsborough MA, Borowicz LM et al. (1997) Predictors of stroke risk in coronary artery bypass patients. Ann Thorac Surg 63:516–21
42. McKibbin DW, Bulkley BH, Green WR et al. (1976) Fatal cerebral atheromatous embolization after cardiopulmonary bypass. J Thorac Cardiovasc Surg 71:741–5
43. Mehigan JT, Bush WS, Pipkin RD et al (1977) A planned approach to coexistant cerebrovascular disease in coronary artery bypass candidates. Arch Surg 112:1403–9
44. Mickleborough LL, Walker PM, Takagi Y et al. (1996) J Thorac Cardiovasc Surg 112:1250–58
45. Moody DM, Bell MA, Challa VR et al. (1990) Brain microemboli during cardiac surgery or aortography. Ann Neurol 28:477–486
46. Moody DM, Brown WR, Stump DA et al. (1995) Dog model for cerebrovascular studies of the proximal-to-distal distribution of sequentialy injected emboli. Microvasc Res 50:105–112
47. Murkin JM, Martzke JS, Buchan AM et al. (1995) A randomized study of the influence of perfusion technique and ph management strategy in 316 patients undergoing coronary artery bypass surgery. II Neurologic and cognitive outcomes. J Thorac Cardiovasc Surg 110:349–62
48. Murkin JM (1997) The brain at risk during cardiopulmonary bypass. Cardiovascular Engineering 2:104–12
49. Newman MF, Wolman R, Kanchuger M, et al. (1996) Multicenter preoperative risk index for patients undergoing coronary artery bypass surgery. Circulation 94: Suppl II:II-74-II-80
50. Oka Y, Inoue T, Hong Y et al. (1986) Retained intracardiac air. Transesophageal echocardiography for definition of incidence and monitoring removal by improved techniques. J Thorac Cardiovasc Surg 91:329–38
51. Padayachee TS, Parsons S, Theobold R et al. (1987) The detection of microemboli in the middle cerebral artery during cardiopulmonary bypass: a transcranial Doppler ultrasound investigation using membrane and bubble oxygenators. Ann Thorac Surg 298–302
52. Padula RT, Eisenstat TE Bronstein MH et al. (1971) Intracardiac air following cardiotomy. Location, causative factors, and a method for removal. J Thorac Cardiovasc Surg 62:736–42
53. Pugsley W, Klinger L, Paschalis C et al. (1994) The impact of microemboli during cardiopulmonary bypass on neuropsychological functioning. Stroke 25:1393–9
54. Rao V, Christakis GT, Weisel RD et al. (1995) Risk factors for stroke following coronary bypass surgery. J Card Surg 10:468–74
55. Roach GW, Karrchiger M, Mangano CM et al. (1996) Adverse cerebral outcomes after coronary bypass surgery. N Engl J Med 335:1857–63
56. Ricotta JJ, Faggioloi GL, Castilone A et al. (1995) Risk factors for stroke after cardiac surgery:Buffalo Cardiac-Cerebral Study Group. J Vasc Surg 21:359–64
57. Reed CC, Romagnoli A, Taylor DE et al. (1974) Particulate matter in bubble oxygenators. J Thorac Cardiovasc Surg 68:971–4
58. Robicsek F, Duncan GD (1987) Retrograde air embolization in coronary operations. J Thorac Cardiovasc Surg 94:110–4

59. Rorick MB, Furlan AJ (1990) Risk of cardiac surgery in patients with prior stroke. Neurology 40:835–837
60. Schwartz AE, Sandhu AA, Kaplon RJ et al. (1995) Cerebral blood flow is determined by arterial pressure and not cardiopulmonary bypass flow rate. Ann Thorac Surg 60:165–70
61. Shaw PJ, Bares D, Cartlidge NEF et al. (1985) Early neurological complications of coronary artery bypass surgery. BMJ 291:1384
62. Silverstein A, Krieger HP (1960) Neurologic complications of cardiac surgery. Arch Neurol 5:601–5
63. Slogoff A, Girgis KZ, Keats AS (1982) Etiologic factors in neuropsychatric complications associated with cardiopulmonary bypass. Anesth Analg 61:903–11
64. Smith PLC, Newman SP, Ell Pj et al. (1996) Cerebral consequences of cardiopulmonary bypass. Lancet 1:823–5
65. Sotaniemi KA (1980) Brain damage and neurological outcome after open-heart surgery. J Neurol Neurosurg Psychiatry 43:127–35
66. Sotaniemi KA (1983) Cerebral outcome after extracorporeal circulation: Comparison between prospective and retrospective evaluations. Arch Neurol 40:75–7
67. Sotaniemi KA, Mononen H, Hokkanen TE (1986) Long-term cerebral outcome after open heart surgery: a five year neuro-psychological follow-up study. Stroke 17:410–16
68. Stump DA, Rogers AT, Hammon JW, Newman SP (1995) Cerebral emboli and cognitive outcomes after cardiac surgery. J Cardiothorac Vasc Anesth 10:113–9
69. Taylor KM, Bain WH, Maxted KJ et al. (1987) Comparative studies of pulsatile and nonpulsatile flow during CPB. I Pulsatile system employed and ist hematologic effects. J Thorac Cardiovasc Surg 75:569–73
70. Taylor KM, Wright GS, Reid JM et al. (1987) Comparative studies of pulsatile and nonpulsatile flow during CPB. II. The effects on adrenal secretion of cortisol. J Thorac Cardiovasc Surg 75:574–8
71. The Warm Heart Investigators (1994) Randomised trial of normothermic versus hypothermic coronary bypass surgery. Lancet 343:559–63
72. Theroux P, Waters D, Lam J et al. (1992) Reactivation of unstable angina after the discontinuation of heparin. N Engl J Med 327:141–145
73. Tuman KJ, Mc Carthy RJ, Najafi H et al. (1992) Differential effects of advanced age on neurologic and cardiac risks of coronary artery operations. J Thorac Cardiovasc Surg 104:1510–7
74. Venn GE, Patel RL, Chambers DJ (1995) Cardiopulmonary bypass: perioperative cerebral blood flow and postoperative cognitive deficit. Ann Thorac Surg 59:1331–5
75. Wong DHW (1991) Perioperative stroke part II: Cardiac surgery and cardiogenic embolic stroke. Can J Anesth 38:471–88

Author's address:
Dr. Alexander Albert
Herzzentrum Lahr/Baden
Hohbergweg 2
77933 Lahr

Cardiac surgery and neurological disorders

V. Schuchardt

Neurologische Klinik, Klinikum Lahr, Germany

Introduction

From a neurological point of view, cardiac surgery is important in two aspects: (1) risks of surgery and modifications of surgical procedures due to preexisting neurological disorders, (2) neurological / neuropsychological complications and sequelae after heart surgery. In-hospital mortality is 10-fold in persons with neurological complications and 5-fold in patients with neuropsychological complications. Duration of intensive care, hospital stay after surgery, and the rate of discharge to care facilities is higher in patients with complications (28). The neurologist's task is to find out or rule out a neurological disorder, to estimate the individual risk, and to diagnose and treat specific neurological complications.

Preexisting neurological diseases

Any surgical procedure might be unfavorable in certain diseases of the nervous system because of the stress of general anesthesia and the operation itself, relaxation, disruption of long-term medication, and provocation of exacerbations. In cardiac surgery, there are additional factors possibly contributing to a higher risk in neurological patients: cardio-pulmonary bypass with decreased systemic blood pressure, hypothermia, anticoagulation, clamping of the aorta. For elective heart surgery, only a limited number of chronic neurological disorders is discussed here.

Parkinson's disease is a disorder mainly of the elderly; about 1% of the population is affected. Lack of dopamine in the basal ganglia causes a typical clinical picture. It consists of stooped posture, stiffness and slowness of movements, and tremors. Interruption of therapy, essentially L-DOPA, may provoke a crisis with complete immobility. Therefore, pharmacological therapy should be maintained up to the morning of surgery and resumed as soon as possible. Drugs potentially causing extrapyramidal symptoms should be withheld, such as phenothiazines, butyrophenone derivates (droperidol). For a crisis, intravenous amantadine is useful.

Epilepsy is one of the most frequent neurological disorders, present in 1% of humans worldwide. As control of seizures depends on a strictly regular medication, oral therapy should be interrupted for the shortest time possible. Epileptic fits are known to complicate cardiac surgery (10, 28); thus, it may be assumed that cardiac surgery might aggravate epilepsy. Anesthesia should be initiated, if possible, with an I.V. barbiturate. If resumption of oral therapy is delayed, I.V. barbiturates, hydantoin (if possible), or benzodiazepines are effective, depending on the type of seizures (30).

Multiple sclerosis has a prevalence of about 50–60 in 100,000 inhabitants. The majority of courses is characterized by exacerbations and remissions. Clinical signs may vary with respect to severity and affected functions. Typical are paresis, spasticity, cerebellar signs, visual deficits, and sphincter disturbances. It has been discussed that stress, accident, surgery, and anesthesia might cause exacerbations, yet evidence is lacking. An elevation of body temperature may aggravate symptoms (Uthoff's phenomenon), but little is known about the effects of hypothermia. The situation is unclear and must be discussed with the patient. If an exacerbation should occur, unless explained by fever, oral methylprednisolone 500 mg/day for 5 days is indicated.

Myasthenia gravis though a rare condition (3 in 100,000 inhabitants), may cause important problems. In this autoimmune disease, the neuro-mucular junction is blocked by auto-antibodies causing a progressive muscular weakness with exertion, in rare instances myasthenic crisis with respiratory failure and disturbed swallowing. Sedative premedication may be tolerated poorly: induction of anesthesia can well be done with an I.V. barbiturate and the smallest doses of muscle relaxants (depolarizing or non-depolarizing) should be used, if needed. Postoperative ventilatory assistance is frequently required, and a even myasthenic crisis may develop after any kind of surgery (22). If oral pyridostigmine therapy must be interrupted for several hours, continuous intravenous application is performed with initially 1/30 of the oral dose. Should crisis develop after heart surgery, plasma exchange or intravenous immunoglobulin therapy is needed (16, 31).

Cerebro-vascular disease poses very large problems for heart surgery, both with regard to carotid stenosis or completed stroke as preexisting risk factors as with regard to stroke as complication of heart surgery. In known carotid stenosis, stroke frequency increases in a graded fashion. Dashe and coworkers (6) found 1.4% strokes in the 0–24% stenosis subgroup, 4.1% strokes in patients with 25–49% stenosis, 10.4% in patients with 50-65% stenosis, and as much as 50% in the 70–99% group. Much lower figures have been given by Furlan and Craciun (11) in their angiographic study: 1.1% stroke rate in the 50-90% stenosis group compared to 6.2% in the group with greater than 90% stenosis. Following Di-Tomaso et al. (8), in non-symptomatic stenosis of the internal carotid artery (i.e. no history of stroke, no transient ischemic attacks), endarterectomy is recommended if stenosis is 70% or more. Symptomatic stenosis (preceding TIAs or completed stroke) should be operated if the vessel diameter is reduced by 50%. If myocardial revascularization is needed, simultaneous endarterectomy of the internal carotid artery and heart surgery, before or during cardio-pulmonary bypass, is strongly advocated by many authors, but not generally accepted (17). Di Tomaso et al. (8) describe only 2 cases of mild cerebral edema in 17 simultaneously operated patients. Christenson and coworkers (5) did simultaneous surgery in 92 cases, 77 of them with non-symptomatic stenosis. 3 patients had transient and 4 permanent deficits, 5 died. On the other hand, following Cernaianu et al. (4), the simultaneous intervention is complicated by cerebrovascular accidents in 18.2%. The question, whether to operate simultaneously or staged, will be discussed in the following paper. Known carotid occlusion is another risk factor for cardiac surgery with 11% perioperative strokes (survey in 6). In their own study, Dashe et al. (6) describe stroke in 2 patients out of 25 with preexisting carotid occlusion undergoing coronary artery bypass, in both ipsilateral to the occlusion. The remaining patients, 4 with bilateral occlusion, did not develop cerebrovascular complications.

Neuropsychological and psychiatric complications of cardiac surgery

Neuropsychological and psychiatric dysfunctions seem to be by far the most frequent complications in patients undergoing heart surgery, so-called diffuse encephalopathy (17). Their frequency varies in the literature with a median of 30% (up to 100%). Precipitating factors are age, preexisting neurological, psychiatric, or pulmonary diseases; hypertension, drugs, excessive consumption of alcohol; perfusion time, hypothermia, hypotension, duration of ventilation (28, 33). In their prospective study in 24 U.S. institutions, Roach et al. (28) found only 55 cases of intellectual function deterioration in 2108 patients after coronary bypass surgery, 2.6% (with additionally 8 cases of epileptic seizures and another 66 cases with cerebrovascular complications). Walzer et al. (33) performed a prospective investigation on 70 patients undergoing myocardial revascularization. They did a comprehensive neuropsychological assessment including orientation, word fluency, arithmetic, memory, and visuoconstructive tasks preoperatively, 2–3, and 5–9 days postoperatively. Ten patients (14%) displayed cognitive impairment (6 delirious patients included) 2–3 days after surgery. The affected patients were older, had required a greater number of defibrillations, and had lower cardiac indices postoperatively. Preoperatively, they had a lower verbal memory, word fluency, and clock orientation. Therapy of psychiatric deterioration, namely delirium, is symptomatic including neuroleptics like haloperidole, benzodiazepines, and (in alcohol withdrawal) clomethiazole, and clonidine.

Neurological complications of cardiac surgery

The frequency of neurological complications varies in different publications. In prospective studies the figures are 68 of 2107 = 3.2% (25), 74 of 2108 = 3.5% (28), 8 of 38 = 21% (19). Fallon et al. (10) did a retrospective study on 523 children with surgery for congenital heart disease and reported 31 cases with neurological complications, 6%. As complications of heart surgery in the literature mostly strokes, or transient ischemic attacks (TIAs) are reported and in a few instances epileptic seizures and persistent stupor or coma.

Cerebral insults obviously are the most common neurological complications in adults, with a high mortality. Egloff et al. (9) reported 68 strokes in 3593 cardiosurgical patients (2%): 41 were minor, 14 major, and 13 lethal. Stroke mainly followed embolism from the aorta or a cardiac valve (n = 11), cardiac arrest (n= 4), preoperatively unknown carotid stenosis (n = 3), embolism with air, cerebral hemorrhage, etc. Roach et al. (28) described 2108 patients, of whom 65 (3.1%) suffered stroke: 8 were lethal, 55 severe, 2 transient ischemic attacks. Newman et al. (25) found in a large prospective multicenter US study on 2107 patients 68 cases of stroke, TIA, or coma, 3.2%. Libman et al. (20) underline that stroke manifests by day 2 in 61%, but that the risk continues and the other 39% develop stroke up to day 9. Following these authors, 70% of strokes cause hemispheric syndromes, 14% brainstem and cerebellar syndromes, and 16% lacunar. Only 29 of 44 patients in Libman's study showed new infarcts in computed tomography.

Main clinical predictors are age, history of previous neurological diseases, diabetes, history of vascular disease, coronary artery surgery, unstable angina, and pulmonary disease (25). Nevertheless, cardiac surgery in carefully selected nonagenarians can be performed with acceptable results (29). Additionally, patients suffering periperatively from acute stroke more often have atheromatous material of the aortic arch, longer periods of CPB and of aortic cross clamping, and simultaneous myocardial revascularization with carotid endarterectomy, longer ICU treatment (4, 28). The history of previous stroke as a risk factor for unfavorable courses was keenly investigated by Redmond et al. (27). In 71 patients with previous stroke, compared to 142 controls without, time to awake and to extubate were longer. More frequent were reintubation, postoperative confusion, a new focal neurological deficit, the latter 43.7% vs. 1.4%. Mortality was higher in persons with previous stroke compared with controls, 7 vs. 0.7%. A laboratory predictor of a severe course after stroke might be the neurone specific enolase (NSE). Isgro et al. (18) measured low NSE (medium 11.1 ng/ml) preoperatively, indicating elevated NSE in 16 of 17 patients with neurological complications with the highest levels in those with the most severe findings, namely TIA and stroke. Similar information might also be obtained from the elevated astroglia-protein S 100 (19).

Procedure If an acute focal neurological deficit is noticed shortly or up to several days after the cardiac intervention, a stroke is probable. A thorough neurological examination must be completed to define the affected cerebral region. At once a CCT should be performed to exclude a cerebral hemorrhage (first radiological signs of ischemic stroke might be seen as early as a few hours after stroke by the very experienced neurologist). As most ischemic strokes after cardiac surgery are supposed to be embolic, from a theoretical point of view, systemic rt-PA-Lysis should be considered. Two large prospective multi-center studies in Europe and the U.S. have proven rt-PA to be beneficial after 3-6 hours after spontaneous ischemic stroke (13, 24). Cardiac surgeons will have to decide, if and at what time after surgery, this procedure might be performed in patients suffering from stroke after heart surgery. Otherwise, systemic heparin could be helpful – if possible. Every stroke-patient after cardiac surgery is to be treated in ICU. The most important rules are no hypotonia, no hyperthermia, no hypo- or hyperglycemia. Especially young stroke patients and those with large territorial infarctions might develop malignant brain edema. Adequate therapy consists of osmotherapy and controlled hyperventilation, and if intracranial pressure is monitored, additional I.V. barbiturate or THAM-buffer. Decompressive craniotomy, though still experimental, must be considered in developing brain edema (14).

Epileptic seizures seem to be rare events in adults after cardiac surgery. In a prospective study, Roach et al. (28) report 8 patients with newly onset seizures out of 2108 after coronary bypass surgery, 0.4%. In children postoperative epilepsy might be somewhat more frequent. Fallon et al. (10) described neurological complications in 31 of 523 children having surgery for congenital heart disease. Three percent 16 children suffered from seizures. In the latter study, the percentage of patients with preexisting epilepsy was not reported. On the other hand, the risks of coronary bypass versus open heart procedures in the two studies might not be comparable. Perhaps seizures are underrepresented in the literature; this is probably because of the retrospective nature of many papers. Therapy of isolated seizures is best done with intravenous single-dose diazepam or other benzodiazepines; rectal diazepam seems to be equivalent. An epileptic status may be treated with repeated doses or continuous infusion of benzodiazepines or barbiturates. Hydantoin bears the risk of cardiac arrhythmia. After every epileptic seizure a meticulous neurological examination including EEG, CCT/MRI, perhaps CSF-tap, is needed, as serious cerebral complications must be ruled out like hemorrhage, infarction, and meningitis.

Diaphragmatic paralysis usually on the left side, rarely bilateral, is due to cryogenic lesions of the phrenic nerve and can be avoided by using only intracoronary cold solution without topical cooling with ice solutions (23).

Rhabdomyolysis with non-anuric renal failure will not appear with indirect cannulation of the femoral artery (21).

Critically ill polyneuropathy is an unusual complication of any intensive care, mainly after sepsis. It is characterized by an axonal damage, causing flaccid paralysis and difficulty in weaning. Therapy is purely symptomatic; the prognosis is favorable (1,3).

What to do?

History Preoperatively a thorough history must be elicided in every patient including preexisting neurological, psychiatric, cardiological, pulmonary diseases, alcohol, and drug consumption. The patient must explicitly be asked about stroke, transient neurological symptoms (TIAs), impaired vision, epileptic seizures. Doppler ultrasound of the extracranial arteries is essential in every patient before cardiac surgery, if possible, additionally transcranial ultrasound.

Examination A complete neurological exam is to be done, if there is a suspicion of neuropsychiatric abnormalities, cardiovascular attacks, or seizures (15, 27). The neurological exam should include the clinical evaluation of mental status, neuropsychological function, cranial nerves, motor system, sensory system, deep tendon and primitive reflexes, and gait and station.

Additional investigations Extracranial ultrasound, if possible Duplex and transcranial sonography, is recommended for every patient undergoing coronary artery bypass, since vessel pathology may not be restricted to cardiac arteries but might affect cerebral vessels, too. Electroencephalography is recommended if epilepsy is suspected; CCT or better MRI if a former stroke must be discussed or focal neurological signs are present.

Modification of procedures Anesthesia could be induced with a barbiturate in cases of preexisting cerebral pathilogy. Following Pascoe et al. (26), the incidence of stroke is lower with barbiturates compared to opioids. But with barbiturates, time until extubation and the ICU stay are longer. Transesophageal echocardiography (TEE) is an adequate tool to diagnose aortic arch atheromas (32). Better results are achieved when TEE is combined with intraoperative epiaortic ultrasound (7). If so, the surgical intervention could be modified and complemented by aortic arch atherectomy. It is not yet clear, if the use of neuroprotective agents will yield any advantage. Grieco et al. (12) report a non-signifcant difference favoring the use of GM1 ganglioside. If acute anticoagulation in patients with acute perioperative stroke is beneficial with regard to the risk of large pericardial effusions, this should be investigated (20).

References

1. Alhan HC, Cakalagaoglu C, Hanci M, et al. (1996) Critical illness polyneuropathy complicating cardiac operation. Ann Thorac Surg 61:1237–1239
2. Barbut D, Gold JP (1996) Aortic atheromatosis and risks of cerebral embolization. J Cardiothorac Vasc Anesth 10:24–29

3. Bolton C (1994) Critical illness neuropathy. In: Hacke W (ed) Neuro Critical Care. Springer, Berlin Heidelberg New York
4. Cernaianu AC, Vassilidze TV, Flum DR, et al. (1995) Predictors of stroke after cardiac surgery. J Card Surg 10:334–339
5. Christenson JT, Maurice J, Simonet F, et al. (1996) Should heart surgery and thrombendarterectomy of the carotic artery be done simultaneously? Swiss Surg Suppl; Suppl 1:19–22
6. Dashe JF, Pessin MS, Murphy RE, Payne DD (1997) Carotid occlusive disease and stroke risk in coronary artery bypass graft surgery. Neurology 49:678–686
7. Davila-Roman VG, Phillips KJ, Daily BB, et al. (1996) Intraoperative transesophageal echocardiography of the thoracic aorta. J Am Coll Cardiol 28:942–947
8. Di-Tomaso L, Caputo M, Ascione R, et al. (1995) Carotid endarterectomy and myocardial revascularisation. A single stage procedure. Minerva Cardioangiol 43:11–12
9. Egloff L, Laske A, Siebenmann R, et al. (1996) Cerebral insult in heart surgery. Schweiz Med Wochenschr 126:477–482
10. Fallon P, Aparicio JM, Elliott MJ, et al. (1995) Incidence of neurological complications of surgery for congenital heart disease. Arch Dis Child 72:418–422
11. Furlan AJ, Craciun AR (1985) Risk of stroke during coronary artery bypass graft surgery in patients with internal artery disease documented by angiography. Stroke 16:797–799
12. Grieco G, d'Hollosy M, Culliford AT, et al. (1996) Evaluating neuroprotective agents for clinical anti-ischemic benefit using neurological and neuropsychological changes after cardiac surgery under cardiopulmonary bypass. Methodological strategies and results of a double-blind placebo-controlled trial of GM1 ganglioside. Stroke 27:858-874
13. Hacke W, Kaste M, Fieschi C, et al. (1995) Intravenous thrombolysis with recombinant tissue plasminogen activator for acute hemispheric stroke. JAMA 274:1017–1025
14. Hacke W, Schwab S, De Georgia M (1997) Intensive care of acute ischemic stroke. In: Ennker J, Coselli JS, Treasure T (eds) Cerebral Protection in Cerebrovascular and Aortic Surgery. Steinkopff, Darmstadt
15. Heyer EJ, Adams DC (1996) Neurologic assessment and cardiac surgery. J Cardiothorac Vasc Anesth 10:99–104
16. Hohlfeld R, Toyka KV (1993) Therapies. In: Myasthenia Gravis. CRC Press, Boca Raton, Ann Harbor, London
17. Hornick P, Smith PL, Taylor KM (1994) Cerebral complications after coronary bypass grafting. Current Opinion in Cardiology 9:670–679
18. Isgro F, Schmidt C, Pohl P, et al. (1997) A predictive parameter in patients with brain related complications after cardiac surgery. Eur J Cardiothorac Surg 11:640-644
19. Johnson P, Lundquist C, Lindgren A, et al. (1995) Cerebral complications after cardiac surgery assessed by S-100 and NSE levels in blood. J Cardiothorac Vasc Anesth 9:694–699
20. Libman RB, Wirkowsky E, Neystat M, et al. (1996) Stroke associated with cardiac surgery. Determinants, timing and stroke subtypes. Arch Neurol 54:83–87
21. Maccario M, Fumagalli C, Dottori V, et al. (1996) The association between rhabdomyolysis and acute renal failure in patients undergoing cardiopulmonary bypass. J Cardiovasc Surg Torino 37:153–159
22. Martz DG, Schreibman DL, Matjasko MJ (1990) Neurological disorders. In: Katz J, Benumof J, Kadis LB (eds) Anesthesia in uncommon diseases. Saunders, Philadelphia
23. Mazzoni M, Solinas C, Sisillo E, et al. (1996) Intraoperative phrenic nerve monitoring in cardiac surgery. Chest 109:1455–1460
24. National Institute of Neurological disorders and Stroke rt-PA Stroke Study Group (1995) Tissue plasminogen activator for acute ischemic stroke. N Engl J Med 333:1581–1587
25. Newman MF, Wolman R, Kanchuger M, et al. (1996) Multicenter preoperative stroke risk index for patients undergoing coronary artery bypass graft surgery. Multicenter study of perioperative ischemia. Circulation 94 (Suppl):II74–80
26. Pascoe EA, Hudson RJ, Anderson BA, et al. (1996) High-dose thiopentone for open-chamber cardiac surgery: a retrospective review. Can J Anaesth 43:a575–579
27. Redmond JM, Greene PS, Goldsborough MA, et al. (1996) Neurological injury in cardiac surgical patients with a history of stroke. Ann Thorac Surg 61:42–47
28. Roach GW, Kanchuger M, Mangano CM, et al. (1996) Adverse cerebral outcomes after coronary bypass surgery. N Engl J Med 335:1857–1863
29. Samuels LE, Sharma S, Morris RJ, et al. (1996) Cardiac surgery in nonagenarians. J Card Surg 11:121–127

30. Schmidt D (1993) Epilepsien. In: Brandt T, Diener J, Dichgans HC (eds) Therapie und Verlauf neurologischer Erkrankungen. Kohlhammer, Stuttgart Berlin Köln
31 Schuchardt V, Hund E, Rieke K (1995) High-dose immunoglobulins in neurocritical care. Intensivmed 32:642–650
32. Trehan N, Mishra M, Dhole S, et al. (1997) Significantly reduced incidence of stroke during coronary artery bypass grafting using transesophageal echocardiography. Eur J Cardiothorac Surg 11:234–242
33. Walzer T, Herrmann M, Wallesch CW (1997) Neuropsychological disorders after coronary bypass surgery. J Neurol Neurosurg Psychiatry 62:644–648

Author's address:
Prof. Dr. Volker Schuchardt
Neurologische Klinik des
Klinikum Lahr
Klostenstraße 19
77933 Lahr

Cardiac surgery and the obese patient

V. Schusdziarra

Department of Internal Medicine II, Technical University of Munich, Germany

Obesity is a disease with increasing prevalence. Of the German population 40% are overweight (BMI 25–30 kg/m^2), 15% are obese (BMI 30–40 kg/m^2), and 1% are morbidly obese (BMI > 40 kg/m^2). Obesity predisposes to a number of severe diseases such as diabetes mellitus, hypertension, gallstone disease, coronary artery disease, myocardial infarction, and stroke (12).

Accordingly, there is an increasing chance that cardiac surgery has to be performed on obese subjects and it is a conventional preconception that obesity is also a risk factor for surgical interventions including cardiac surgery.

A number of studies evaluating several thousand patients after cardiac surgery have shown that obesity clearly increases the risk of minor wound infections as in all other types of surgical procedures. Three groups reported no increase in operation mortality in obese patients following coronary artery bypass grafting (CABG) and other types of cardiac surgery (8, 10, 11). Prasad et al. (11) demonstrated an increased frequency of respiratory problems, arrhythmias, sternal dehiscence, and postoperative myocardial infarction, while others showed no cardiopulmonary complications (8, 10). Josa et al. found obesity to be a risk factor for the development of pulmonary embolism after cardiac surgery (6). From those 33 patients, 14 were reported to be obese. Furthermore, 6 patients died but only 2 of them being obese. Thus, by looking closely at the data the conclusion of the authors is somewhat difficult to understand. All studies agree that obesity is a risk factor for the development of minor complications such as superficial sternal wound infection, leg infection, atrial arrhythmias, or respiratory infections.

In view of these data the necessity of preoperative weight reduction remains controversial. Since obesity does not favor major complications, one could ignore this problem. On the other hand, it might be possible to reduce even minor complications by preoperative reduction of body weight. To approach this problem further, it is necessary to analyze the time course of weight reduction and compare it with the potential time period over which cardiac surgery could be postponed without augmenting complications by the underlying disease per se. Several controlled weight reduction trials have shown a decrease in body weight by a mean of 6–10 kg in six months. This does not exclude that certain patients lose 20 kg over this time period. During the first 3 months a loss of 5 kg is a reasonable result (4, 5).

Depending on the degree the patient is overweight, this magnitude of weight loss does not promise to reduce too many of the more or less minor problems following cardiac surgery. In most patients cardiac disease has reached a severe state when cardiac surgery is clearly indicated, and therefore, it is more reasonable to perform surgery ignoring the weight problem. When surgery is postponed due to body weight, the chance is much greater that the patient dies as a result of the underlying cardiac disease rather than of postoperative complications due to obesity as supported by the available data.

Considering that most of the operations are coronary artery bypass grafts (CABG), which are necessary as the result of artherosclerosis, and the development of which is triggered substantially by obesity it seems to be much more important to treat obesity postoperatively to prevent a relapse.

This has been examined by Prasad et al. (11) who were able to show that over a follow-up period of 3 years obesity was associated with a greater incidence of recurrent angina in combination with further weight gain. This was significant already 12 months after surgery.

According to these data it is necessary to take care of all risk factors especially in CABG patients which means that obesity must be treated vigorously and with the same intensity as high blood glucose and cholesterol levels.

Treatment of obesity should consist of a multimodal approach combining hypocaloric diets with modifications of eating behavior, psychological treatment (if necessary), and increased physical activity (3). Drugs such as centrally acting serotoninergic agonists (dexfenfluramine, sibutramine) or peripherally acting inhibitors of pancreatic lipase (reducing fat digestion and absorption) can be helpful for a successful treatment (2, 5, 9). Since obesity treatment is a long-term problem, only those drugs should be used that can be considered safe even when taken for many years. Side effects such as pulmonary hypertension and cardiac valvular disease have to be considered carefully (1, 2, 9).

In conclusion the existing data do not justify postponement of cardiac surgery because of obesity. However, it seems to be important to treat obesity postoperatively to prevent relapse especially in CABG patients.

References

1. Abenhaim L, Moride Y, Brenot F (1996) Appetite-suppressant drugs and the risk of primary pulmonary hypertension. N Engl J Med 335: 609–16
2. Cannistra LB, Davis SM, Baumann A (1997) Valvular heart disease associated with dexfenfluramine. New Engl J Med no. 337
3. Ellrott Th, Pudel V (1997) Adipositastherapie. Thieme, Stuttgart
4. Guy-Grand B, Apfelbaum M, Crepaldi G, Gries A, Lefebvre P (1989) International trial of long-term dexfenfluramine in obesity. Lancet 2: 1142–5
5. James WPT, Avenell A, Broom J, Whitehead J (1997) A one-year trial to assess the value of orlistat in the management of obesity. Int J Obesity 21 [Suppl 3]: 24–30
6. Josa M, Siouffi SY, Silverman AB, Barsamain EM, Khuri SF, Sharma GVRK (1993) Pulmonary embolism after cardiac surgery. JACC 21: 990–996
7. Kelly F, Wade AG, Jones SP, Johnson SG (1994) Sibutramine hydrochloride vs dexfenfluramine: Weight loss in obese subjects. Int J Obesity 18 [Suppl. 2]: Abstract 0235, p 61
8. Koshal A, Hendry P, Raman SV, Keon WJ (1985) Should obese patients not undergo coronary artery surgery? Cam J Surg 28: 331–334
9. McMurray J, Bloomfield P, Miller HC (1986) Irreversible pulmonary hypertension after treatment with fenfluramine. BMJ 292: 239–40
10. Moulton MJ, Creswell LL, Mackey ME, Cox JL, Rosenbloom M (1996) Obesity is not risk factor for significant adverse outcomes after cardiac surgery. Circulation 94 (suppl II): 87–92
11. Prasad US, Walker WS, Sang CTM, Campanella C, Cameron EWJ (1991) Influence of obesity on the early and long term results of surgery for coronary artery disease. Eur J Cardio-thorac Surg 5: 67–73
12. Von Itallie ThB, Lew EA (1993) Estimation of the effect of obesity on health and longevity. In: Stunkard AJ, Wadden TA (eds) Obesity: Theory and Therapy. Raven Press, New York pp 219–230

Author's address:
Prof. Dr. med. V. Schusdziarra
Leitender Oberarzt der II. Medizinischen Klinik
Klinikum rechts der Isar
Ismaninger Straße 20
81675 München, Germany

Obesity – A risk factor in coronary artery surgery?

J. Ennker, F. Schoeneich, A. Lichtenberg

Heart Institute Lahr/Baden, Germany

In the Federal Republic of Germany 40% of the population is overweight, 16% are obese, and 1% super obese. Therefore, in comparison Germany shows the highest prevalence of obesity in the world (10). On the one hand obesity is a known risk factor for coronary artery disease (1, 4); on the other hand the coincidence of other risk factors for coronary artery disease in obese persons, such as diabetes mellitus, hypertension, and hyperlipidaemia are increased (7). Consecutive a high rate of obese patients must undergo coronary artery bypass graft (CABG) surgery.

Overweight is still regarded as a significant risk factor for CABG surgery, therefore the majority of the German heart institutes will not accept patients for CABG procedures unless the patient reduced the body weight. In our experience this applies also to patients with left main stem stenosis and patients symptomatic on low exercise level. The following article analyzes our experience regarding open heart surgery in severely and super obese patients and evaluates whether a preoperative reduction of weight is justified or not. Between 1 March 95 and 31 December 97 we performed 5092 open heart procedures using the cardio-pulmonary bypass. 81.6% (4154) were CABG procedures and 2.5% (103) of these patients had a Body-Mass-Index of more than 35.

Classification of obesity

The cardio-pulmonary syndrome of severely and super obese patients has been described after the novel figure coachman Joe of the Pickwick Tales from Charles Dickens. Particular characteristics are an alveolar hypoventilation with arterial hypoxemia, respiratory acidosis, polycytemia, and somnolence.

Scientifical classification of obesity is increasingly defined by the Body-Mass-Index (BMI): weight in kg / height in meters^2. The Broca-Index defined as the body height in cm minus 100, only facilitates accurate values in persons with a height between 160–180 cm. Normal weight persons are classified with a Body-Mass-Index from 20–25. A Body-Mass-Index under 20 signals underweight, values of greater than 30 indicate obesity (Table 1).

Preoperative reduction of weight?

A preoperative reduction of weight in order to reduce the perioperative risk has been constantly demanded so far, although the current literature only knows of one investigation regarding this point. An evaluation of a preoperative weight reduction of 14.6 ± 5.3 kg in 105 patients within 5.4 ± 3.1 weeks did not show a statistically significant difference regarding perioperative morbidity (2).

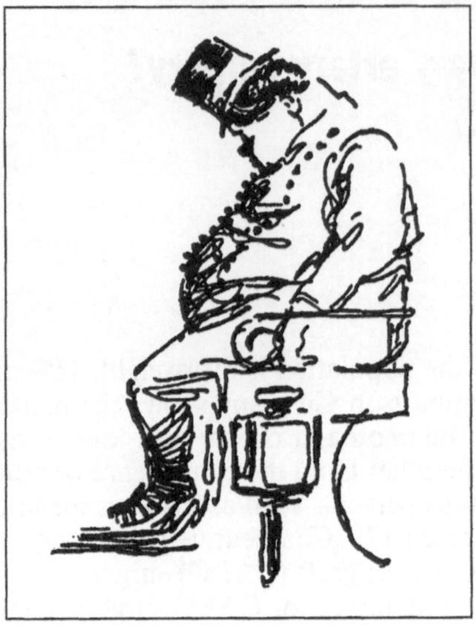

Fig. 1. Pickwick-Syndrom

Table 1. Classification of obesity (1)

Body-Mass-Index (kg/m^2)	
Underweight	< 20
Normal weight	20–25
Overweight	25–30
Obesity	30–35
Severely obesity	35–40
Super obesity	> 40

There are adverse psychological consequences of dieting, such as, depression, nervousness, weakness, and irritability (8). An investigation by Wadden et al. (9) showed significant short-term complications associated with inappropriate dieting: water and electrolyte problems (a loss of sodium and potassium), orthostatic hypotension with vertigo, increased uric acid concentrations, muscle cramping, headache, gastrointestinal distress, and a loss of immunologic activity. Long-term complications of very-low-calorie diets include the risk of severe therapy resistant ventricular arrhythmias with increased QT intervals, which were identified as cause of death. Inappropriate calorie intake at any time during adherence to a very-low-calorie diet may also be associated with attacks of cholecystitis and pancreatitis (3, 12).

Obesity associated health hazards can, nevertheless, be positively influenced by weight reduction such as insulin sensivity increases, insulin secretion by the islet cells improves, hepatic glucose production decreases, and glucose disposal improves. Pulmonary function improves, as hypertension and dyslipidemia with a decrease of the LDL/HDL ratio (11, 12).

Nevertheless, there is a lack of meaningful epidemiological studies in patients, who underwent longer-term weight loss to verify a decrease in mortality rates as well as a provable reduction of risk factors. A control result within the Framingham-Study clarified that severe fluctuations in body weight even increased the coronary mortality as well as the total mortality (yo-yo effect) (4).

Patients and methods

At the Heart Institute Lahr/Baden a total of 5092 open heart operations were performed between March 1 1995 and December 31, 1997. 81.6% (4154 patients) operations of these cases were CABG procedures.

19.0% (791) of the patients who underwent CABG surgery showed a preoperative BMI from 30 to 35, 2.3% (95) of the patients showed values from 35 to 40, and 0.2% (8) values from over 40. The patients preoperative BMI data are listed in Table 2.

The analysis was designed to compare severe / super obese patients (BMI > 35) and non-obese patients (BMI 20–25) who formed the control group.

Data was collected retrospectively from preoperative, operative, and postoperative patient case records, perfusion records, cardiology follow-up records, and letters from general practitioners. The long-term follow-up data was obtained from telephone interviews with the patients themselves or their GP: the current body weight, sternal dehiscence, and NYHA functional classification were recorded. The retrospective analysis of data was designed to evaluate the preoperative risks, perioperative complications, and post-operative morbidity. Therefore, patients were observed up to the time of their discharge and the following months with regard to events such as perioperative myocardial infarction, sternal dehiscence, mediastinitis, and respiratory insufficiency. To investigate the perioperative mortality, every death occurring within 30 days of surgery was documented.

The operative procedures were performed – according to the standard protocol of the Department – under cardioplegic arrest with crystalloid cardioplegic solution (Kirsch/Haes) and under moderate hypothermia (32 °C) with local surface cooling, recently with normotherme blood cardioplegic solution. Membrane oxygenation with a linear flow (roller pumps) were used for the cardiopulmonary bypass. Most patients had a complete revascularization, 93.2% of the patients had left internal mammary artery grafts plus saphenous vein grafts. The average total bypass time, the aortic clamp time, number, and type of bypass-grafts were documented. All patients were placed on aspirin therapy postoperatively; those patients with fat metabolism dysfunction were placed on lipid-blocking medication.

Table 2. Preoperative patients BMI data n = 4154

BMI (kg/m^2)	N	%
< 20	60	1.4
20–25	1063	25.6
25–27.5	1136	27.4
27.5–30	1001	24.1
30–35	791	19.0
35–40	95	2.3
> 40	8	0.2

Results

The preoperative clinical characteristics from severely and super obese patients (BMI > 35) patients in comparison with the group of normal weight patients (BMI 20-25) showed significantly elevated incidences of diabetes mellitus ($p < 0.05$), triple vessel disease ($p < 0.02$) and hypertension ($p < 0.00001$). With an average age of 62.1 ± 9.4 years, the investigated group was clearly younger than the patients with normal weight (65.9 ± 9.5 years) and had better LV function (58.6 ± 14.8% versus 53.0 ± 16.3%) (Table 3).

In contrast to the results of Fasol et al. and Prasad et al. (3, 9) there was no significant higher incidence of hyperlipidaemia (66% versus 58.5%) and main stem stenosis (22.3% versus 23.7%) in our data.

The analysis of surgical data in the obese patient group showed a significantly longer operation time ($p < 0.05$). Concerning the total bypass time, the aortic clamp time, implantation of IABP, and number and type of implanted grafts no significant difference could be detected (Table 4).

Compared with the control group, obese patients had an increased postoperative morbidity, but no significantly increased mortality. The ventilation time ($p < 0.02$) was longer with a more frequent respiratory insufficiency ($p < 0.05$) and obese patients required reintubation significantly more frequent than non-obese patients ($p < 0.02$). The obese group had also a higher incidence of mediastinitis ($p < 0.01$) and sternal dehiscence ($p < 0.005$). As a result of increased respiratory insufficiency

Table 3. Preoperative data

	BMI > 35 n = 103 (100%)	BMI 20–25 n = 1063 (100%)	P value
Age	62.1 ± 9.4	65.9 ± 9.5	< 0.001
LV-function (EF)	58.6 ± 14.8	53.0 ± 16.3	< 0.02
NYHA	3.4 ± 0.7	3.4 ± 0.8	NS
Diabetes mellitus	34 (33.0%)	267 (25.1%)	< 0.05
Hypertension	87 (84.4%)	631 (59.4%)	< 0.00001
Hyperlipidaemia	68 (66.0%)	622 (58.5%)	NS
Angiography			
Left main stem	23 (22.3%)	252 (23.7%)	NS
Single vessel	2 (1.9%)	53 (4.9%)	NS
Double vessel	16 (15.5%)	202 (19.0%)	NS
Triple vessel	65 (63.1%)	602 (56.6%)	< 0.02

Table 4. Operative data

	BMI > 35 n = 103 (100%)	BMI 20–25 n = 1063 (100%)	P value
Operation time (min)	215.0 ± 45.3	203.3 ± 56.3	< 0.05
Total bypass time (min)	98.9 ± 31.1	94.1 ± 37.1	NS
Aortic clamp time (min)	52.8 ± 15.9	50.5 ± 17.7	NS
Mean number of grafts	3.1 ± 0.7	3.0 ± 0.8	NS
LIMA/RIMA-grafts (n %)	96 (93.2%)	977 (91.9%)	NS
IABP (n, %)	7 (6.8%)	49 (4.6%)	NS

Table 5. Postoperative data

	BMI > 35 n = 103 (100%)	BMI 20–25 n = 1063 (100%)	P value
Blood loss (ml)	554.4 ± 540.2	670.8 ± 641.0	NS
IPP ventilattion (days)	2.7 ± 6.7	1.4 ± 4.5	< 0.01
Days on the ICU	4.9 ± 8.0	3.0 ± 5.0	< 0.001
Resp. insuff. (n, %)	15 (14.6%)	88 (8.3%)	< 0.05
Reintubation	9 (8.7%)	41 (3.9%)	< 0.02
Myocardial infarction (n, %)	4 (3.9%)	19 (1.8)	NS
Mediastinitis (n, %)	3 (2.9%)	1 (0.1%)	< 0.002
Sternal dehiscense (n, %)	3 (2.9%)	2 (0.2%)	< 0.005
Mortality (n, %)	3 (2.9%)	24 (2.3%)	NS

Table 5. Long term results

	Perioperative data	actual	P value
Body weight (kg)	101.3 ± 12.9	98.9 ± 14.2	NS
BMI (kg/m²)	36.8 ± 2.1	35.8 ± 3.2	NS
NYHA	3.4 ± 0.7	2.1 + 0.6	< 0.05
Mortality (n, %)	3 (2.9%)	3 (2.9%)	

Table 7. Literature comparison (2, 5, 6)

	Heart Institute Lahr/Baden n = 103 BMI > 35 1.3.95–31.12.97	Th Rohs Michigan n = 28 BMI > 35 1984–1992	U.S. Prasad Edinburgh n = 248 > 20% of ideal weight 1984–1987	R. Fasol Freiburg n = 343 > 12% of ideal weight 1990
Myocardial Infarction %	3.9	7.6	–	6.1
Would infection %	5.4	8.0	25.0	2.6
Sternal dehiscence %	1.4	9.2	15.0	1.9
Respiratory insuff. %	14.6	27.6	45	14.0
Mortality	3 (2.9%)	1 (3.6%)	2 (0.8%)	5 (1.4%)

the obese group had on average with 4.9 ± 8.0 days a longer stay on the ICU than the non-obese controls with 3.0 ± 5.0 days ($p < 0.001$). Nevertheless, there was no significant difference in incidence of mortality between the obese group (2.9%) and the non-obese group (2.3%), (Table 5).

For the long-term follow-up, we could collect data from 84 out of 103 investigated patients The mean postoperative follow-up time was 25.3 months (range 2-35 months). The degree of effort tolerance was measured by NYHA-grading in comparison with perioperative data. At the follow-up time the exercise level of 84 patients (BMI > 35) was with an average NYHA value of 2.2 clearly improved, compared with perioperative data of 3.4 ($p < 0.05$). Table 6 lists the assessed data.

Discussion

It is known that overweight itself is an important risk factor for coronary artery surgery. In our experience severely obese and super obese patients did not undergo routine operations in other departments until a previous reduction of body weight. However, the analysis of the Framingham Heart Study by Lissner et al. (4) indicated a higher risk of coronary artery disease and a higher total mortality in patients whose body weight fluctuates often or within a wide range than in patients with a stable body weight. Obesity associated health hazards, as hypertension, diabetes mellitus, and hyperlipidaemia can be positively influenced by preoperative dieting (11, 12), nevertheless, a decreased morbidity could not be confirmed (2). The inappropriate side effects of very low calorie diets, such as loss of immunologic activity, cardiac arrhythmias, water and electrolyte problems, etc., which can cause intraoperative complications should also be taken in consideration.

The expected increased mortality rate in cardiac bypass surgery under accumulation of risk factors associated with obesity could not be confirmed by the results of our own investigation. Our results did not reveal any significant difference concerning mortality between both groups: the obese group of 103 patients with a BMI > 35 had a mortality rate of 2.9%, the group of 1063 normal weight patients a mortality rate of 2.3%. Similar results from studies, dealing with this subject, have been described by Th. Rohs, U.S. Prasad and R. Fasol (Table 7). The operative data of the obese group did not show any significant differences compared to the control group of normal weights, apart from a longer operation time (215.0 min ± 45.3 min versus 203.3 min ± 56.3 min $p < 0.05$).

The peri- and postoperative morbidity was increased. Obese patients required IPP ventilation significantly longer than non-obese patients (2.7 ± 6.7 d versus 1.4 ± 4.5 d; $p < 0.01$), and had a higher incidence of respiratory insufficiency (14.6% versus 8.3%; $p < 0.05$)

Therefore, the obese group spent more days on the ICU (4.9 ± 8.0 d versus 3.0 ± 5.0 d; $p < 0.001$). Further perioperative complications as mediastinitis (5.4% versus 1.0%; $p < 0.01$) and sternal dehiscence (2.9% versus 0.2%; $p < 0.005$) were statistically increased.

As a conclusion of our results, it is not justified to defer symptomatic severely and super obese patients from cardiac surgery for reasons of preoperative weight reduction. The analysis of data did not show a significant difference in the postoperative course of severely obese and super obese patients with a previous preoperative weight reduction in comparison with overweighed patients without preoperative dieting (2). Our experiences have shown that overweight patients with coronary artery disease can undergo coronary bypass surgery without a statistically increased mortality rate.

References

1. Bray GA (1995) Complications of obesity, Ann Int Med 103: 1052–62
2. Fasol R (1992) The influence of obesity on perioperative morbidity: retrospective study of 502 aortocoronary bypass operations, J Thorac Cardiovasc Surg 40: 126–29
3. Isner JM, et al (1979) Sudden, unexpected Death in Avid Dieters Using the Liquid-Protein-Modified-Fast Diet, Circulation 60, N° 6: 1401–12
4. Lissner L, et al (1991) Variability of Body Weight and Health Outcomes in The Framingham Population, The New Eng J Med 26: 1839–44

5. Prasad US (1991) Influence of obesity on the early and long term results of surgery for coronary artery disease, Eur J Cardio-Thorac Surg 5: 67–73
6. Rohs TH, et al (1995) Early Complications and Long-Term Survival in Severely Obese Coronary Bypass Patients,The Am Surgeon 61: 949–953
7. Royal College of Physicians of London, Obesity. Report, J R Coll Physicians London (1983) 17: 5–65
8. Wadden TA, Stunkard AJ (1985) Social and Psycological Consequences of Obesity, Ann Intern Med 103 (6 pt 2): 1062–67
9. Wadden TA, et al (1990) Responsible and irresponsible use of very-low-calorie diets in the treatment of obesity, JAMA 263: 83–5
10. Wechsler GJ, et al (1995) Konsensusgespräch der Deutschen Adipositas-Gesellschaft, München
11. Wolf RN, et al (1983) Influence of weight reduction on plasma lipoproteins in obese patients, Arteriosclerosis 3: 160–9
12. Xavier F, Pi-Sunyer (1993) Short-Term Medical Benefits and Adverse Effects of Weight Loss, Ann Intern Med 119 (7 pt 2): 722–726

Author's address:
J. Ennker, M.D.
Heart Institute Lahr/Baden
P.O.B. 1340
D-77933 Lahr, Germany

Obesity – A risk factor in the postoperative course?

J. Rötker, N. Röder, A. Reimann, H.H. Scheld

Thoracic and Cardiovascular Surgery, Westphalian Wilhelms-University, Münster, Germany

Background

The significance of obesity as a concomitant disease according to the postoperative course is in dispute.

Methods, Results

2753 patients operated on for coronary artery disease from Jan 01, 1994 to April 39, 1997 were investigated for 30 day mortality and adverse events after surgery. All data were acquired prospectively by an on-line computer-based data system. Patients were assigned to four groups according to their body mass index (BMI): group I: BMI < 20 (1.2% of patients), group II: BMI 20 < 25 (33.4%), group III: BMI 25 < 30 (60.3%), and group IV: BMI ≥ 30 (5.0%).

There were no differences according to age, ejection fraction, NYHA classification, end diastolic pressure in the left ventricle, operating time, bypass time, and x-clamp time. More than 60% of patients had a body mass index of more than 25. 30-day mortality was not different for all groups. Patients with a BMI > 30 had significantly more events of respiratory failure in the postoperative course than patients with no obesity ($p < 0.05$; relative risk: 2.0). The risk of sternal wound infection was increased in patients with an BMI > 25 compared to patients without obesity ($p < 0.005$; relative risk: 2.48).

Conclusions

Obese patient who undergo coronary artery bypass surgery have an increased risk of respiratory failure and sternal wound infection after surgery; 30-day mortality is not increased. Obese patient should use their time waiting for the electively scheduled operation to decrease their body weight.

Author's address:
Jürgen Rötker, M.D.
Thoracic and Cardiovascular Surgery
Westphalian Wilhelms-University,
Albert-Schweitzer-Str. 33
48129 Münster, Germany

Coronary artery bypass grafting in severe obese patients

U. Schindel, H. E. Zeplin

Cardio Clinic Frankfurt, Frankfurt/Main, Germany

Introduction and purpose

Severe obesity is defined as a Body Mass Index (Quetelet Index) > 30 kg/m^2. Many surgical centres refuse to accept obese patients for open heart surgery and insist on weight reduction prior to surgery, claiming an unacceptable operative risk. At present there is little information available concerning the risk of obese patients in cardiac surgery. Therefore, this study was performed retrospectively to help estimate the operative risk in obese patients undergoing coronary artery bypass grafting (CABG).

Design and patient population

From January 1994 to December 1996 we accepted 166 patients for CABG though their Body Mass Index (BMI) was 30 kg/m^2 or more (mean 33 kg/m^2 range 30–49.3). The operative data and postoperative complication rate was compared to the results of 1122 normal weight patients (mean BMI 25.2, range 19.2–29.9) during the same period after CABG.

Since most obese patients came for urgent (57%) or emergency (34%) CABG no preoperative weight reduction was attemped. The elective ones (9%) failed all their attempts of weight reduction suffering from angina.

Risk factors were hypertension 70.5% (non-obese 65%), hyperlipidaemia 44.6% (40%), and diabetes 25.6% (26.3%). Decompensated low output failure or recent recompensation occured in 45% (51%) of the pts. CABG was performed by midsternotomy in all pts. LIMA was used in 48% (68%).

Operative data

Mean operation time was 104 min (non-obese 107 min). Mean Bypass time: was 54 min (53 min), and mean aortic X-clamping time was 27 min (26 min). The intraoperative sight shows that obese women have small heart sizes. Thus, the size of heart seems to correlate more with body height than body mass. The extent epicardial fat was less than expected.

Postoperative course and results

Intensive care unit stay was 1.9 days (non-obese 2.3 days). Sternal infection, 0.6% (0.3%), and sternal refixation, 4.8% (2.6%). The mean blood loss was 691 ml (789 ml). Bank blood requirement was unavoidable in 28.9% (34%).

The mean postoperative mechanical ventilation time took 7 h (9 h) when weaned beginning with a core temperature > 36.5 °C. A low output syndrome with indication for IABP occured in 2.4% (1.8%). The mortality within 30 days was 4.2% (non-obese 3.7%). Mortality of the obese patients was 0% elective, 4.2% urgently and 5.3% emergency intervention.

Conclusion

Regarding the acquired results, it is not justified to refuse obese patients especially in case of urgent and emergency priority. We recognized that patients, who were denied for surgical treatment at other hospitals showed enormous motivation after finally being accepted for operation. Postopertive compliance is raised and patients are very cooperative in mobilization.

Author's address:
Ulrike Schindel, M.D.
Cardio Clinic Frankfurt
Fachkrankenhaus für Herzchirurgie
Usinger Str. 5
60389 Frankfurt/Main, Germany

Cardiac surgery in adult patients with congenital heart and severe concomitant disease

I. Dähnert, F. Berger V. Alexi-Meskishvili, U. Bauer, S. Dittrich, B. Stiller, Y. Weng, H. Kuppe, R. Hetzer, P. E. Lange

Deutsches Herzzentrum Berlin, 13353 Berlin, Germany

Introduction

Congenital heart disease (CHD) today is treated surgically and/or interventionally during infancy or childhood. Nevertheless, an increasing number of adults with CHD is admitted to hospitals dedicated to the care of such patients (5). During the last 4 years at the Deutsches Herzzentrum Berlin, 30% of the patients operated for congenital heart disease were older than 16 years (Fig. 1). Cardiac operations in such patients may be needed because the malformation was not detected earlier (7, 9) or it was not considered severe enough to warrant surgery during childhood (10). Some patients require definitive corrective repair (17, 26, 27), and others repair of residual, and/or for new lesions (2, 6, 14, 16–18), as well as additional palliative procedures.

Concomitant diseases, however, have not been addressed systematically in a larger group of such patients. Thus, we retrospectively analyzed concomitant diseases associated with or related to congenital heart disease in 763 patients operated at the Deutsches Herzzentrum Berlin one or more times during the period 1988 to 1997 (Fig. 2).

Patients and methods

In 763 patients with congenital heart disease (CHD) older than 16 years in whom 827 operations were performed between May 1988 and May 1997 at the Deutsches Herzzentrum Berlin, concomitant diseases (Fig. 2) were analyzed retrospectively with respect to operative risk factors. The diagnoses and the age distribution are depicted in Fig. 1a–d for the 4 groups ventricular volume overload, ventricular pressure overload, cyanosis, as well as one with miscellaneous rare CHD.

Operations were separated into conventional operations and transplantations (n = 28, Fig. 3). Out of 827 operations 792 were corrections and 35 palliations. Included were 1 patient with severe coronary heart disease and atrial septal defect (ASD) who died after aorto-coronary-vein bypass and ASD-closure as well as 2 patients with ASD/partial abnormal pulmonary venous drainage and severe grade IV Heath-Edwards pulmonary hypertension, who died 2 and 3 weeks postoperatively. Both were not tested preoperatively in the cardiac catheterization laboratory as has been our routine for many years now (12, 22, 24).

Concomitant diseases were divided into cardiac (arrhythmias, myocardial insufficiency, coronary heart disease), cardiac dependent (collaterals, cyanosis, pulmonary hypertension) and non cardiac (Fig. 2). Some patients had more than one concomitant disease (Fig. 4).

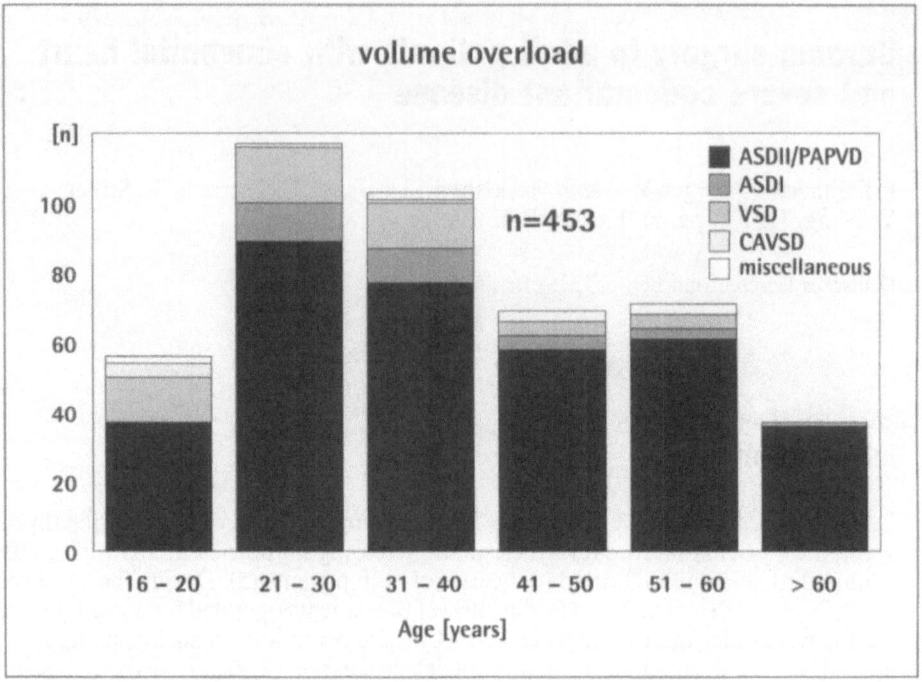
volume overload
[n]
100
80
60
40
20
0
ASDII/PAPVD
ASDI
VSD
CAVSD
miscellaneous
n=453
16 – 20
21 – 30
31 – 40
41 – 50
51 – 60
> 60
Age [years]

a

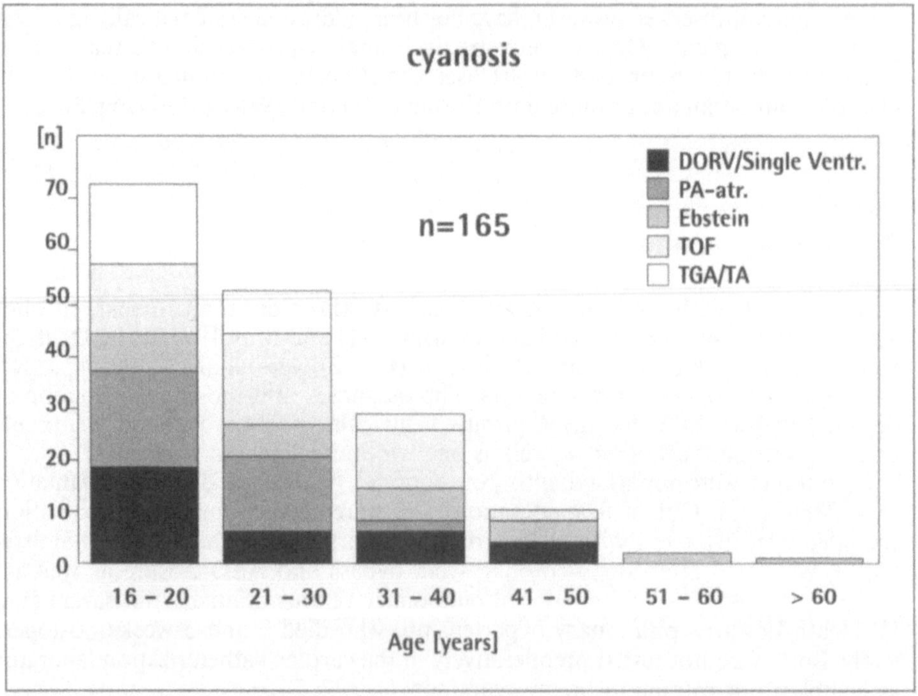
cyanosis
[n]
70
60
50
40
30
20
10
0
DORV/Single Ventr.
PA-atr.
Ebstein
TOF
TGA/TA
n=165
16 – 20
21 – 30
31 – 40
41 – 50
51 – 60
> 60
Age [years]

b

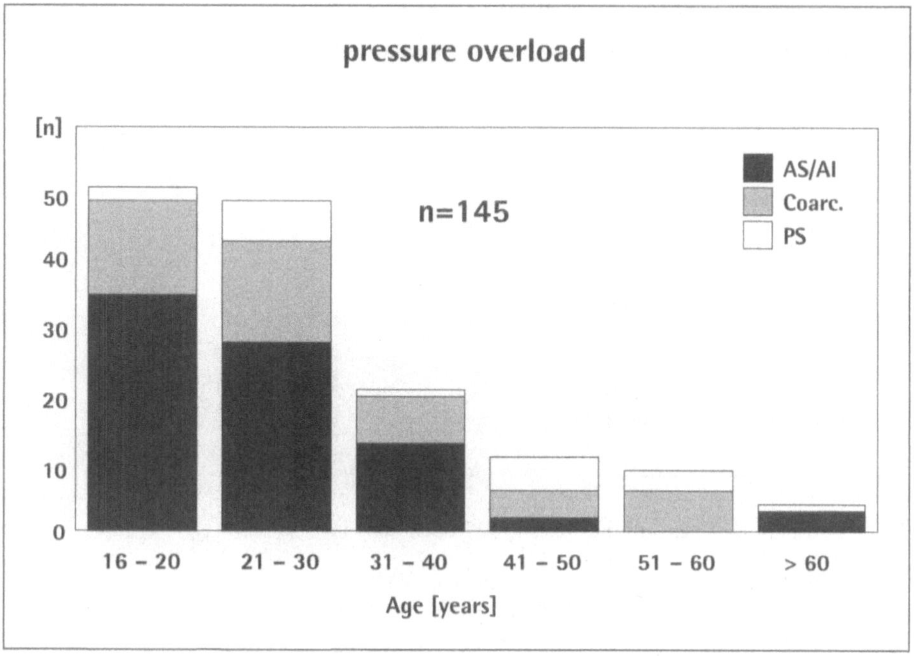

c

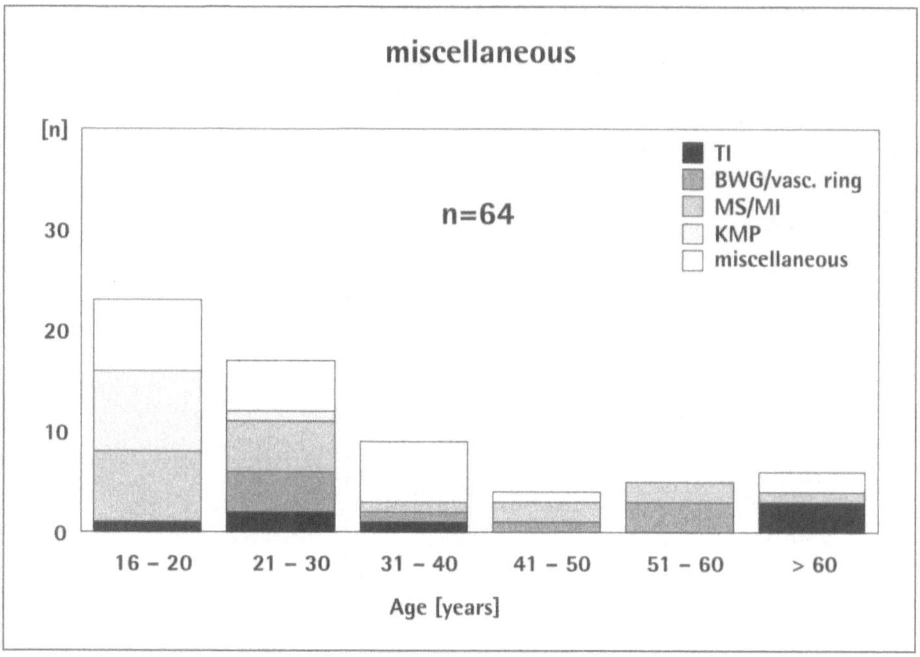

d

Fig. 1a–d. Concomitant diseases in 827 operations in adult patients with congenital heart disease. Cardiac: arrhythmias, myocardical insuffiency, coronary heart disease. Cardiac dependent: collaterals, cyanosis, pulmonary hypertension. Non cardiac: see Fig. 4

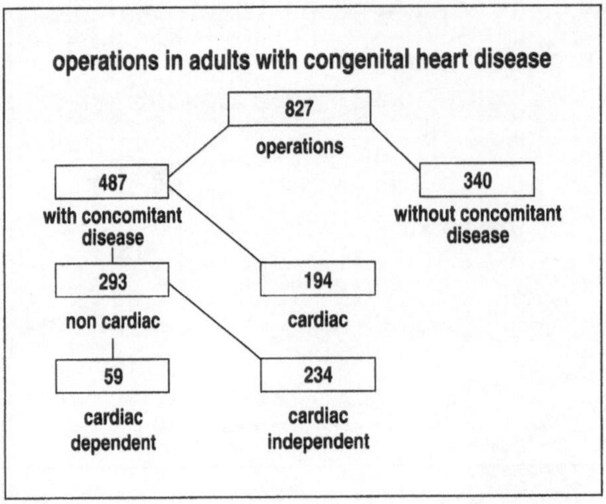

Fig. 2. Distribution of age and diagnosis in 827 operations in 463 adult patients with congenital heart diseases.
ASD II: atrial septal defect of the secundum type; PAPVD: partial anomalous pulmonary venous drainage; ASDI: atrial septal defect of the primum type; CAVSD: complete atrioventricular septal defect; AS: aortic stenosis; AI: aortic insufficiency; Coarc: coarctation of the aorta; PS: pulmonary stenosis; DORV: double outlet right ventricle; Single ventricle: single ventricle; PA-atr.: pulmonary atresia; Ebstein: Ebstein's anomaly; TOF: tretralogy of Fallot; TGA: transposition of the great arteries; TA: tricuspid atresia; TI: tricuspid insufficiency; BWG: Bland-White-Garland syndrome; MI: mitral insufficiency; KMP: cardiomyopathy. The mortality was 1.1% (volume overload), 2.8% (pressure overload), 10.9% (Cyanosis), and 4.9% (miscellaneous)

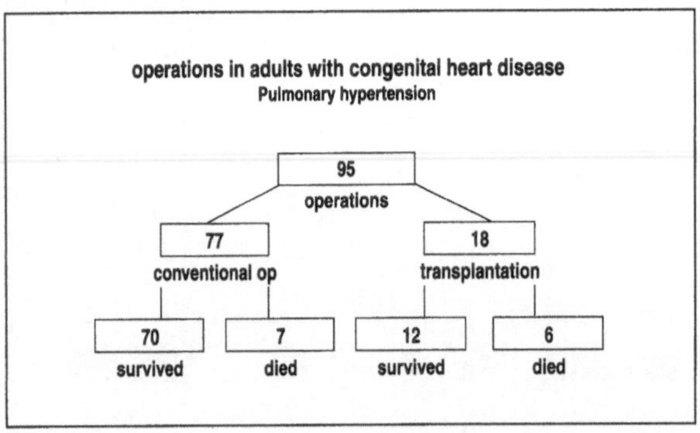

Fig. 3. Pulmonary hypertension was a risk factor for corrective and palliative operations in adult patients with congenital heart disease. All patients, who did not survive transplantation, received single/double lungs or heart-lungs

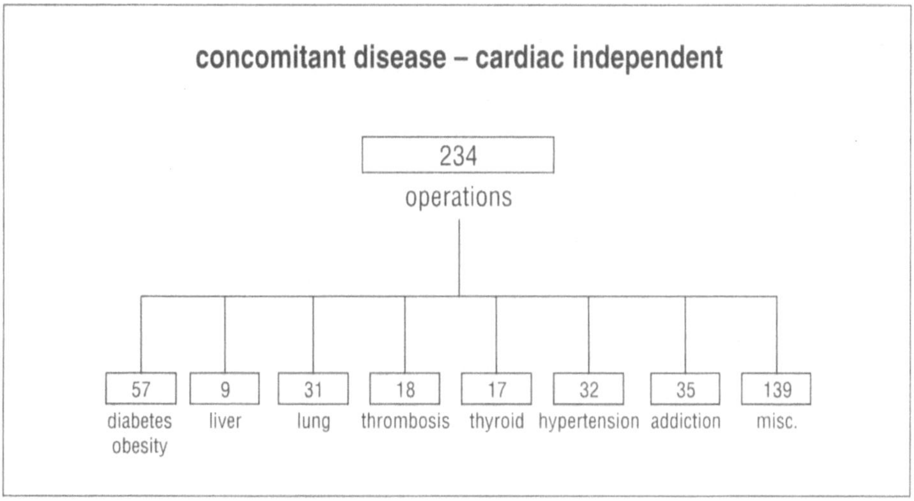

Fig. 4. Cardiac independent concomitant disease was not a risk factor for corrective and palliative operations in adult patients with congenital heart disease

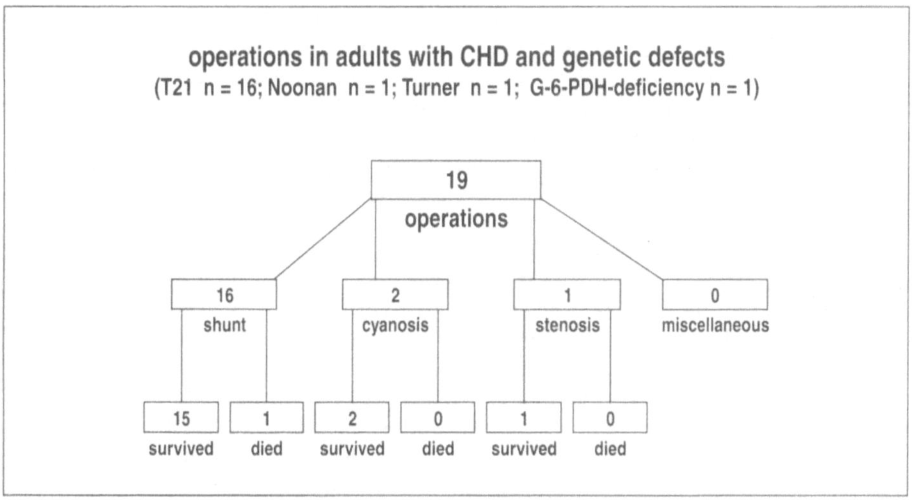

Fig. 5. A genetic defect was not a risk factor for corrective and palliative -operations in adults with congenital heart defect (CHD)

Results

The results are summarized in the Fig. 1–5. The overall hospital mortality was 3.9% for conventional operations and 28.5% (8 out of 28) for transplantation, all of them in patients after lung or heart/lung transplantation. For the subgroups (Fig. 1) the mortality was 1.1% (volume overload, n = 453), 2.8% (pressure overload, n = 145), 10.9% (cyanosis, n = 165), and 4.9% (miscellaneous, n = 64).

A genetic defect was not a risk factor (Fig. 5). One out of 19 patients (a 19 year old patient with Down's syndrome, complete atrio-ventricular defect and pulmonary hypertension) died during a pulmonary hypertensive crisis. Non cardiac concomitant disease (Fig. 5) and coronary heart disease (1 out of 23 patients; 4.3%) did not influence hospital mortality. In 8 out of 23 patients with concomitant coronary heart disease (median age 55 years) bypass operations were performed at the time of repair of CHD.

Cyanosis and pulmonary hypertension were risk factors, the hospital mortality being 10.9% (13 out of 106 operations) and 9.1% (7 out of conventional 77 operations) (Fig. 3).

An increasing mortality was noted with increasing numbers of reoperations (1st op: 2.6%, 2nd op: 6.4%, 3rd op: 8.6%, 4th op: 13.3%, 5th op: 16.6%). Age was only a risk factor in the patients with cyanosis (16–20 years: 9.9%, 21–30 years: 11.8%, 31–40 years: 14.3%, 41–50 years: 0%, 51–60 years: 25%).

Discussion

For decades surgery for congenital heart disease (CHD) has been associated with infants and children. Surgery in adults with CHD has received some attention only in recent years (1, 4, 8, 13, 14, 16, 18, 25, 27). Problems of adult patients with CHD are usually quite different from those during childhood (3–5, 9–11, 15, 17, 25, 27). Besides concomitant diseases typical for older persons without CHD (Fig. 4), one has to deal with sequelae of the original CHD, residual postoperative defects, and consequences of previous operations.

The limitations of this study are the retrospective analysis of patient data as well as the fact that many of the patients were only seen by us during their hospital admission for the operation. This referal pattern of special patients to a specialized center may also explain the unusual high incidence of 58% of concomitant diseases – cardiac and/or non cardiac (Figs. 2–5). Meaningful statements and conclusions about the severity of the concomitant diseases, however, were not possible retrospectively.

The small number of genetic disorders (Fig. 5) among our patients like the Down's syndrome – especially in conjunction with pulmonary hypertension – appears to indicate that these patients were operated earlier because of symptoms or cannot be operated anymore because of Eisenmenger's disease. This probably contributes also to the finding that genetic disorders (Fig. 5) were not an operative risk factor. Risk factors, however, were cyanosis, pulmonary hypertension or reoperation.

Cyanosis is usually the consequence of a complex CHD, requiring complex surgery with its sequelae. In addition cyanosis leads to alterations of all organs especially the myocardium (11) and the kidneys (3). Of the 165 originally cyanotic patients 55 were reoperated, reoperation being a known risk factor (5). Our mortality of 12.2% is similar to the 18%, reported recently for such patients by Dore et al. (5).

Pulmonary hypertension as a cardiac dependent concomitant disease (Fig. 3) is a very well – known risk factor even in infants and children. The pulmonary hypertensive crisis immediately after the operation in the intensive care unit (20, 21, 23) may be the limiting pressure overload for the right ventricle (20, 23) especially in the adult with CHD and longstanding volume/pressure overload. The mortality of 9.1% in 77 conventional operations (Fig. 3) is too high. Routine testing of the pulmonary vascular reagibility (12, 22, 24) and, thus, characterization of an agent or a combination of agents which can be helpful immediately postoperatively (20, 23, 24) seem to have improved our surgial results in children and adults with CHD in recent years. Preferable, however, is an operation during infancy or childhood. The well – known fact that reoperations carry a higher operative risk (1, 5) was also true in our adult patients with CHD. The more reoperations the higher the mortality was. It increased from 2.6% for the first operation to 6.4%, 8.6%, 13.3% and 16.6% for the second, third, fourth and fifth operation, respectively. Since in our opinion reoperations will increasingly be required in the future in such patients with operated complex CHD reaching adulthood, further investigations are necessary to decrease their risk.

Coronary heart disease is seemingly rare is patients with CHD. This may be at least in part due to the relatively young age of most of the observed patients (Fig. 1). However, in 23 of our patients with a median age of 55 years such diagnosis was established during cardiac catheterization, eight requiring a bypass operation at the time of correction of the CHD. Cardiac concomitant diseases like rhythm disturbances or myocardial failure (Fig. 2) were no operative risk factors but caused increased immediate postoperative morbidity and longer hospital stays. Other noncardiac concomitant diseases like kidney, liver, or thyroid insufficiency did not alter the risk of operation in the analyzed groups (Fig. 4). Renal function, however, requires special attention in these patients. In the cyanotic ones a more detailed preoperative evaluation appears advisable (3). The age independent low mortality in patients with ventricular volume (Fig. 1) and pressure overload speaks in favor of present surgical and anesthesiologic techniques as well as postoperative management. The increasing mortality with increasing age in the group of patients with cyanosis has to be expected. Although all organs are involved, myocardial fibrosis (11) seems to be decisive. Thus, CHD should be operated during infancy or childhood although palliative and corrective surgery in adults with CHD can be performed with an acceptable risk of an overall mortality of 3.9%. On the other hand continuing further studies are necessary since an increasing number of patients with operated complex CHD will reach adulthood as chronic cardiac patients with very special problems, which vary according to the very variable CHD as well as to the different surgical methods applied over the last years.

References

1. Albertucci M, Wong K, Petrou M, Mitchell A, Somerville J, Theodoropoulos S, Yacoub M (1994) The use of unstented homograft valves for aortic valve reoperations: Review of a twenty-three-year experience. J Thorac Cardiovasc Surg 107: 152–161
2. Danielson GK, Anderson BJ, Schleck CD, Ilstrup DM (1995) Late results of pulmonary ventricle to pulmonary artery conduits. Semin Thorac Cardiovasc Surg 7: 162–167
3. Dittrich S, Haas N, Müller C, Bührer C, Alexi-Meskishvili V, Lange PE (1998) Die "zyanotische" Nephropathie bei unkorrigiertem Vitium cordis – Risiko für die Entwicklung eines akuten Nierenversagens nach kardiopulmonalem Bypass. Z Herz Thorax Gefäßchir 12: 1–7
4. Dittrich S, Dähnert I, Uhlemann F, Berger F, Weng Y, Alexi-Meskishvili V, Hetzer R, Lange PE (1996) Ergebnisse nach Korrektur der Fallotschen Tetralogie im Erwachsenenalter. Z Kardiol 85(Suppl 2): 94
5. Dore A, Glancy L, Stone S, Menashe V, Somerville J (1997) Cardiac surgery for grown-up congenital heart patients: survey of 307 consecutive operations from 1991 to 1994. Am J Cardiol 80: 906–913
6. Driscoll DJ, Offord KP, Feldt RH, Schaff HV, Puga FJ, Danielson GK (1992) Five- to fifteen-year follow-up after Fontan operation. Circulation 85: 469–496
7. Glancy DL, Morrow AG, Simon AL, Roberts WC (1983) Juxtaductal aortic coarctation. Analysis of 84 patients studied hemodynamically, angiographically, and morphologically after age 1 year. Am J Cardiol 51: 537–551
8. Hoffmann JIE (1987) Incidence, mortality and natural history. In: Anderson RH, Macartney FJ, Shinebourne EA, Tynan M (eds) Pediatric Cardiology. Churchill Livingstone, Edinburgh, pp 4–14

9. Horvath KA, Burke RP, Collins JJ, Cohn LH (1992) Surgical treatment of adult atrial septal defect: Early and long-term results. J Am Coll Cardiol 20: 1156–1159
10. Kitchiner D, Jackson M, Walsh K, Paert I, Arnold R (1993) The progression of mild congenital aortic valve stenosis from childhood into adult life. lnt J Cardiol 42: 217-223
11. Krymsky LD (1965) Pathologic anatomy of congenital heart disease. Circulation 32: 814–827
12. Lange PE, Berger F, Gorenflo M, Schulze-Neick I, Kampmann C, Hausdorf G, Alexi-Meskishvili V, Weng Y, Loebe M, Hetzer R, Vogel M, Bein G, Uhlemann F (1994) Pulmonale Hypertension bei angeborenen Herzfehlern. Z Herz Thorax Gefäßchir 8: 231–239
13. Lindenau KF, Torka M, Schneider A, Hacker RW (1997) Operative Behandlung angeborener Herzfehler im Erwachsenenalter. Z Herz Thorax Gefäßchir 6: 263–269
14. Lundstrom U, Bull C, Wyse RK, Somerville J (1990) The natural and "unnatural" history of congenital corrected transposition. Am J Cardiol 65: 1222–1229
15. Martinez JE, Mohiaddin RH, Kilner PJ, Khaw, K, Rees S, Somerville J, Longmore DB (1992) Obstruction in extracardiac ventriculopulmonary conduits: Value of nuclear magnetic resonance imaging with velocity mapping and Doppler echocardiography. J Am Coll Cardiol 20: 338–334
16. Pome G, Rossi C, Colucci V, Passini L, Morello M, Taglieri C. Pezzano A, Figini A, Pellegrini A (1992) Late reoperations after repair of tetralogy of Fallot. Eur J Cardiothorac Surg 6: 31–35
17. Presbitero P, Demarie D, Aruta E, Villani M, Disumma M, Ottino GM, Orzan F, Fubini A, Spinnler MT, Conte MR, Morea M (1996) Results of total correction of tetralogy of Fallot performed in adults. Ann Thorac Surg 61: 1870–1873
18. Sampson C, Kilner PJ, Hirsch R, Rees RS, Somerville J, Underwood SR (1994) Venoatrial pathways after the Mustard operation for transposition of the great arteries: anatomic and functional MR imaging. Radiology 193: 211–217
19. Sampson C, Martinez J, Rees S, Somerville J, Underwood R, Longmore D (1990) Evaluation of Fontans operation by magnetic resonance imaging. Am J Cardiol 65: 819–821
20. Schulze-Neick I, Bültmann M, Werner H, Gamillscheg A, Ichihashi K. Uhlemann F, Vogel M, Rossaint R, Alexi-Meskishvili V, Hetzer R, Lange PE (1996) Quantitative Echokardiographie des rechten Ventrikels zur Beurteilung der Therapie mit inhalativem Stickmonoxyd bei der postoperativen Betreuung von Patienten mit angeborenen Herzfehlern. Z Herz Thorax Gefäßchir 10: 107–111
21. Schulze-Neick I, Nürnberg J, Igde H, Haas N, Uhlemann F, Berger F, Lange PE (1996) Pulmonary hypertensive crisis (PHTC) is associated with acute changes of pulmonary function. Chest 110 (Suppl): 41S
22. Schulze-Neick I, Nürnberg J, Haas N, Igde H, Dähnert I, Hofstadler G, Uhlemann F, Berger F, Opitz C, Kleber FX, Lange PE (1996) Evaluation des Lungengefäßwiderstandes bei Patienten mit angeborenen Shuntvitien und primärer pulmonaler Hypertension. Monatsschr Kinderheilkd 144 (Suppl 1): S38
23. Schulze-Neick I, Bültmann M, Werner H, Gamillscheg A, Vogel M, Rossaint R, Hetzer R, Lange PE (1997) Right ventricular function in patients treated with inhaled nitric oxide after cardiac surgery for congenital heart disease in newborns and children. Am J Cardiol 80: 360–363
24. Schulze-Neick I, Uhlemann F, Nürnberg J, Bültmann M, Haas N, Dähnert I, Alexi-Meskishvili V, Opitz C, Pappert D, Rossaint R, Kleber FX, Hetzer R, Lange PE (1997) Aerosolisiertes Prostacyclin zur praeoperativen Evaluation und postkardiochirurgischen Behandlung von Patienten mit pulmonaler Hypertension. Z Kardiol 86: 71–80
25. Somerville J (1996) The adult with surgically corrected congenital heart disease: long term care. Cardiol Rev 4: 57–64
26. Stewart S, Alexson C, Manning J, Oakes D, Eberly SW (1988) Long-term palliation with the classic Blalock-Taussig Shunt. J Thorac Cardiovasc Surg 96: 117–121
27. Warnes CA, Somerville J (1986) Tricuspid atresia in adolescents and adults: Current state and late complications. Br Heart J 56: 535–543

Author's address:
Dr. med. Ingo Dähnert
Deutsches Herzzentrum Berlin
Abteilung für angeborene Herzfehler / Kinderkardiologie
Augustenburger Platz 1
13353 Berlin, Germany

The role of heart transplantation and assist devices in patients with severe concomitant diseases

M. Loebe, M. Hummel, R. Hetzer

Deutsches Herzzentrum Berlin, Dept. of Thoracic and Cardiovascular Surgery, Berlin/Germany

Introduction

Some 30 years ago when Christiaan Barnard first started using orthotopic human heart transplantation as a treatment for end stage heart failure, this attempt was followed by tremendous press coverage and a rapidly expanding number of operations performed worldwide. But while a number of surgeons all over the world were eager to follow the technique Barnard used in this operation, it instantly turned out that the knowledge of immunology, immunosuppression, and the like was not developed sufficiently at that point of time to make the procedure a successful one (33). In the following years extensive basic research paved the way for a resurrection of heart transplantation as a decent type of treatment for end stage heart failure. At Stanford University, N. Shumway and his coworkers achieved this in no small part by introducing very strict selection criteria for both patients put on the heart transplant waiting list and acceptable donor organs (19). Using these criteria and gaining more and more insight into allograft rejection, the Stanford-group was able to increase 1 year survival rates from less than 30% in 1968 to a more acceptable survival rate of over 60% in the late seventies (19). Of course the greatest step forward was then the introduction of cyclosporine as a new immunosuppressive treatment in heart transplantation in the early 1980s (23). But when contemplating about the role of concomitant diseases in heart transplantation one should keep in mind that from early on strict criteria in recipient selection were mandatory for bringing cardiac transplantation to a point were results allowed the more widespread use of this treatment.

Today more than 40000 heart transplant recipients are listed in the data base of the International Society for Heart and Lung Transplantation (16). Medium and long-term results obtained with this treatment are extremely good with up to 60% of patients surviving for more than 10 years (38). At the Deutsches Herzzentrum Berlin we have performed more than 1000 orthotopic heart transplant procedures since 1986. The long-term survival is given in Fig. 5.

These extremely good long-term results were obtained in a group of transplant candidates that from the start included a number of patients who presented with concomitant diseases commonly regarded as contraindications to heart transplantation according to the Stanford criteria (19,22). Since the initiation of our transplant program it has been our policy to rather include than exclude patients from a lifesaving procedure such as heart transplantation. We have rather searched for ways to reduce the risks arising from conditions such as patients comorbidity (24). This allows us today to draw some conclusions from our long-term experience in so-called borderline heart transplant recipients. The first part of this chapter covers our own experience in the field as well as discusses some recent reports in the literature on heart transplantation and concomitant disases.

The second part is dedicated to the use of mechanical assist devices in patients with comorbidity. Also ventricular assist devices were first developed aiming at permanent replacement of the failing heart; they gained widespread use when implanted as a bridge to heart transplantation (40). Today growing attention is focused on using those devices as an alternative to heart transplantation in patients presenting with concomitant diseases that may negatively affect the outcome of heart transplantation (39). Based on our experience at the Deutsches Herzzentrum Berlin with more than 350 ventricular assist devices implanted over the last 10 years we will discuss some of the aspects concerning permanent replacement as well as the recovery of secondary organ dysfunction under mechanical support and its influence on myocardial recovery.

Heart transplantation

Several factors correlating with mortality rates in patients with congestive heart failure have been identified in the past (8, 30, 36, 44) (Table 1). Based on these findings the indication for heart transplantation is given when the patient has an estimated chance of survival time below 12 months and no alternative treatment is available. Of course the main indication for heart transplantation is severe activity limiting heart failure under full medical management. The age usually should be less than 65 years, which is already an extension of the classic Stanford Criteria where the upper age limit for heart recipients was 45 years (8).

Irreversible secondary organ damage such as renal and hepatic dysfunction, severe chronic pulmonary disease, non-reversible elevated pulmonary hypertension, diabetes with important end-organ damage, severe peripheral and cerebrovascular disease, active infection or malignancies, cardiac involvement as part of a systemic disease, severe obesity, and psychosocial instability or noncompliance to medical treatment have been considered as contraindications to heart transplantation

Table 1. Factors correlating with mortality rates in patients with congestive heart failure (modified from Costanzo (7))

Clinical	
	Heart disease etiology
	Heart disease duration
	Gender
	Progression of cachexia
Hemodynamic	
	Left ventricular ejection fraction
	Right ventricular ejection fraction
	Pulmonary artery wedge pressure
	Stroke work index
Functional capacity	
	NYHA class
	Oxygen consumption at peak exercise (V02 max)
	Distance covered during 6min. walk
Neurohumoral	
	Plasma norepinephrine
	Zytokine-levels
Arrhythmias	

(Table 2) (2, 7, 8, 15). The list can certainly be extended. Nevertheless, in most major centers a number of patients who presented with one or several of those exclusion criteria have been transplanted in the past and their outcome was quite successful (14,22). Recurrent reports of extended recipient criteria can be found in the literature (5, 6, 11, 19, 23, 32). In our view it is more important to develop strategies for reducing the posttransplant risk associated with certain comorbidities than to have an anecdotal patient who survived the procedure despite concomitant conditions generally regarded as contraindications. We believe that except for active infection and malignant diseases all these so-called contraindications for heart transplantation rather have to be considered as risk factors for posttransplant complications than as mere exclusion criteria for the treatment. One must of course carefully weight the risks caused by comorbidity and the benefit the patient may gain from the transplant procedure. This thoughtful evaluation forms the basis of patient counseling before heart transplantation. If there is the option of an alternative treatment that offers a fair and near equal chance of survival and quality of live for this given patient, then this alternative should be suggested to the patient and his family.

From the American registry of heart transplanted patients (2, 16) there is an extensive analysis available about risk factors influencing the postoperative course

Table 2. Conditions which may affect morbidity and mortality after cardiac transplantation

Age
Coexistent systemic illness with poor prognosis
Myocardial infiltrative and inflammatory disease
Irreversible pulmonary arterial hypertention
Irreversible pulmonary parenchymal disease
Acute pulmonary thromboembolism
Severe peripheral/cerebrovascular disease
Irreversible renal dysfunction
Irreversible hepatic dysfunction
Active peptic ulcer
Active diverticulosis or diverticulitis
Insulin-dependent diabetes with end-organ damage
Severe obesety
Active infection
Coexisting neoplasm
Psychosocial instabiliy
Substance abuse

Table 3. Risk factors for 1 year mortality after heart transplantation in the USA (UNOS-database)

Preoperative Variable	odds ratio	p-value
Repeat Tx	3.51	< 0.0001
Ventilator dependent	2.39	<0.0001
Donor age 60	2.21	< 0.0001
Recipient age 70	1.92	< 0.0001
Small transplant center	1.29	0.0002
Donor female	1.22	< 0.0001
ICU/ Assist device dependent	1.21	0.001

Table 4. Risk factors for acute renal failure after heart transplantation; Deutsches Herzzentrum Berlin-Multiple step regression analysis

Variable	p-value
Infection	0.0015
Adrenaline	0.0019
Gender(female)	0.0026
Cyclosporine preop	0.0097

(Table 3). But again mostly those related to the acute severity of cardiogenic shock were statistically significantly predicting one year mortality. Patients who were ventilator dependent, in ICU, and on mechanical support had an unfavorable outcome, while those factors one would expect to have an impact according to the exclusion criteria mentioned before did not reach high statistical significance. Nevertheless, chronic comorbidity does of cause influence patients posttransplant course and to some extent his or her long-term outlook. But only very few comorbid conditions have the tendency to worsen under immunosuppressive treatment. A patient with generalized arterial occlusive disease, for example, will have a great chance to encounter some problems arising from this co-condition (10), but there is no scientific evidence that the progression of systemic arteriosclerotic disease is by any means influenced by the posttransplant medication. The same holds true for diabetes, which may improve or worsen under cyclosporine treatment (32). Some factors, however, do influence the perioperative course dramatically, and they will be discussed here.

Renal disease

About 20% of patients develop renal dysfunction after heart transplantation according to the combined UNOS and ISHLT registry (16). As in most of the secondary organ dysfunction it is sometimes hard to distinguish between acute renal failure after surgery when cyclosporine is given in high dosage and preexisting chronic irreversible impairment of renal function. A number of risk factors have been identified at the Deutsches Herzzentrum Berlin, influencing the incidence of acute renal failure in heart transplant recipients early after the procedure (Table 4) (17). During perioperative patient treatment the damaging effect of cyclosporine can be adjusted by iv administration and careful cyclosporine level monitoring (24). But it seems to be more important to administer drugs which protect the kidney. We have been very successful in using Urodilatin, a human atrial natriuretic hormone analogon, to prevent acute renal failure (18).

Age

If one looks at age there is a statistically significant decrease of 1 year survival in patients older than 70 years (16). In these patients mortality is doubled compared with candidates around 50 years of age or quadrupled compared to a recipient who is in his 30s. But this means that 1 year survival drops from about 95% to around 85%, and it seems to be unjustifiable to us to exclude patients from a lifesaving treatment that carries a risk of 15% mortality within the first year after surgery. A number of publications have been presented recently from centers who increased the upper age limit from 54 up to 70 years and everybody reported quite favorable results (6, 11, 23). In our own experience when comparing patients above 55 years of age, at the time of transplantation and those below 55 years of age there was virtually no difference in mid- and long-term outcome. For more than 10 years we have extended the indication criteria for our recipients and liberally accepted patients over the age of 55. Today these patients account for about 1 quarter of the total number of patients transplanted at our institution.

Nevertheless, these patients had an increased risk to attract infectious and renal complications in the early posttransplant period (22, 42). This is certainly due to concomitant diseases present in the elderly transplant recipient who mostly presented with ischemic cardiomyopathy. Therefore, general arteriosclerosis was more common in this group as well as chronic pulmonary diseases, rendering these patients more prone to attract lung infections. To overcome these problems we have modified the immunosuppression over the years for this subgroup of patients. We avoid the application of monoclonal antibodies (OKT) for rejection prophylaxis, and we reduced the use of polyclonal antibodies (ATG)(24). We now try to keep older patients on a immunosuppressive regime free of steroids when ever possible. In addition immunosuppression in the first few weeks after transplantation highly relies on immunologic monitoring. A much more individualized approach for each patient depending on his or her immunocompetence and state of immunologic activation allowed us widely to abolish overimmunosuppression in older patients. Cyclosporine is already started preoperatively intravenously. The use of urodilatin was very helpful in protecting renal function which is of particular importance in the older age group. Infectious prophylaxis for legionella, CMV, and toxoplasma seems to have as well helped to improve results over the years. Finally a non-invasive day by day monitoring of rejection via intramyocardial electrocardiogram after the patient is discharged home had a very positive impact on providing individualized immunosuppressive treatment, therefore, reducing the risk of infection and secondary organ dysfunction due to immunosuppression or recurrent rejection (46, Table 5).

Psychosocial behavior and non-compliance

Undoubtedly heart transplantation requires a secure social background for the patient to cope with several problems arising from both waiting time and the procedure itself. Chronic intake of medication is mandatory, and the patient and his or her caregiver must understand the importance of rejection surveillance and regular hospital contacts. We have relied on the support of psychotherapists who form an

Table 5. Improvements in postoperative care for heart transplant recipients; Deutsches Herzzentrum Berlin

– Modified immunosuppression No monoclonal antibodies, reduced use of polyclonal antibodies, reduced or no induction therapy)
– Protection of renal function Use of urodilatin
– Prophylaxis of infection Legionella, CMV, Toxoplasma
– Daily non-invasive rejection monitoring

Table 6. Factors that may influence morbidity and mortality after assist device implantation

Irreversible secondary organ dysfunction
Active infection
Coagulopathy
Previous cardiac surgery
Mechanical heart valves
Intraventricular thrombi
Age
Right heart failure
Severe peripheral vascular disease
Insulin-dependent diabetes with end-organ damage

Table 7. Transplantability score; Deutsches Herzzentrum Berlin

One point for
– liver failure (OT> 100 U/l)
– renal failure (CREA> 2.5 U/l)
– loss on conciousness
– infection
– respirator dependent

important part of the transplant team (1). The patients as well as their caregivers undergo psychological evaluation before putting the patient on the waiting list. However, this is not meant to exclude noncompliant patients from the procedure than rather to identify early possible sources of complications. These problems are than actively addressed and taken into consideration when planing patients posttransplant treatment.

Elevated pulmonary vascular resistance

Pulmonary vascular resistance remains the major obstacle in heart transplantation as far as extended recipient criteria are concerned (8). There are several approaches and a number of medications to take care of this problem. However, a pulmonary vascular resistance above 6 Wood unit increases the risk of the procedure to a intolerable extent. From the Stanford heart transplant experience Costard-Jaeckle and coworkers (9) have collected data that demonstrate how patients outcome depends on the degree of preexisting pulmonary vascular resistance. Heart transplant candidates were classified according to the response of their pulmonary vascular resistance to treatment. Patients, who had either no increased PVR or in whom PVR could be normalized by medication without compromising systemic blood pressure, had a favorable posttransplant course. However, in the group of patients where the pulmonary vascular resistance could only be decreased for the cost of decreased systemic systolic pressure midterm survival was significantly reduced. In patients where the high pulmonary vascular resistance measured preoperativly was refractory to all kinds of medications, one year survival was reduced to 40%. Patients with increased pulmonary vascular resistance did to a lesser extent do die from overt right heart failure but more commonly due to a higher incidence of infectious complications and other problems. This is probably related to their extended stay in the intensive care unit with extended periods of respirator dependency.

Our approach to a patient with increased pulmonary vascular resistance is to test pulmonary vascular reagibility by administration of prostaglandine (E1 or E2). If the pulmonary vascular resistance is reduces and the transpulmonary gradient is lower than 12 mmHg, the patient is classified as a responder and listed for heart transplantation. In patients with a transpulmonary gradient above 12 mmHg NO inhalation is applied at the time of heart transplantation. The non-responders undergo a prolonged treatment with prostacyclin and positive inotropic drugs over several days or even weeks and are re-tested. Some are put on intravenous catecholomines and then retested and reevaluated. Nevertheless, in this subgroup of patients the risk of recurrent right heart failure after heart transplantation is increased compared to responders and patients with low pulmonary vascular resistance. Increased PVR still remains a serious problem for heart transplant recipients. But as long as no alternative treatment is available (except for heart lung transplantation, which in the midterm survival carries a risk nearly equal to isolated heart transplantation in this patients subgroup), it is only justified to exclude candidates from heart transplantation who have a PVR above 6 Wood units and do not respond to PVR-testing.

Diabetes, cachexia, and previous malignancies

From our experience and that of others diabetes mellitus can not be regarded as a contraindication to heart transplantation. Long-term survival in this subgroup is very much comparable to what we see in non-diabetic recipients (32, (Fig. 1). Nevertheless, the degree of end-organ damage due to diabetes has to be assessed and will influence the posttransplant course. The same is true for cachectic and severely obese patients (Fig. 2) although in our experience patients with a high body mass index had a somewhat impaired survival. This may be surprising as

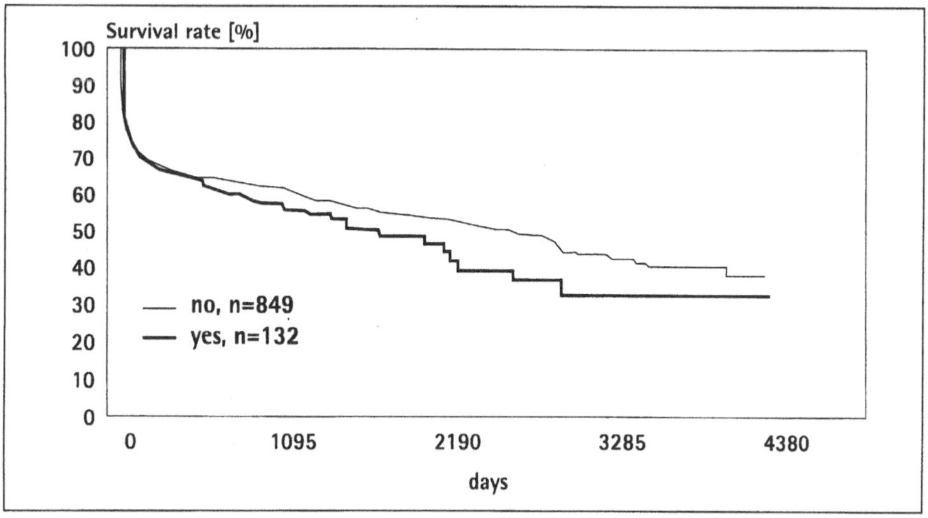

Fig. 1. Survival after heart transplantation depending on diabetes mellitus; Deutsches Herzzentrum Berlin experience

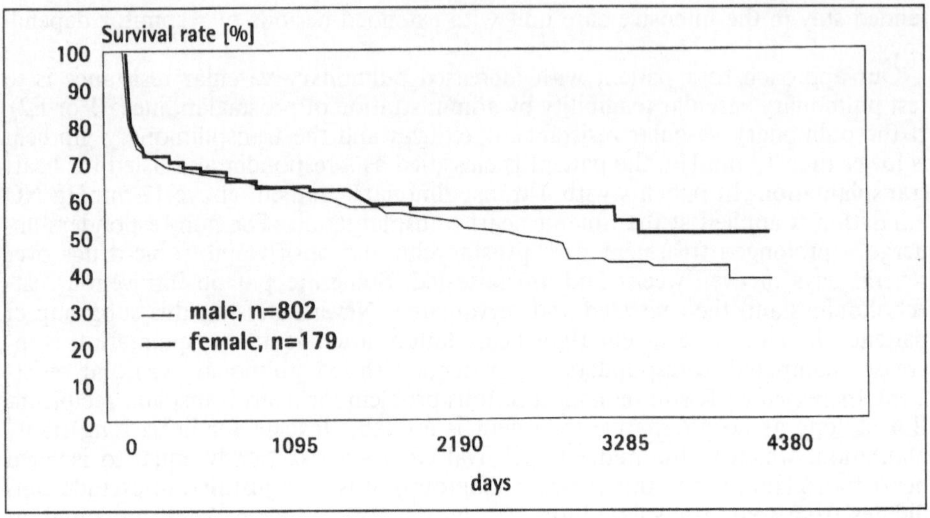

Fig. 2. Survival after heart transplantation depending on obesity and cachexia; Deutsches Herzzentrum Berlin experience

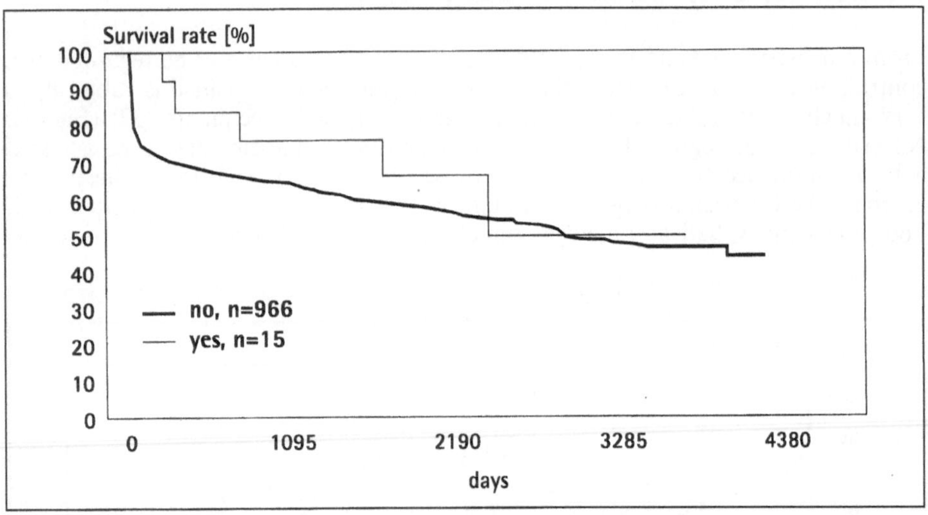

Fig. 3. Survival after heart transplantation depending on history of malignancy; Deutsches Herzzentrum Berlin experience

recent evidence from the literature shows that cachexia is a strong predictor of unfavorable outcome in heart failure patients (4). Judging from our experience, reestablishing adequate hemodynamics after heart transplantation and subsequent rehabilitation reverses this process.

A few patients who had a history of previous malignancies have been transplanted at the Deutsches Herzzentrum Berlin very successfully (Fig. 3). M. Musci (33) has reported in more details about our approach in this subgroup of patients. Again, tailored individualized immunosuppression forms the basis of posttransplant treatment. Today there is no evidence that the risk of tumor reoccurrence is increased in this subgroup of transplant recipients (20, 33).

For most of the concomitant diseases traditionally considered as contraindications for heart transplantation, we now have measurements to control and adapt treatment. Renal insufficiency can mostly be prevented by the prophylactic administration of Urodilatin. The risk arising from impaired pulmonary function, previous carcinomas, and diabetes can at least be reduced by avoiding overimmunosuppression (Fig. 4). The posttransplant risk related to elevated pulmonary vascular resistance can be overcome at least in part by the application of inhaled nitric oxide perioperatively. Severe acute secondary organ dysfunction before transplantation can be resolved by the use of ventricular assist devices with later on transplanting the patient in much better general conditions.

Patients psycho-social problems are addressed by intensive psychological guidance and social worker support.

Looking again at the combined UNOS and ISHLT registry (16) one realizes that donor specific comorbidity like donor age, the demand of catecholamines, gender, center experience in heart transplantation, and (to very little extent) ischemic time do influence the postoperative outcome more than recipient related comorbidity. Matching the heart donor and heart transplant recipient remains a very difficult task to achieve (41, 47). Should one assign the marginal donor organ to a marginal recipient? Would this then not add up the risks in both parts of the procedure? As far as outcome is concerned, is it not more helpful to give a ideal donor organ to a marginal recipient to reduce the accumulative risk? But one may also argue that a patient who would have been excluded for his comorbidity may then receive a marginal donor organ with acceptable risks compared to his fate when completely excluded from the treatment. In any case one should carefully value the increasing risks when assigning a marginal donor organ to a non optimal recipient.

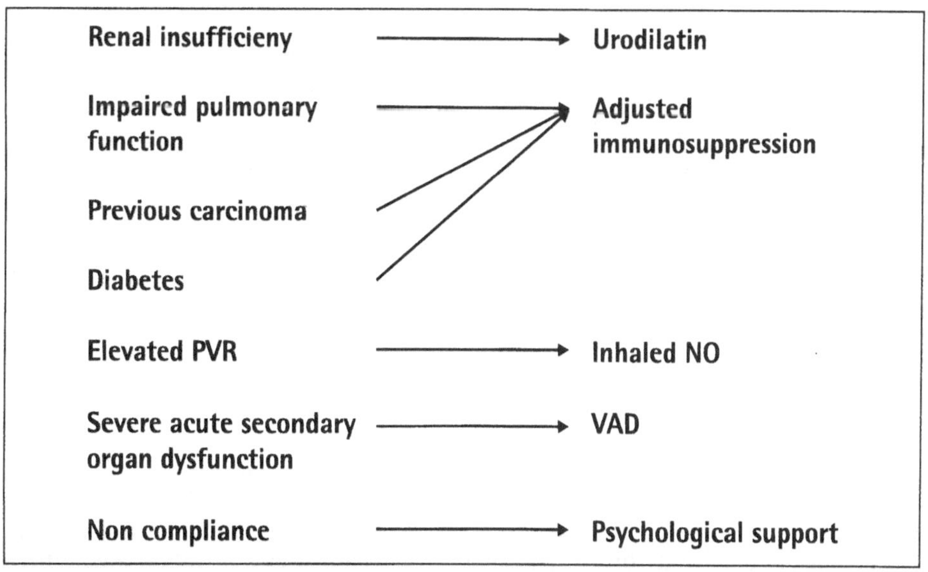

Fig. 4. Improvements in postoperative care for high risk heart transplant recipients

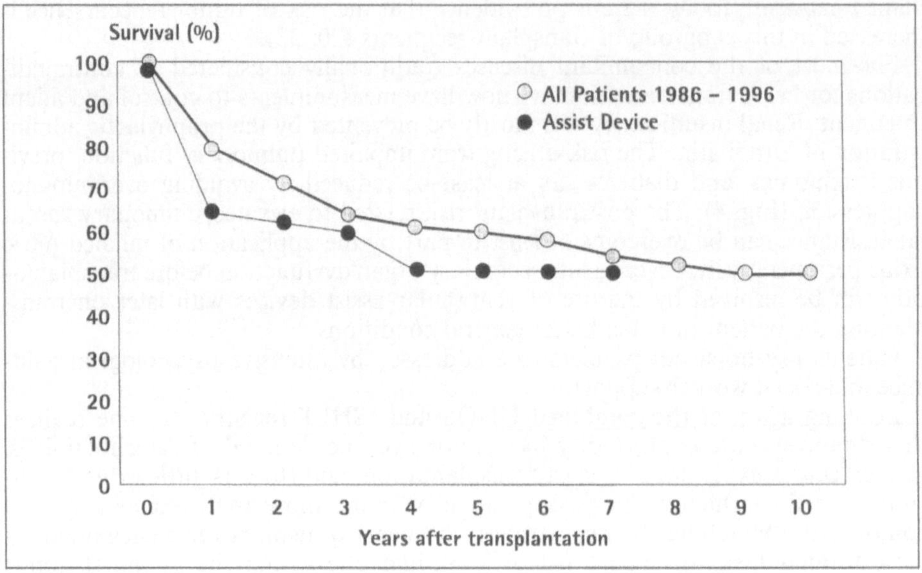

Fig. 5. Survival after heart transplantation depending on previous use of mechanical assist device; Deutsches Herzzentrum Berlin experience

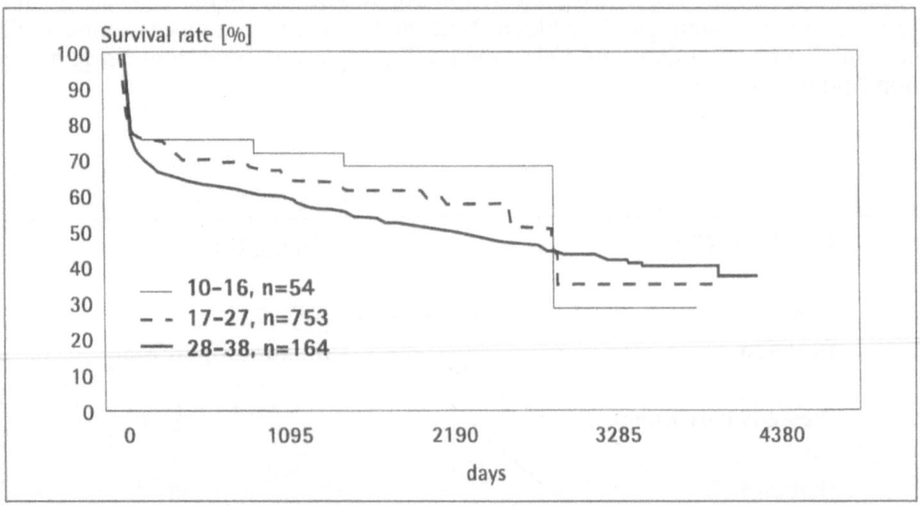

Fig. 6. Survival after heart transplantation depending on recipients gender; Deutsches Herzzentrum Berlin experience

Also recipient criteria can be easily extended (41); the number of donor hearts available will continue to limit a wider use of this surgical approach to heart failure. The major problem is the lack of donor organs with an increasing waiting time and increasing death rate on the transplant list. While one can widely extend indications for transplant recipients, the acceptance of donor organs can only be broadened to a limited extend. From very early on we have been successful in using older and marginal donor hearts. Nevertheless, these approaches have not let us to sufficiently increase the total number of donor organs available; therefore, the total number of patients saved by organ transplantation has not increased substantially over recent years. If one looks at the evolution of the number of transplant procedures in Germany, there is no increase between 1989 and 1995. Therefore, a tremendous number of patients in end stage heart failure cannot be helped by heart transplantation.

One consequence is to extend the indications for organ saving procedures such as revascularization or valve replacement or the use of medical treatment in patients with impaired ventricular function (37). This leaves heart transplantation to a admittedly rather sick group of patients (27). The use of coronary artery revascularization in patients with severely reduced left ventricular function has increased at our institution over the years. Mid- and long-term results of patients with highly impaired left ventricular function in coronary bypass surgery are well comparable to those obtained in heart transplantation. Other chapters in this book will address high risk conventional heart surgery in more detail.

The second part of this paper will touch on the issue of mechanical circulatory support and its relation to comorbidity. Mechanical circulatory support today may

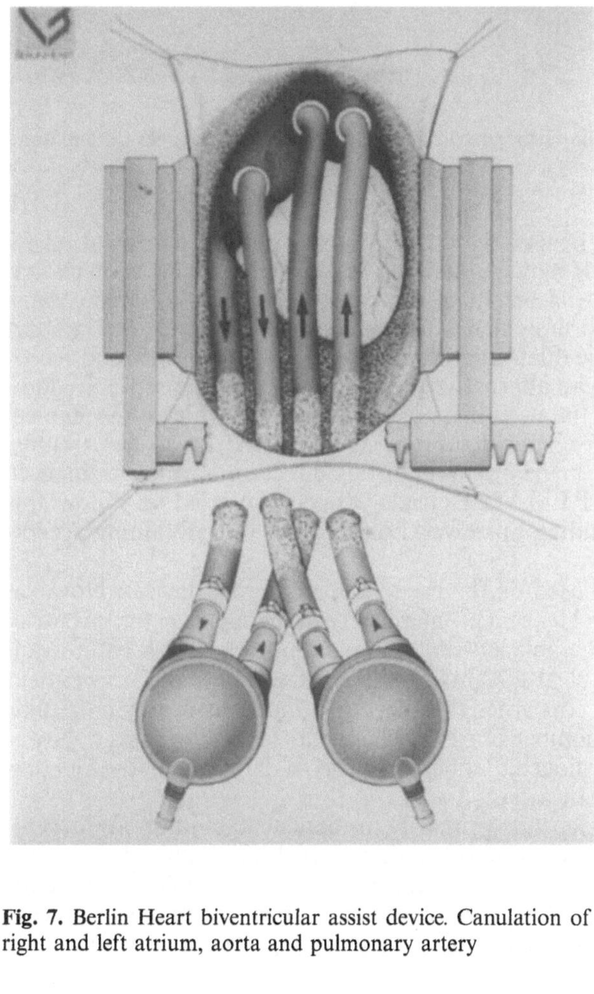

Fig. 7. Berlin Heart biventricular assist device. Canulation of right and left atrium, aorta and pulmonary artery

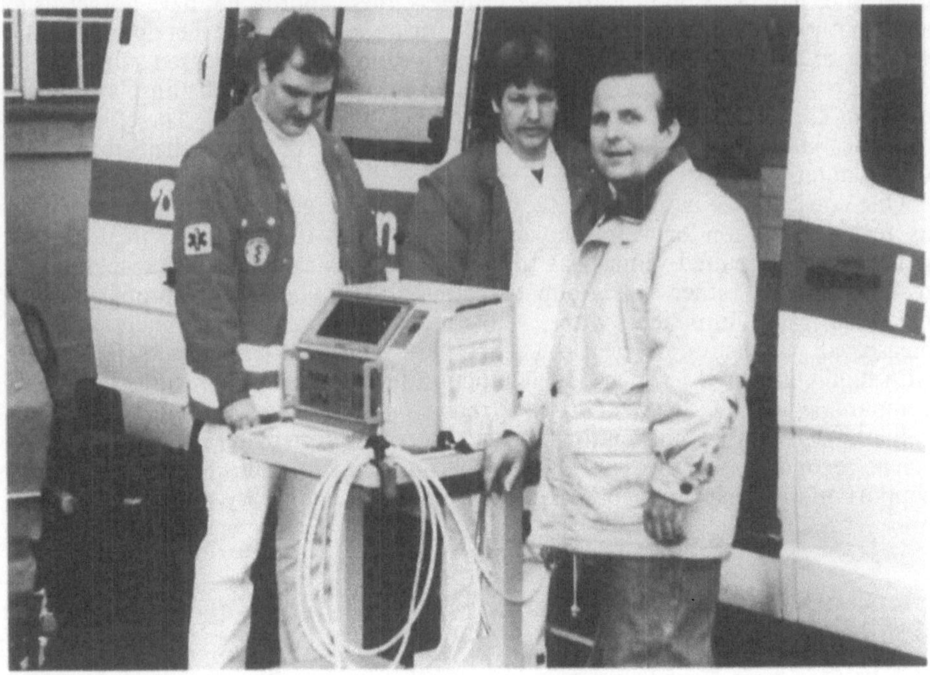

Fig. 8. Patient ambulatory with Berlin Heart biventricular assist device and Heimes driving unit

have several goals (35). It may be used as postcardiotomy support aiming at recovery of the patients own heart. It may be intended as a bridge to heart transplantation and lead to the natural replacement of the patients heart by a human transplant. Recently, we were able to show that extended mechanical circulatory support in some patients with idiopathic dilated cardiomyopathy leads to myocardial recovery and, therefore, can become an alternative to heart transplantation (31). In addition one may speculate about the usefulness of the presently available mechanical assist devices as permanent mechanical support as an alternative to heart transplantation (39). Most recently some attempts in this direction have been made in the USA by introducing the REMATCH trial. Others who tried to follow this direction some years ago, including ourselves, however, failed in obtaining acceptable midterm results (25).

Our experience in Berlin is based on the use of three different devices: Novacor, TCI HeartMate, and the Berlin Heart. The later has been mainly used for biventricular support (Fig. 7–9). The wearable left ventricular support devices became available to us in 1995. Despite the clear advantages these systems have as far as patient mobility and rehabilitation is concerned, we have continued to use biventricular assist devices in a substantial number of cases. These patients were in severe biventricular heart failure and cardiogenic shock with secondary organ dysfunction when they presented at our institution.

The selection of the device depends primarily on patients condition and, therefore, on concomitant organ dysfunction other than (left) heart failure. In the situation of rapidly progressing cardiogenic shock, it is mostly impossible to differentiate between chronic organ dysfunction and acute impairment secondary to recent malperfusion. As heart failure itself is more and more regarded as a whole body

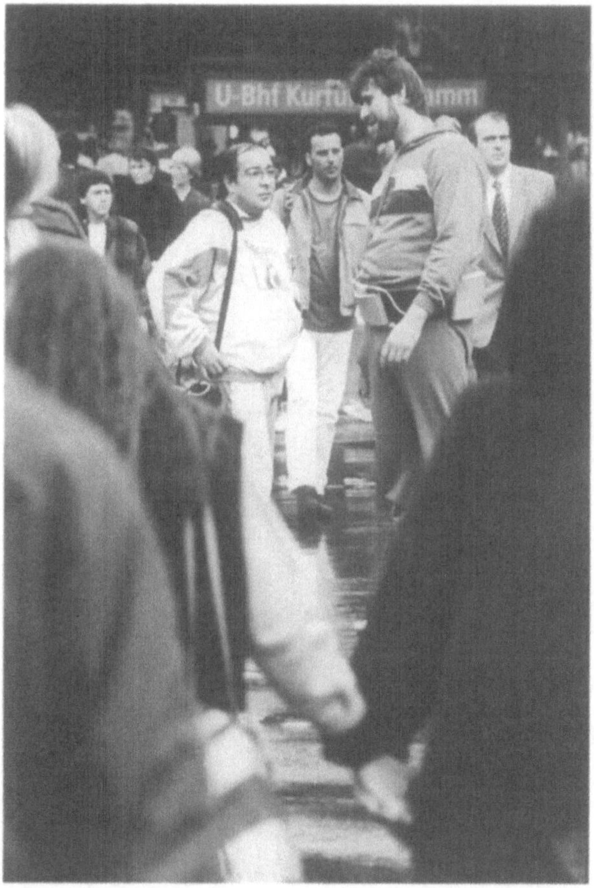

Fig. 9. Two patients with wearable Novacor assist devices

inflammatory syndrome (4, 36) reversal of end-organ dysfunction and peripheral tissue ischemia may also have a tremendous impact on myocardial recovery. The great advantage of biventricular support is the complete replacement of both right and left ventricular function by the support system. But the somewhat bulky driving units to a great extent do restrict the patients ability to walk around and be mobile. The advantage of nearly complete rehabilitation with the wearable LVADs therefore, has to be considered.

Survival of heart transplantation after extended mechanical circulatory support is equal to primary heart transplantation (12, 28), and actually survival after bridging by LVADs has been 96% in the last two year at our institution.

The literature reports a number of exclusion criteria for mechanical circulatory support (29, 40). Severely impaired renal function has been regarded as a contraindication. Of cause severe cerebrovascular disease, cancer, hepatic disease, and severe infections resistant to treatment have been listed as contraindications.

Our experience in the extensive use of assist devices taught us that for many of the dysfunctions listed above it is hard to identify whether they are of chronic

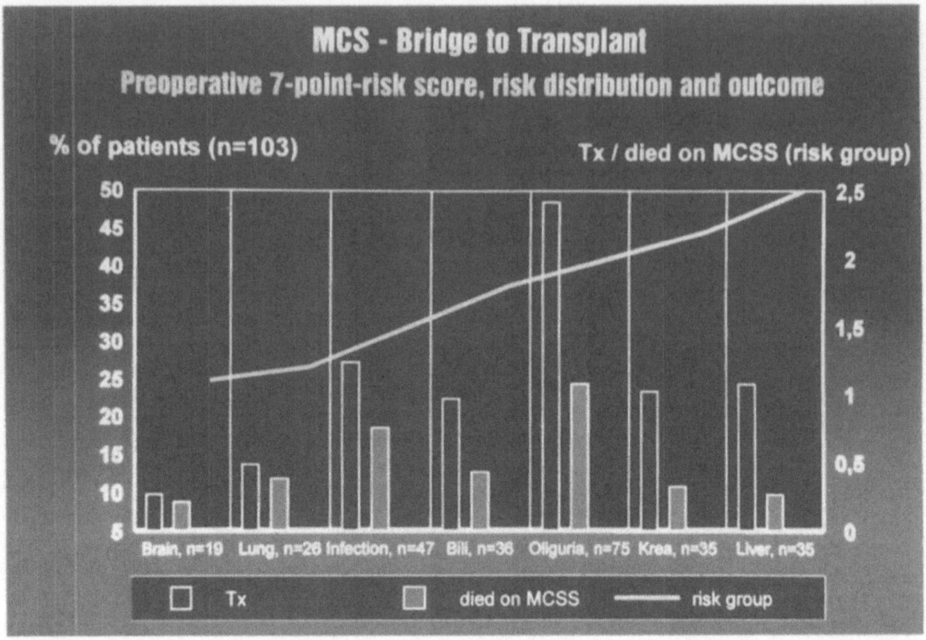

Fig. 10. Preoperative risk evaluation in patients receiving biventricular Berlin Heart support. Note the increased risk with impaired brain and lung function before device implantation while renal and liver dysfunction had comparable little influence on further course

or acute origin in patients presenting with end stage heart failure. The question therefore, is which risk one is willing to take to save the patient's life (Fig. 10).

It has to be kept in mind that the patient will go through several phases when placed on mechanical support (22,25). During the first phase his or her life is saved by reestablishing sufficient hemodynamics. Then follows the recovery from secondary organ dysfunction. During this period of time it is determined whether liver, renal or other organ dysfunctions are reversible or not. While going through this period the patient, in addition to his preexisting conditions, is endangered by complications arising from mechanical circulatory support as well as complications due to non-sufficiently recovered organ function or newly attracted organ dysfunction (13). After successfully passing the first phases the patient has to wait for a suitable donor organ. He is exposed to the problems of chronic mechanical circulatory support. In case myocardial recovery takes place, the patient may be weaned from the device and the device can be removed.

In the light of long-term mechanical support due to the extensive waiting time on the transplant list, one prefers to use wearable implantable devices whenever possible. These systems enable the patients to walk around freely and to be discharged from the hospital (26, 39). Therefore, it is important to predict exactly the risk of right heart failure after isolated left ventricular assist device implantation (45). One aspect that influences the patients post-implant outcome essentially is the inflammatory response caused by chronic heart failure. Tumor necrosis factor alpha (TnF-a) as well as blood urea level (BUN) seem to be quite good indicators for a chronic body malperfusion (Fig. 11). Patients who recovered under isolated

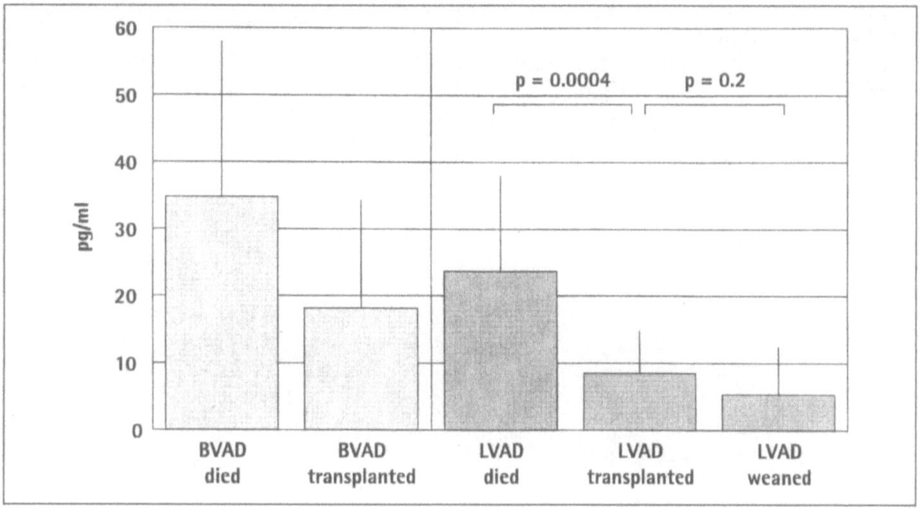

Fig. 11. Tumor necrosis factor predicts patients course after assist device implantation. Note that patients surviving to transplantation on LVAD had significantly lower TnF levels before implantation than those dying

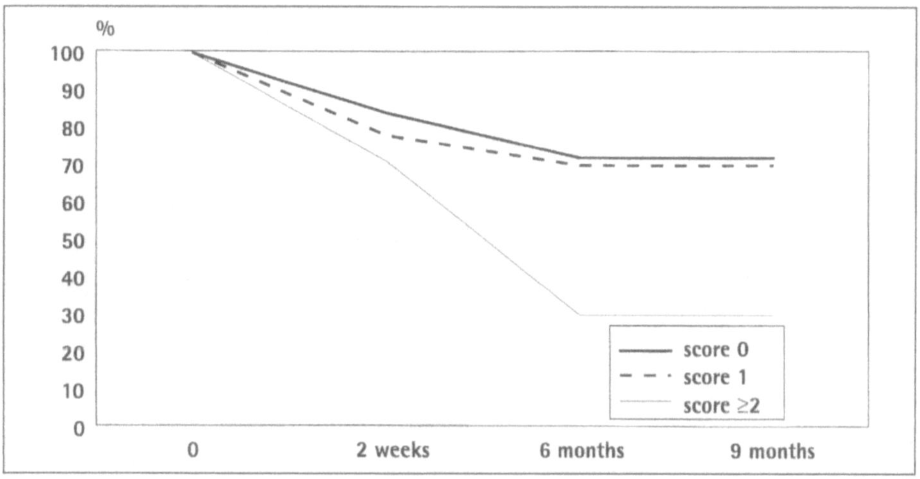

Fig. 12. Survival after heart transplantation in patients with previous mechanical support. Survival depended on degree of recovery from secondary organ dysfunction according to transplantatbility score

left ventricular support had a rather low level of preimplant TNF-a, while those who died on left ventricular support had clearly elevated TNF-a levels. At the same time patients with elevated TNF-a levels were saved by biventricular assist device implantation. Nevertheless, those with extremely high TNF-a levels before implantation had a risk of increased mortality even when put on biventricular support. Since TNF-a is more an expression of the systemic inflammatory response to severe heart failure, this systemic response to heart failure is a major indicator for progression and reversibility of heart failure in both medical treatment and after assist device implantation.

After establishing sufficient circulatory function, it turns out that the liver function becomes of major influence in predicting the further course of the patient. Those patients who recovered from liver dysfunction within the first two weeks after device implantation had a much more favorable outcome compared to those

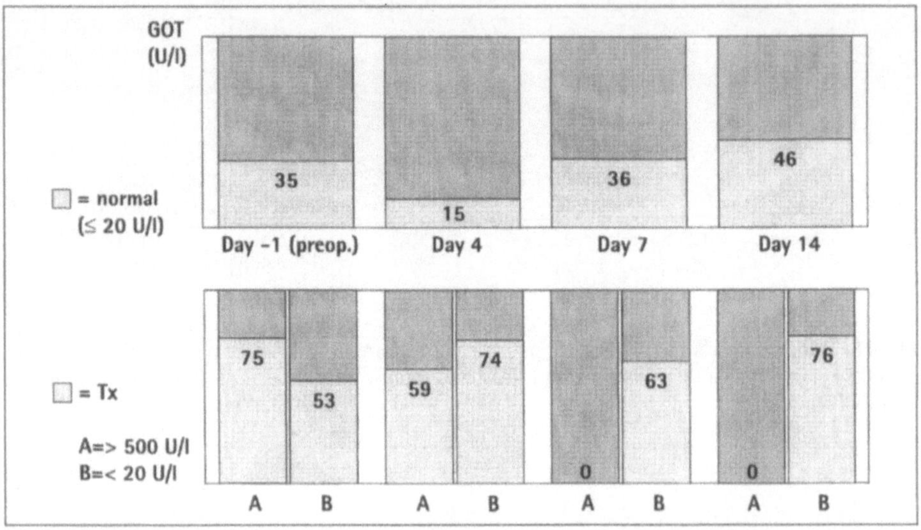

Fig. 13. Recovery of liver function in patients on biventricular Berlin Heart support; after two weeks of support none of the patients with persistent severe liver dysfunction reached transplantation

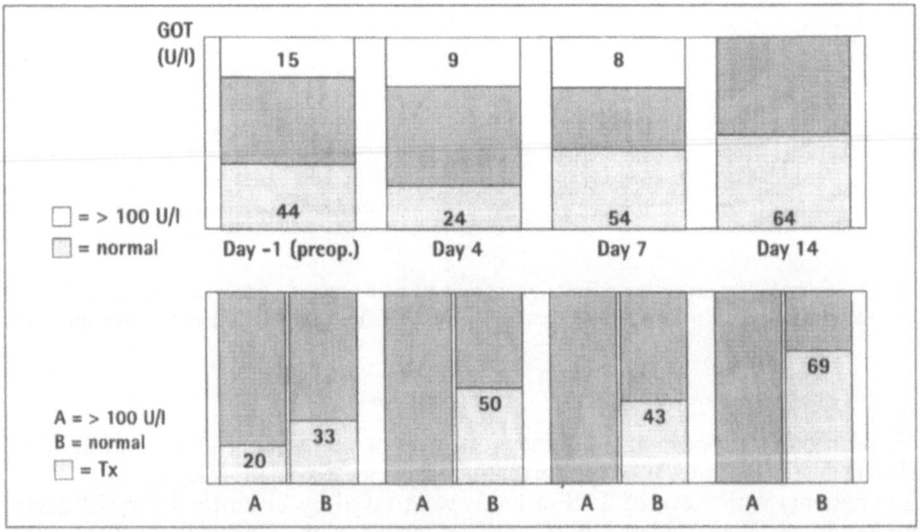

Fig. 14. Recovery of liver function in patients on left ventricular assist devices; none of the patients with persistent severe liver dysfunction after assist implantation reached transplantation

with ongoing liver dysfunction (Figs. 13, 14). This applies to patients supported with left ventricular as well as biventricular assist devices. The recovery of immunocompetence during resolving cardiogenic shock is an additional important predictor. Patients who died on the support system continued to have highly impaired immunocompetence after device implantation. HLA-DR expression on circulating monocytes was markedly reduced in these patients (Fig. 15). Zytokine levels as

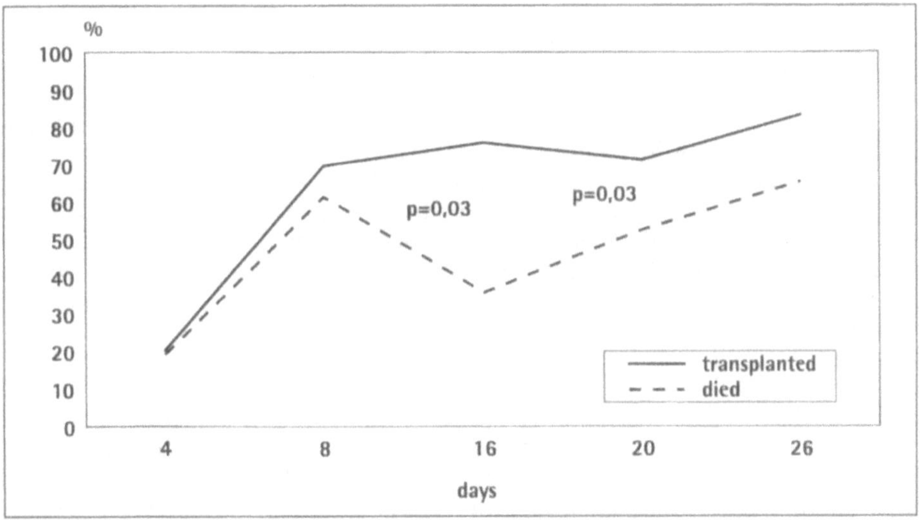

Fig. 15. Recovery of immuno-competence in BVAD patients. Patients dying while on device continued to expose reduced immuno-competence

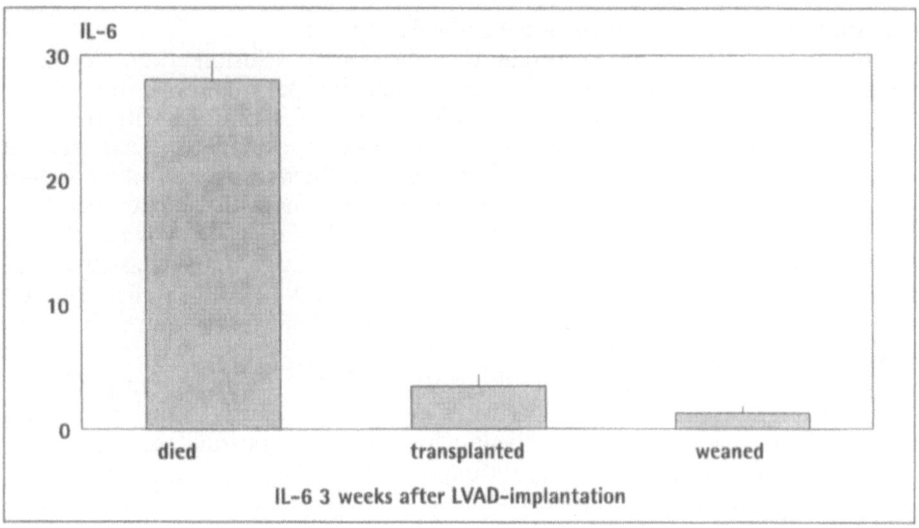

Fig. 16. Recovery from proinflammatory reaction in patients on LVAD support. Patients who did not overcome inflammatory reaction within the first three weeks after device implantation had an unfavorable prognosis

well could to some extent predict the further course of a patient (Fig. 16). Three weeks after implantation patients who later on died on the device continued to have highly elevated interleukin-6 levels, while those who subsequently reached transplantation had clearly overcome the inflammatory situation of heart failure.

Complete rehabilitation of the patients is, therefore, extremely important in gaining acceptable results in heart transplantation after mechanical circulatory support. It is also extremely important to notice that only complete termination of whole body inflammatory reaction gives room for recovery of the patients own heart (3, Fig. 12).

The rather favorable experience gained in bridge to transplant patients led us to include patients who were considered as being no candidates for heart transplantation due to concomitant diseases into a program of permanent mechanical circulatory assistance. Over a couple of years we have implanted ten patients with LVADs as an alternative to heart transplantation. All patients in this group were older than 60 years, had diabetes, and severe peripheral vascular disease as well as a long history of disabling cardiac disease. Rapidly these patients turned out to be in extremely sick conditions. Therefore, their rehabilitation after implantation of the devices was very slow and difficult. One of the patients later on was weaned and transplanted. All others died within one year after LVAD implantation although some of them had regained substantial physical activity, and three were actually discharged home for short periods of time.

We do not feel that the presently available devices are able to provide permanent support with acceptable risks. They are still struck with a number of severe side effects and complications. Their long-term use is limited by the durability of the device components. One of our patients, who was equipped with a LVAD for 795 days, had recurrent episodes of gastrointestinal infections. He later developed endocarditis on the biological valve prosthesis of his Novacor (26). The patient was successfully weaned and the device explanted. Diagnosing valve or system malfunction poses a difficult task and makes timely intervention nearly impossible. Thrombembolic events, bleeding, device infection, and technical failure have to be addressed when contemplating mechanical assist devices as an alternative to heart transplantation in patients with severe comorbidity.

Looking back at what has been said when discussing exclusion criteria for heart transplantation, it is very hard in our view to define a patient who is too sick for heart transplantation but still good enough to have a fair outlook with the presently available mechanical circulatory support devices. Certainly these patients will do better with LVAD support than with medical treatment alone. But the question will not be answered how these patients would have done with heart transplantation. Age as the only limiting factor for heart transplantation today is not acceptable anymore. Furthermore, including older patients as permanent assist device recipients is in contradiction with information from the Novacor as well as the TCI devices database, indicating at least tendency of higher mortality and morbidity in patients over the age of 55 (35, 43).

According to our present experience the only real alternative to heart transplantation when using assist devices is the perspective of myocardial recovery during mechanical support. We now have observed 19 patients who exhibited myocardial recovery during a support period of mostly more than 100 days, mainly with the Novacor device. These patients were explanted and remained in stable conditions except for 5 who had recurrent myocardial failure and underwent subsequent heart transplantation. Two patients have died after explantation from noncardiac cause.

All these patients with signs of myocardial recovery followed a strict protocol of weaning. Due to life threatening device related complications, however, we have explanted some patients who did not fulfill all criteria for weaning. The five patients who exhibited myocardial deterioration after explantation and had to be transplanted belonged in the later group.

Conclusion

The indication for heart transplantation can be extended to include patients with severe secondary diseases without a negative impact on the overall heart transplant outcome. This can be achieved with individualized posttransplant treatment according to the patients needs, but it often produces extended stays on intensive care unit, recurrent hospital admissions, and increased cost. It does not increase, however, the number of patients saved by heart transplantation, since the lack of donor organs is the major limiting factor for a widespread use of heart transplantation.

Alternative procedures for heart transplantation, therefore, have to be used extensively and we at our institution would prefer to use high risk coronary bypass surgery over heart replacement.

As far as assist devices are concerned today one can state that assist devices are safe and reliable. Long-term VAD support is a reality, recovery of secondary organ dysfunction is achievable with these devices, and it is mandatory before heart transplantation is feasible. Reversibility of secondary organ dysfunction depends on duration and severity of cardiac failure and the degree of systemic body inflammatory response to heart failure.

Myocardial recovery in dilated cardiomyopathy is possible. Today this is the only real alternative to heart transplantation when using mechanical assist devices. Permanent assist devices may be an option in the future.

References

1. Albert W, Kiekbusch S, Köller K, Hetzer R (1997) Quality of life with ventricular assist devices. In: Hetzer R, Hennig E, Loebe M (eds.) Mechanical circulatory support, Steinkopff Verlag, Darmstadt, pp. 191–205
2. American Heart Association (1995) selection and treatment of candidates for heart trasnplantation. A statement for health professionals from the committee on heart failure and cardiac transplantation of the council on clinical cardiology Circulation 92:3593–3612
3. Andresen B, Loebe M, Friedel N, Harke C, Ullmann H, Hetzer R (1997) Verlauf von Elastase, Komplementfaktor C3a und Endotoxin bei Patienten mit mechanischen extrakorporalen Kreislaufunterstützungssystemen Typ Berlin Heart. Z. Herz-, Thorax-, Gefäßchir 11:100–107
4. Anker S, Coats AJ (1996) Metabolic, functional and hemodynamic staging for CHF? Lancet 348:1530–31
5. Baker AM, Levine TB, Goldberg AD, Levine AB (1992) Natural history and predictors of obesity after orthotoptic heart transplantation J Heart Lung Transplant 11:1156–1159
6. Blanche C, Matloff JM, Denton TA, Czer LS, Fishbein MC, Takkenberg JJ, Trento A (1996) Heart transplantation in patients 70 years of age or older: initial experience. Ann Thorac Surg 62:1731-1736
7. Bourge RC, Naftel DC, Costanzo-Nordin MR, Kirklin JK, Young JB, Kubo SH, Olivari MT, Kasper EK (1993) Pretransplantation risk factors for death after heart transplantation: a multiinstitutional study. J Heart Lung Transplant 12:549–62
8. Costanzo MR (1996) Selection and treatment of candidates for heart transplantation Seminars in Thoracic and Cardiovascular Surgery 8:113-125
9. Costard-Jäckle A, Hill I, Schroeder JS (1991) The influence of preoperative patient characteristics on early and late survival following cardiac transplantation. Circulation 84:III-329–34

10. Erdoes LS, Hunter GC, Venerus BJ, Hall KA, Bull DA, Berman SS, Pallos LL, Copeland JC (1995) Prospective evaluation of peripheral vascular disease in heart transplant recipients J Vasc Surg 22:434–440
11. Everett JE, Djalilian AR, Kubo SH, Kroshus TJ, Shumway SJ (1996) Heart transplantation for patients over age 60. Clin Transplant 10:478–481
12. Frazier OH, Rose EA, MacManus Q, Burton Na, Tector A, Levin H, Kayne HL, Poirer VL, Dasse KA (1995) Improved mortality and rehabilitation of transplant candidates treated with a long-term implantable left vetricular assist system. Ann Surg 222:327–336
13. Friedel N, Viazis P, Schiessler A, Warnecke H, Hennig E, Tritin A, Bottner W, Hetzer R (1992) Recovery of end-organ failure during mechanical circulatory support. Europ J Cardio-thorac Surg 6:519–523
14. Hauptman PJ, Kartashov AI, Couper GS, Mudge GH Jr.,Aranki SF, Cohn LH, Adams DH (1995) Changing patterns in donor and recipient risk: a 10-year evolution in one heart transplant center. J Heart Lung Transplant 14:654–8
15. Haywood GA, Rickenbacher PR, Trindalde PT, Gullestad L, Jiang JP, Schroeder JS, Vagelos R, Oyer P, Fowler MB (1996) Analysis of deaths in patients awaiting heart transplantation: impact on patient selection criteria. Heart 75:455–462
16. Hosenpud JD, Bennett LE, Keck BM, Fiol B, Novick RJ (1997) The registry of the International Society for Heart and Lung Transplantation: fourteenth official report-1997. J Heart Lung Transplant 16:691–712
17. Hummel M, Warnecke H, Schüler S, Luding K, Hetzer R (1991) Risiko der Nebennierenrindeninsuffizienz nach Herztransplantation. Klin Wochenschr 69:269–273
18. Hummel M, Kuhn D, Bub A, Mann B, Schneider B, von Eickstedt KW, Forssmann WG, Hetzer R (1992) Urodilatin, a new therapy to prevent kidney failure after heart transplantation. J Heart Lung Transplant 12:209–218
19. Jamieson SW, Oyer PE, Reitz BA, Baumgartner WA, Bieber CP, Stinson EB, Shumway NE (1982) cardiac transplantation at Stanford. Heart Transplantation 1:86–91
20. Koerner MM, Tenderich G, Minami K, Mannebach H, Koertke H, zu Knyphausen E; El-Banayosy A, Baller D, Kleesiek K, Gleichmann U, Meyer H, Koerfer R (1997) results of heart transplantation in patients with preexisting malignancies. Am J cardiol 79:988–991
21. Kormos RL, Borovetz HS, Gasior T, Antaki JF, Armitage JM, Pistas JM, Hardesty RL, Griffith BP (1990) Experience with univentricular support in mortally ill cardiac transplant candidates. Ann Thorac Surg 49:261–272
22. Loebe M, Schüler S, Spiegelsberger S, Matheis G, Warnecke H, Hetzer R (1990) Infektionen nach Herztransplantationen. Z. Herz-, Thorax-, Gefäßchir 4:196–204
23. Loebe M, Hetzer R, Schüler S, Hummel M, Friedel N, Weng Y, Schiessler A (1992) Herztransplantation-Indikation und Ergebnisse. Zentrbl. Chir 117:681–688
24. Loebe M, Hummel M, Musci M, Sodian R, Grauhan O, Hetzer R. (1995) Aktuelle Aspekte der Immunsuppression nach intrathorakalem Organersatz. Transplantationsmedizin 4:200–204
25. Loebe M, Hennig E, Müller J, Spiegelsberger S, Weng Y, Hetzer R (1997) Long-term mechanical circulatory support as a bridge to transplantation, for recovery from cardiomyopathy, and for permanent replacement. Europ J Cardio-thorac Surg 11 Suppl:S18–24
26. Loebe M, Weng Y, Müller J, Dandel M, Halfmann R, Spiegelsberger S, Hetzer R (1997) Successful mechanical circulatory support for more than two years with a left ventricular assist device in a patient with dilated cardiomyopathy. J Heart Lung Transplant 16:1176–9
27. Manzcini DM, Howard E, Kussmaul W. (1991) Value of peak exercise oxygen consumption for optimal timing of cardiac transplantation in ambulatory patients with heart failure. Circulation 83:778–786
28. Massad MG, McCarthy PM, Smedira NG, Cook DJ, Ratliff NB, Goormastic M, Vargo RL, Navia J, Young JB, Stewart RW (1996) Does successful bridging with the implantable left ventricular device affect cardiac transplantation outcome? J Thorac Cardiovasc Surg. 112:1275–1283
29. Mehta SM, Aufiero TX, Pae WE Jr, Miller CA, Pierce WS (1995) Combined registry for the clinical use of mechanical ventricular assist pumps and the total artifical heart in conjunction with heart transplantation: sixth official report-1994. J Heart Lung Transplant. 14:584–593
30. Mudge GH, Goldstein S, Addonizio LJ, Caplan A, Mancini D, Levine TB, Ritsch ME Jr.,Stevenson LW(1993) 24th Bethesda conference: cardiac transplantation. Task force 3: recipients guidlines/priorization. J Am Coll Cardiol 22:21–31

31. Müller J, Wallukat G, Weng Y, Dandel M, Spiegelsberger S, Semrau S, Brandes K, Theodoridis V, Loebe M, Meyer R, Hetzer R (19997) Weaning from mechanical cardiac support in patients with idiopathic dilated cardiomyopathy. Circulation 96:542–549
32. Munoz E, Lonquist JL, Radovancevic B, Baldwin RT, Ford S, Duncan JM, Frazier OH (1992) Long-term results in diabetic patients undergoing heart transplantation. J Heart Lung Transplant 11:943–949
33. Musci M, Loebe M, Grauhan O, Weng Y, Hummel M, Lange P, Hetzer R. (1997) Heart transplantation for doxorubicin-inducedcongestive heart failure in children and adolescents. Transplant Proc. 578–9
34. National Heart Institute ad hoc task force on cardiac replacement (1969) Cardiac replacement: medical, ethical psychological and economical implications. US goverment printing office
35. Noon GP (1993) Clinical use of cardiac assist devices. In: Akutzu T, Koyanagi H (eds) Heart Replacement: Artifical Heart 4, Tokyo, Japan: Springer-Verlag pp.195–205
36. Packer M (1992) treatment of chronic heart failure. Lancet 340:92–95
37. Packer M, Bristow MR, Cohn JN, Colucci WS, Fowler MB, Gilbert EM, Shusterman NH (1996) The effect of carvedelol on morbidity and mortality in patients with chronic heart failure. N Engl J Med 334:1349–1355
38. Pasic M, Loebe M, Hummel M, Grauhan O, Hofmeister J, Weng Y, Hetzer R (1996) Heart transplantation: a single-center experience. Ann Thorac Surg 62:1685–90
39. Rose EA, Goldstein DJ (1996) Wearable long-term mechanical support for patients with end-stage heart disease: a tenable goal. Ann Torac Surg 61:399–402
40. Schiessler A, Friedel N, Weng Y, Heinz U, Hummel M, Hetzer R (1994) Mechanical circulatory support and heart transplantation. ASAIO J 40:M476–481
41. Schüler S, Matschke K, Loebe M, Hummel M, Fleck E, Hetzer R (1993) Coronary artery disease in patients with hearts from older donors: morphologic features and therapeutic implications. J Heart Lung Transplant 12:100–106
42. Smart FW, Naftel DC, Constanzo MR, Levine TB, Pelletier GB, Yancy CW, Hobbs RE, Kirklin JK, Bourge R (1996) risk factors for early, cumulative and fatal infections after heart transplantation: a multiinstitutional study. J Heart Lung Transplant 15:329–41
43. Smedira NG, Dasse KA, Patel An, Vargo RL, Massad MG, McCarthy PM (1996) Age related outcome after implantable left ventricular assist system support. ASAIO J 42:M570-M573
44. Torre-Amione G, Kapadia S, Schort D, Young JB (1996) Evolving concepts regarding selection of patients for cardiac transplantation- assessing risks and benefits. Chest 109:223–32
45. Wagner F, Dandel M, Günther G, Loebe, M, Schulze-Neick I.,Laucke U, Kuhly R, Weng Y, Hetzer R (1997) Nitric oxide in the treatment of right ventricular dysfunction following left ventricular assist device implantation. Circulation 96 (supplII):II-291-II-296
46. Warnecke H, Schüler S, Götze H, Matheis G, Süthoff U, Müller J, Tietze U, Hetzer R (1986) Noninvasive monitoring of cardiac allograft rejection by intramyocardial electrogram recordings. Circulation 74:III72-76
47. Young JB, Naftel DC, Bourge RC, Kirklin JK, Clemson BS, Porter CB, Rodeheffer RJ, Kenzora JL (1994) Matching the heart donor and heart transplant recipient. Clues for successful expansion of donor pool: a multivariable, multiinstitutional report. J Heart Lung Transplant 13:353–64

Author's address:
M Loebe, M.D.
Deutsches Herzzentrum Berlin
Augustenburger Platz 1
13353 Berlin

Cardiac surgery in solid organ transplant recipients with functioning allografts

Surindra N. Mitruka, Bartley P. Griffith, Robert L. Kormos, Brack G. Hattler, Frank Pigula, Ron Shapiro, John J. Fung, Si M. Pham

University of Pittsburgh School of Medicine, Department of Surgery, Pittsburgh, Pennsylvania, USA

Introduction

Since 1986, at the University of Pittsburgh, 602 heart transplants, 316 lung transplants, 4347 liver transplants, and 2323 kidney transplants have been performed. As the population of transplant survivors has aged, the number of patients developing symptomatic cardiovascular disease has risen. The first reported case of cardiac surgery performed on an organ transplant survivor was in 1974 by Menzoian and colleagues (3). Since that time, there have been numerous case reports and small series supporting the performance of cardiac surgery in solid organ transplant recipients (4, 7, 9, 16). There remains however, no comprehensive assessment of the management issues that must be considered when approaching these unique patients.

The management of cardiopulmonary bypass (CPB), immunosuppression, antibiotic prophylaxis, and the administration of particular medications is poorly defined in these patients. Additionally, outcome measures such as incidence of graft loss, renal dysfunction, major infectious and bleeding complications, rejection, and overall mortality are not well documented.

In this large transplant series, we report our experience with the management techniques and subsequent outcomes of cardiac surgery on solid organ transplant recipients with functioning allografts. We additionally sought to assess the role of specific transplant allografts as risk factors for major complications and mortality. We excluded patients who were on active hemo- or peritoneal dialysis, and additionally excluded those patients who underwent a concurrent cardiac procedure and organ transplant.

Material and methods

Patient demographics

By computerized search of the databases for each transplant population, the charts of 64 patients were identified who had functioning allografts and subsequently required a cardiac surgical procedure (Table 1). The mean interval from transplant to cardiac surgery was 53 months (range 1 day to 220 months). Sixty-six cardiac operations were performed in these 64 patients as outlined in Table 2.

Table 1. Patient demographics

	Kidney (n = 40)	Liver* (n = 17)	Thoracic (n = 7)	Total (n = 64)
Age	51 (29–77)	56 (19–75)	57 (44–63)	53 (19–77)
Male	26 (65%)	13 (76%)	7 (100%)	46 (72%)
Female	14 (35%)	4 (24%)	0	18 (28%)
IDDM	17 (43%)	8 (47%)	3 (43%)	28 (44%)
Hypertension	39 (98%)	16 (94%)	7 (100%)	62 (97%)
MI	12 (30%)	6 (35%)	1 (14%)	19 (30%)
CHF	10 (25%)	1 (6%)	1 (14%)	12 (19%)
Endocarditis	6 (15%)	1 (6%)	0	7 (11%)
NYHA III	14 (35%)	8 (47%)	2 (29%)	24 (38%)
NYHA IV	26 (65%)	9 (53%)	5 (71%)	40 (62%)

CHF – congestive heart failure
IDDM – insulin dependent diabetes mellitus
MI – myocardial infarction
NYHA – New York Heart Association
* – includes one combined liver/kidney transplant recipient

Table 2. Operative procedures

	Kidney (n = 40)	Liver (n = 17)	Thoracic (n = 7)	Total (n = 64)
CABG	18 (2*)	11 (1*)	1	30
Valve	16 (1#)	5	3	24
CABG/valve	3 (1#)	0	0	3
Aorta	3 (3*)	0	1	4
Cardiectomy	0	0	1	1
Pericardiectomy	1	1	1	3
TMLR	1	0	0	1
Total	42	17	7	66

mean interval from transplant to cardiac surgery = 53 months
(range 1 day-220 months)
(N* = emergency operation) (N# = redo operation)
CABG – coronary artery bypass grafts
TMLR – trans-myocardial laser revascularization

The native cardiectomy was performed in a patient following heterotopic heart transplantation, who subsequently developed hemodynamically significant arrhythmias in the native heart. Two patients required re-operations. The first was a 65 year old female who received a renal transplant in 1992 for diabetes induced nephropathy. She required a four vessel CABG six months later for coronary artery disease and an aortic and mitral valve replacement with a single vessel CABG three years later for progressive cardiac symptoms. The second patient was a 37 year old m ale who underwent kidney transplantation in 1989 and developed bacterial endocarditis four years later. He initially underwent aortic valve repair for significant aortic insufficiency but required a reoperation with aortic valve replacement three months later for continued disease progression.

Immunosuppresive regimen

The maintenance immunosuppressive regimen consisted of oral cyclosporine (CsA)(6 mg/kg/day : range 400–900 mg/day) or tacrolimus (0.30 mg/kg/day : range 2–20 mg/day), azathioprine (Imuran)(2 mg/kg/day : range 100–250 mg/day), and prednisone (15–20 mg/day). Serum CsA levels approximated 1000 ng/ml (polyclonal immunoassay, TDX, Abbott Laboratory, Abbott Park, IL), and serum tacrolimus levels were maintained at approximately 1.0 ng/ml (enzyme linked immunosorbent assay). The normal oral immunosuppressive medications were administered the morning of surgery in all transplant patients undergoing cardiac operations. The dose the day following surgery was administered orally if the patient was extubated, or by nasogastric tube if the patient continued to be ventilated. At the time of surgery, stress doses of steroids were initiated, consisting of hydrocortisone 100 mg IV every 8 hours for 24 hours or Solumedrol 25 mg IV every 6 hours for 24 hours. Serum drug levels of CsA or tacrolimus were monitored in the perioperative period as a routine, and if the levels were noted to be abnormally low in the post-operative period, the dose was supplemented intravenously. If the drug levels were elevated, the immunosuppression was held or reduced until the levels returned to baseline. Likewise, if acute allograft failure was suspected, based on a falling urine output or a rising serum creatinine level, the immunosuppression was reduced until the graft dysfunction had resolved.

Surgical management

Routine cardiac narcotic anesthesia and standard cardiopoulmonary bypass (CPB) techniques were utilized in all patients. High flow CPB at 2–4 liters/min/m^2, adjusted for calculated body surface area and mixed venous oxygen saturations, with cooling to 32 °C was maintained. Cold blood potassium cardioplegia was administered to all patients as is the routine practice at this institution. Activated clotting times were maintained between 500–600 seconds for the kidney and thoracic transplant patients, and 400–500 seconds for the liver transplant recipients. For all groups, the perfusion pressures were maintained in the 60–90 mmHg range, and use of vasoconstrictive drugs was avoided when possible. Postoperatively, inotropic support was administered as needed, and intravenous dopamine (3–5 µg/kg/min) was routinely utilized in kidney transplant recipients to maximize renal perfusion. Intravenous mannitol (25 gm) and furosemide (20–40 mg) were administered at the conclusion of the operation in renal transplant recipients to encourage allograft diuresis. No hemostatic adjuncts, such as aminocaproic acid or aprotinin, were routinely used, as many of these patients had marginal renal function that may have been exacerabated by the use of these agents.

Medical management

The medical management of these patients was relatively uniform throughout the peri-operative period. An effort was made to minimize alterations in the patient's routine pre-operative period. An effort was made to minimize alterations in the patient's routine pre-operative medications. If possible, medications were administered orally the morning of surgery, and again orally or through nasogastric tubes the morning following surgery. In the immediate post-operative period, normal blood pressure and cardiac outputs were supported with dopamine and dobutamine. Hypertension was treated with IV nitroprusside or nitroglycerine to achieve mean arterial blood pressures in the target range. Close attention was paid to the intravascular volume status to maintain hydration during the peri-operative period. Furosemide or bumetinide were judiciously administered as a bolus or continuous infusion to maintain a urine output of 0.5 to 1.5 mg/kg/hr, yet, assure adequate hydration and graft perfusion. Certain medications were avoided in the peri-operative period such as non-steroidal anti-inflammatory drugs (e.g., ibuprofen) and captopril, or other nephrotoxic and hepatotoxic medications.

Fifty-five of 64 (86%) patients were prophylaxed with broad spectrum antibiotics pre-operatively consisting of 1 gram IV vancomycin and 1 gram IV ceftriaxone (Rocephin). Seven of 64 (11%) received cefamandole (Mandol) 1 gram IV, and 2 of 64 (3%) patients, with significant documented penicillin allergies and normal renal function, were administered 1 gram of vancomycin with 1–1.5 mg/kg IV gentamycin.

Monitoring of allograft function and rejection

Preoperative laboratory values included: hematocrit, total white blood cell with differential leukocyte and platelet count, prothrombin time, electrolytes with BUN and creatinine. Additionally, liver function tests were performed in liver transplant recipients. Laboratory values were determined again, as a minimum, on the first postoperative day and before discharge. Fluid intake, urine output, and renal function were closely monitored in all patients. Suspected episodes of graft rejection were addressed by immediate biopsy and histologic analysis followed by pulse steroids with 1 gram of IV methylprednislone (Solumedrol) daily for three days if rejection was proven by biopsy or strongly suspected clinically.

Length of stay

Length of stay was assessed by evaluating both intensive care unit length of stay and total length of stay. Notably, the recent advent of clinical pathways have promoted a shorter total length of stay.

Statistical analysis

The chi-square (contingency table) test (Statistica™ Software, 1993 Statsoft Inc. Tulsa, OK) was utilized to determine significant differences in outcomes between groups.

Results

Survival

There were 2 (3%) early deaths (< 30 days) following the cardiac surgical procedures, both in kidney transplant recipients. One patient died of overwhelming pseudomas sepsis seven days after a CABG. This patient was the oldest (77 years)

Table 3. Causes of death

	< 30 days	> 30 days
Kidney		
	sepsis (1)	subdural hematoma (1)
	arrhythmia (1)	sepsis/MSOF (1)
		ESLD/biliary sepsis (1)
		met renal cell CA (1)
		prostate CA (1)
		unknown (1)
Liver		
		sepsis/MSOF (1)
Total	2 (3%)	7 (11%)

values in parentheses represent number of patients
CA – cancer
ESLD – end-stage liver disease
MSOF – multi-system organ failure

in the study and had received her kidney transplant ten years before symptomatic coronary artery disease developed. She had a myocardial infarction two weeks preoperatively, developed postinfarction angina, and was in NYHA Class IV before her operation. Her allograft functioned well with a pre-operative creatinine level of 1.9 mg/dl. The second early death involved a 50 year old female with IDDM and a 12-year-old kidney allograft with a baseline creatinine level of 2.0 mg/dl. She developed symptomatic aortic stenosis with a measured valve gradient of 44 mmHg and a surface area of 0.6 cm^2. She underwent an aortic valve replacement and had an uncomplicated postoperative course. However, she died suddenly of an arrhythmia induced cardiac arrest on the ninth postoperative day. Electrolyte levels and renal function were normal the morning of death. Post-mortem examination revealed an undetected perioperative myocardial infarction.

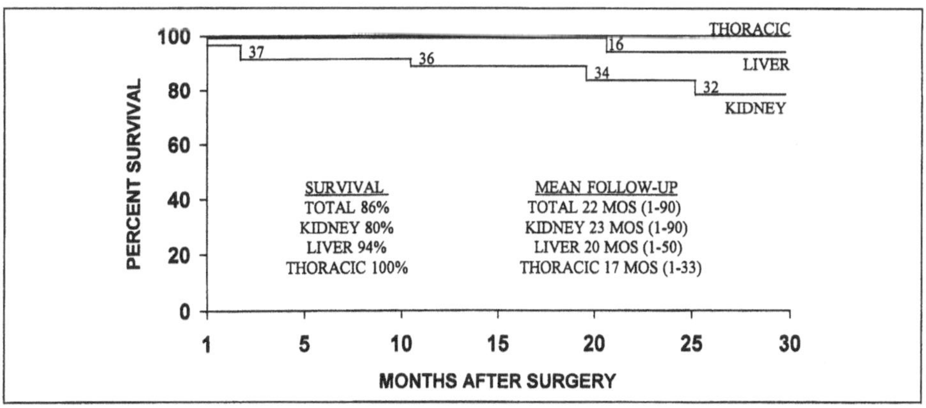

Fig. 1. Actuarial survival curves for each subgroup of transplant patients is displayed. The curves represent the death of patients within each group at the given time point. No censored patient follow-up data was utilized. Total survival at a mean follow-up of 22 months and mean follow-up for each subgroup are likewise displayed in the inserts.

There were seven (11%) late deaths form seven weeks to 26 months following the cardiac operation. None of the late deaths was attributable to the procedure or directly related to a cardiac cause. Six late deaths occurred in kidney transplant recipients (Table 3). There was one late death caused by sepsis and multi-system organ failure in a liver transplant patient 19 months following an aortic valve replacement. Actuarial survival at a mean follow-up of 22 months is displayed in Fig. 1.

Allograft failure

Sixteen of 64 (25%), transplant patients, including thirteen of 40 (33%) kidney transplant recipients, had chronic renal failure pre-operatively (serum creatinine > 3 mg/dl). Of the 13 renal transplant patients, 7 (54%) developed acute graft failure post-operatively, and required hemodialysis (Table 4). These seven patients had 3 CABG, 2 emergent aortic procedures, and 2 valve replacements. The other six patients (47%) had uneventful postoperative courses and were discharged with creatinine levels similar to preoperative levels. Of the 7 patients who had acute renal failure post-operatively, four improved with dialysis by the time of discharge, and required no further treatment, whereas the remaining three patients had permanent allograft loss (Table 5). These three patients had CABG (n = 2) and valve replacement (n = 1) electively. This cohort represents (23% (3/13) of chronic renal allograft failure patients, 7.5% (3/40) of the total kidney transplant population, and 4.7% (3/64) of the total study group. Two of these 3 patients suffered late deaths from sepsis. All had perioperative immunosuppressive drug levels within the therapeutic range. No liver or thoracic organ transplant recipient suffered allograft dysfunction or loss postoperatively.

Table 4. Serum creatinine levels in kidney transplant recipients with postoperative allograft failure

Patient	Serum creatinine (mg/dl)			Comment
	PRE-OP	POD 1	Discharge	
1	3.2	4.3	2	recovery
2	3.1	3.2	3.1	permanent graft failure
3	3.9	3.1	2.3	recovery
4	3.3	4.1	3.8	permanent graft failure
5	3.5	5.5	3.6	recovery
6	4.3	5.3	3.6	recovery
7	3.1	3.5	3.9	permanent graft failure

POD – opst-operative day

Table 5. Allograft failure/rejection

	Kidney (n = 40)	Liver (n = 17)	Thoracic (n = 7)	Total (n = 64)
Graft failure				
temporary	4 (10%)*	0	0	4 (6.3%)
permanent	3 (7.5%)*	0	0	3 (4.7%)
Rejection	2 (5%)*	0	1 (14.3%)	3 (4.7%)

* p = NS; chi-square (contingency table) test

Rejection

Thirty-seven of 64 (58%) patients received tacrolimus based immunosuppression including 17 of 40 kidney, 16 of 17 liver, and 4 of 7 thoracic transplant recipients. Twenty-seven of 64 (42%) patients were treated with CsA-based immunosuppression. Tacrolimus or CsA blood levels displayed minor fluctuations perioperatively that were found to be clinically inconsequential.

There were two (5%) episodes of biopsy proven rejection in kidney recipients (Table 5). One patient with chronic renal failure (serum creatinine, 3.2 mg/dl) underwent an emergency repair of an ascending aortic dissection, and developed rejection 5 weeks post-operatively. He was one of the seven patients who developed acute graft failure, which subsequently improved with hemodialysis. This patient's immunosuppression was reduced postoperatively because of his acute renal failure. The other patient had a baseline creatinine level of 3 mg/dl and initially tolerated an aortic valve replacement, but developed rejection 2 weeks later. However, this patient developed acute tubular necrosis postoperatively that was treated medically (including a reduction in immunosuppression), but had a creatinine of 3.4 mg/dl at the time of discharge. Both cases of rejection were treated with pulsed doses of steroids as previously described with neither resulting in permanent graft loss.

The only other case of acute allograft rejection was recorded in a lung transplant recipient who underwent a pericardiectomy for tamponade one day following a single left lung transplant. He developed acute rejection, documented radiographically and by biopsy findings 11 days, later, and was effectively treated with a three day course of methylprednisolone.

Renal function

The pre- and post-operative blood urea nitrogen and serum creatinine levels were stratified by the type of organ transplanted : kidney, liver (including one combined liver/kidney transplant recipient), and thoracic organ (Table 6). There were no statistically significant alterations observed in the preoperative and postoperative

Table 6. Renal function

	Kidney (n = 40)	Liver (n = 17)	Thoracic (n = 7)	Total (n = 64)
mean pre-op BUN (mg/dl)*	42.7 (11–113)	29.6 (13–56)	40 (10–73)	39 (10–113)
mean post-op BUN (mg/dl)	50.3 (8–97)	36.2 (14–93)	39 (20–56)	45.5 (8–93)
pre-op CRT (mg/dl)*				
< 2	18	14	3	35
2–3	11	1	3	15
> 3	13	2	1	16
mean	2.3 (0.8–4.6)	1.7 (1.3–3.9)	2.2 (0.8–3.7)	2.1 (0.8–4.6)
post-op CRT (mg/dl)				
< 2	16	11	4	31
2–3	12	5	3	20
> 3	14	1	0	15
mean	2.3 (0.6–4.6)	1.8 (0.9–2.5)	1.9 (0.8–2.5)	2.1 (0.6–4.6)

* p = NS; t-test chi square (contingency table) test; pre vs. postoperative values
BUN – blood urea nitrogen
CRT – serum creatinine level

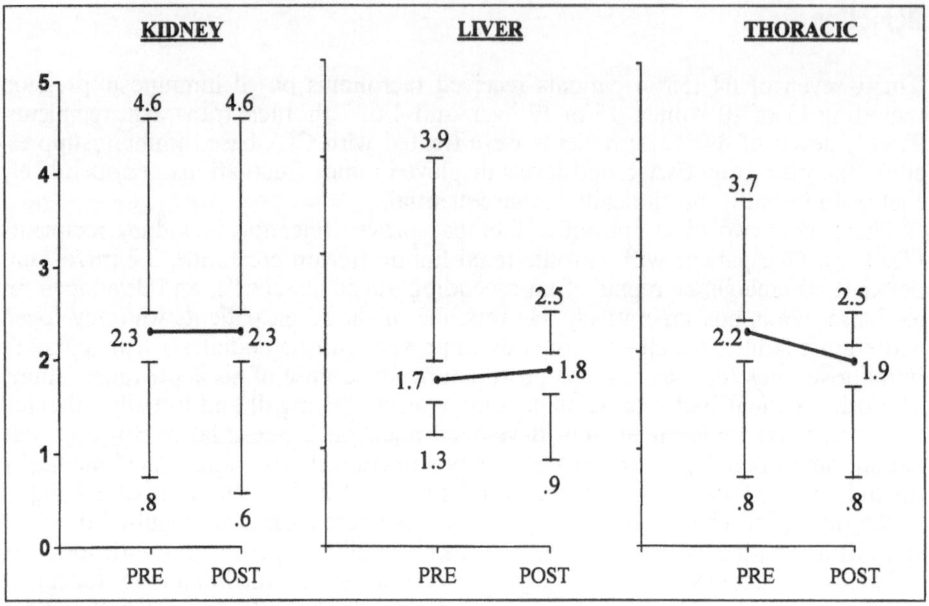

Fig. 2. Mean serum creatinine levels (mg/dl) as a measure of renal function are displayed for subgroup of transplant patients. The range of values pre- and post-operatively are indicated by vertical markers. No statistically significant difference was found between the pre- and post-operative levels in any group.

mean serum creatinine levels in any group (Fig. 2), although there were minor fluctuations in the blood urea nitrogen and creatinine levels of individual patients within each transplant group as indicated in Table 6. The renal group includes the 7 patients who suffered graft failure and required hemodialysis. No patient aside from these seven required hemodialysis regardless of fluctuations in the serum cratinine levels.

Table 7. Incidence of infectious complications

	Kidney (n = 40)	Liver (n = 17)	Thoracic (n = 7)	Total (n = 64)
Major				
mediastinitis	3 (8%)	0	0	3 (5%)
sepsis	4 (10%)	0	0	4 (6%)
pneumonia	3 (8%)	1 (6%)	1 (14%)	5 (8%)
Minor				
leg wound	2 (5%)	2 (12%)	0	4 (6%)
C. diff colitis	2 (5%)	0	1 (14%)	3 (5%)
UTI	2 (5%)	0	0	2 (3%)
Total	16 (41%)	2 (18%)	2 (28%)	21 (33%)

UTI – urinary tract infection

Surgical management

The mean aortic cross-clamp time was 92 min (range 0–190 min) with a mean cardiopulmonary bypass time of 141 minutes (range 47–340 min). The values were uniform between kidney and liver transplant recipients with a mean cross-clamp time of 93 min vs. 86 min and a mean CPB time of 136 min vs. 134 min, respectively. The thoracic transplant group had a longer mean cross clamp time of 104 min with a mean CPB time of 188 min.

Infectious complications

Twelve major infections (19%) were documented including three cases (5%) of mediastinitis (one long term fatality): two due to Staphylococcus aureus and one multiple organism. Four cases (6%) of sepsis, one each with cytomegalovirus, Candida albicans, Pseudomonas aeruginosa (short term fatality), and Staphylococcus aureus were recorded. Five cases (8%) of pneumonia, were effectively treated. Overall, there were 10 major infections in 8 kidney recipients, one in 1 liver recipient, and one in 1 thoracic recipient (Table 7).

Nine (14%) minor infections were recorded including four (6%) leg wound infections/cellulitis (but no wound breakdown) requiring oral antibiotics. Three (5%) cases of Clostridium difficile colitis, and two (3%) urinary tract infections were definitively treated by oral medications with no significant sequelae. Overall, there were six minor infections in 5 kidney recipients, two in 2 liver recipients, and one in 1 thoracic recipient. All infectious complications (major and minor) totaled 16 in 13 kidney recipients, three in 3 liver recipients, and two in 1 thoracic recipient. For the total group of transplant patients, there was a 33% incidence of infectious complications (21 cases) in 26.5% (17/64) of the patients.

Other complications

Ten patients (16%) required re-exploration for mediastinal hematoma with resultant tamponade postoperatively. There was one documented case of intra-operative coagulopathy in a liver transplant recipient that was treated medically. Blood or clotting factor transfusion in the intra- or postoperative period was not considered excessive or unusual in any case. There were no significant alterations in the measured prothrombin times in those patients who required re-exploration, and the activated clotting times were adequately corrected after Protamine administration following CPB. Other major and minor complications are listed in Table 8. Overall, there were 14 major complications (including bleeding) in 13 kidney recipients, four in 4 liver recipients, one in 1 thoracic recipient. There were 17 minor complications in 15 kidney recipients, 12 in 10 liver recipients, and one in 1 thoracic recipient. All complications (major and minor) totaled 31 in 22 kidney recipinets, 16 in 12 liver recipients, and two in 1 thoracic recipient. For the total group of transplant patients, there was a 78% incidence of complications (49 cases) in 55% (35/64) of the patients.

Hospital stay

The intensive care unit and total length of stay are depicted in Fig. 3 for each subgroup and the total group.

Table 8. Incidence of other complications

	Kidney (n = 40)	Liver (n = 17)	Thoracic (n = 7)	Total (n = 64)
Major				
bleeding	7 (18%)	2 (12%)	1 (14%)	10 (16%)
myocardial infarction	1 (3%)	0	0	1 (2%)
CVA	1 (3%)	0	0	1 (2%)
ATN	3 (8%)	1 (6%)	0	4 (6%)
vascular thrombosis	1 (3%)	1 (6%)	0	2 (3%)
GI perforation	1 (3%)	0	0	1 (2%)
Minor				
atrial arrythmia	12 (30%)	6 (35%)	1 (14%)	19 (30%)
pulmonary failure	0	4 (24%)	0	4 (6%)
pleural effusion	4 (10%)	0	0	4 (6%)
encephalopathy	0	1 (6%)	0	1 (2%)
pericarditis	1 (3%)	1 (6%)	0	2 (3%)

ATN – acute tubular necrosis
VCA – cerebrovascular accident
GI – gastrointestinal

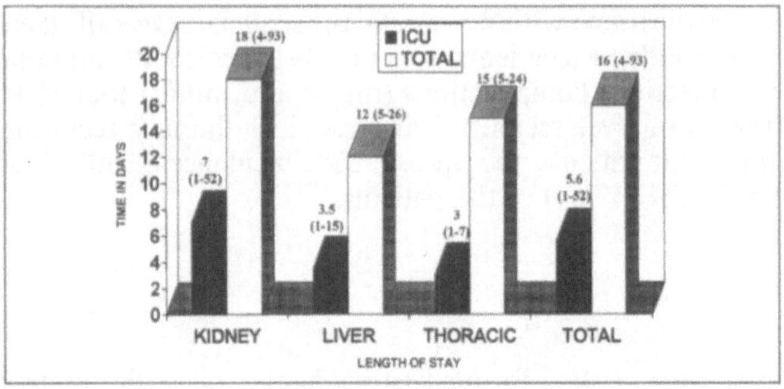

Fig. 3. Length of stay (ICU and total) is shown for each subgroup and as a total. The mean value and range are provided above each bar.

Follow-up

Fifty of 55 surviving patients at a mean follow-up of 22 months (range 1–90 months) are alive and well with no recurrent cardiac symptoms. Five patients were lost to follow-up. At the time of discharge in 61 surviving patients, 55 of 61 (90%) were in NYHA Class I, and 6 of 61 (10%) were in NYHA Class II.

Discussion

As the surviving transplant population ages, the number of patients developing symptomatic cardiovascular disease requiring surgical intervention has increased. Numerous reports have documented the safety and efficacy of performing cardiac surgery in transplant recipinets (2, 4, 7–9, 16). The development of pronounced cardiovascular disease in transplant patients, particularly previous renal failure patients, is well documented. Increased steroids and local immune events are believed to accelerate atheroma formation in coronary arteries (7). In a review by Najarian and colleagues (15), it was found that 29% of deaths after renal transplantation were from cardiovascular causes, with a majority occurring after one year. They additionally found a large disparity between diabetic and non-diabetic recipients of allografts, with the former having an eight-fold higher mortality. Others have reported a 10 to 30% incidence of death from atherosclerotic cardiovascular disease in patients on long-term hemodialysis (3, 5). Our patient population had a mean age of 53 years; yet 44% were insulin dependent diabetics, 97% were hypertensive, 30% had recent myocardial infarctions, and 62% were in NYHA Class IV. The potential morbidity and mortality of performing cardiac surgery in this group of high risk patients prompted a review of the experience at this institution over the past decade.

In our series, the early mortality of 3%, with only one of the two patients expiring from a cardiac cause, was consistent with the mortality of cardiac operations in the non-transplant population (18). The late mortality of 11%, none from a cardiac cause, is arguably consistent with a patient population having numerous co-morbid medical conditions. The occurrence of four late term deaths from sepsis and two from metastatic cancers (renal and prostatic) may represent the unique causes of death that often afflict transplant recipients on chronic immunosuppressive therapy. Notably, neither emergency procedures nor re-operations had a significant impact on outcome. The actuarial 2 year survival for these patients was 86% (Fig. 1). Similar survival statistics have been found in other limited series (2, 6, 8, 20).

Sixteen of 64 (25%) transplant patients had chronic renal failure pre-operatively (creatinine > 3 mg/dl). This included 13 of 40 (33%) kidney, 2 of 17 (12%) liver, and 1 of 7 (14%) thoracic transplant recipients. We observed an overall 5% incidence (n = 3) of permanent allograft loss, all in kidney transplant patients with chronic renal failure. An additional four patients in that subgroup of 13 patients developed post-operative graft dysfunction requiring hemodialysis. The underlying cause of chronic renal failure in kidney transplant recipients may be chronic rejection, whereas the underlying cause of chronic renal failure in liver and thoracic transplant recipients may be long-term immunosuppressive therapy. This basic difference may account for the high failure rate in the kidney transplant population. It is also notable that no patient with a creatinine less than 3 mg/dl pre-operative suffered progressive graft failure. It is reasonable to conclude that renal transplant recipients with chronic renal failure (serum creatinine level > 3 mg/dl) represent a very high risk group for acute renal failure (54%) and permanent graft loss (23%) after cardiac operations.

The preservation of peri-operative renal function in all transplant patients maintained on chronically nephrotoxic immunosuppressive drugs is paramount. Renal function was optimized by adequate hydration, administration of mannitol and furosemide, maintenance of uniform perfusion pressures during CPB, close attention to urine output, and judicious diuresis. Alpha-adrenergic agents were not used, but dopamine was routinely administered, especially to renal transplant recipients. A similar management approach has been taken by Bolman and colleagues (2); however, we did not encounter difficulties related to maintaining perfusion pressures lower than 70 mmHg in these patients. Interestingly, although minor variations existed among individuals within groups, we found no significant difference in the pre- and post-operative mean serum creatinine levels in any group (Table 6, Fig. 2).

Acute rejection developed in 3 (5%) of the 64 patients in this study, including 2 kidney and 1 lung transplant patient. Both renal transplant recipients were in their fifties, and had their allografts in place for over three years. Both, however, had pre-operative creatinine levels greater than 3 mg/dl, and one of the two developed graft failure post-operatively that resolved with hemodialysis, whereas the other patient developed acute tubular necrosis. Both also had a reduction in their immunosuppression regimens post-operatively, which may account for the subsequent development of rejection. The other patient was a pulmonary transplant recipient who developed rejection 11 days following the transplant; a relatively common event in this patient population (90% incidence within the first year at our institution). The overall incidence of acute rejection in this series (4.7%) is evidence that transplanted allografts can manage the stress of major operations. We believe that our management of the immunosuppressive regimen, and fastidious attention in maintaining consistent blood levels of tacrolimus and Cyclosporine was instrumental in ensuring a low rejection rate. We advise checking the blood level the day before surgery, administering the routine dose the morning of surgery, checking the blood level the morning after surgery, and administering the POD 1 dose orally, by nasogastric tube, or intravenously if necessary. Should the blood levels be low on the first postoperative day, the immunosuppressive agent should be administered intravenously to obtain therapeutic blood levels. If the blood levels are found to be elevated or renal impairment is suspected, withholding the scheduled dose and rechecking the blood level on consecutive days is warranted.

The potential infectious and wound healing complications that are concomitant with chronic immunosuppression and systemic steroids is always of concern in the transplant population. Our major infectious complication rate of 19% was considered significant and included three cases of mediastinitis, one of which contributed to overwhelming sepsis and death seven weeks after the cardiac procedure. All three cases occurred in diabetic renal transplant recipients who underwent CABG with a left internal mammary artery anastomosis to the left anterior descending artery. Four cases of sepsis were also a problem in this subgroup of patients, one of which resulted in a death nine days after the patient's procedure. A high incidence of sepsis has been noted in other series (11, 14), despite a similar regimen of prophylactic peri-operative broad spectrum antibiotics. Chronic immunosuppression and bacterial colonization of the airways, GI tract, and skin may play an important etiologic role. Three patients developed leg wound infections without wound breakdown and were effectively treated with antibiotics.

The incidence of re-operations for evacuation of mediastinal hematomas causing tamponade was inexplicably high with 16% of patients requiring this intervention. Similar findings have been noted in other studies with non-transplanted renal failure patients, but not in the transplant population (10, 19). There were no episodes of coagulopathy, no unusual or excessive clotting factor or platelet requirement, and no difficulties reversing heparinization at the conclusion of the procedure in these patients. Additionally, coagulation studies were considered within the normal range perioperatively. Dunton and colleagues (8) found a similar lack of clotting aberrations and normal clotting parameters in their group of three liver transplant patients with no significant bleeding sequelae. The high mediastinal hematoma rate may be due to friable tissue from chronic steroid use, and post cardiotomy platelet dysfunction, particularly in the patients with chronic renal failure. At re-operation, no patient had an identifiable surgical cause for the bleeding. The liberal use of fresh frozen plasma and platelets may circumvent the risk of this complication. The incidence of other major complications was not considered excessive. There was one GI complication in a kidney transplant patient consisting of a perforated viscus requiring exploratory laparotomy and a bowel resection a few days following an AVR. This patient tolerated both procedures with no difficulties. Interestingly, all four patients requiring re-intubation for the management of pulmonary insufficiency were liver transplant patients, whereas all four patients with pleural effusions were renal transplant recipients. The serum albumin levels recorded for three of the 4 liver and two of the 4 kidney transplant patients preoperatively were in the normal range.

Outcome measures that were additionally evaluated in this study included the CPB and cross-clamp times, as one measure of technical complexity, and length of stay, as a measure of the overall physiologic reserve of these patients to compensate for the considerable stress of major operations. The mean cross clamp and bypass times of 92 and 141 min, respectively, were considered acceptable. The thoracic organ transplant group, not unexpectedly, had longer times. The ICU length of stay averaged 5.6 days and was longer than our non-transplant patients, as was the average 16 day total length of stay. The kidney transplant recipients fared worse than the two other subgroups, in both ICU and total length of stay (Fig. 3).

A mean follow-up of two years revealed no patient with recurrent cardiac disease, and all were in NYHA Class I or II. Our excellent long term results are contrary to those found by Shafei and colleagues (17) who found five of their seven patients developed recurrent angina 1 month to 1 year following cardiac surgery with three, of five having myocardial infarctions. Similar outcomes were reported by Beauchamp (1), who found two of three patients with recurrent angina at one year follow-up. Bolman et al. (2) in their series observed similar results to ours. The discrepancy in the recurrence of late cardiac symptoms may be due to patient population differences and progression of cardiovascular disease, which emphasizes the importance of careful and complete follow-up (Fig. 4).

In summary, we have evaluated 64 solid organ transplant recipients with functioning allografts who subsequently underwent cardiac surgical procedures. The

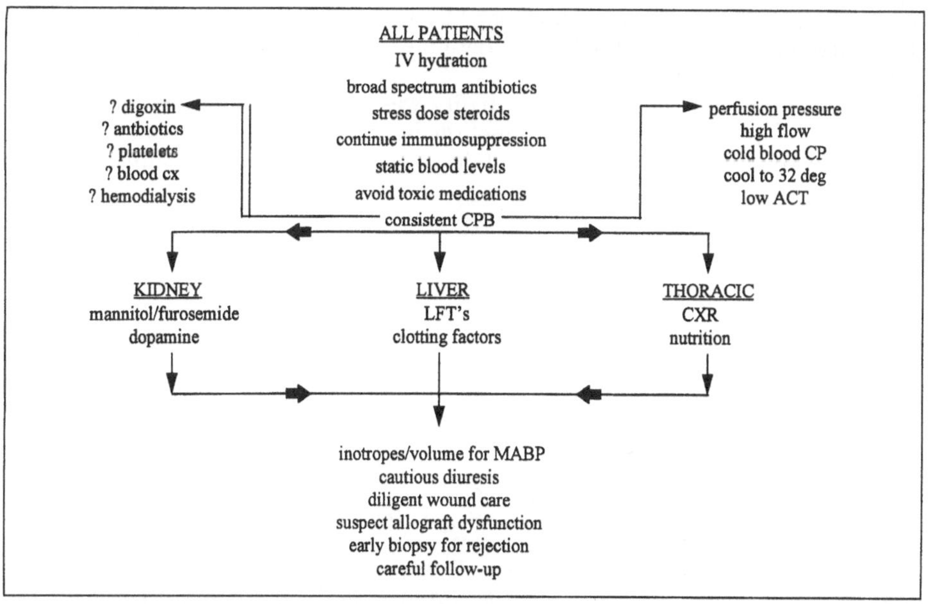

Fig. 4. Management algorithm

incidence of short term infectious and bleeding complications was significant and probably related to chronic immunosuppressive therapy and the presence of co-morbid medical conditions. However, the low incidence of permanent graft failure, rejection, renal impairment, and mortality was consistent with results obtained in the non-transplant cardiac surgery patient population. We propose that these patients be approach with caution and diligence but not undue apprehension.

Summary

Background: We report a single institution's ten year experience with the management techniques and outcomes of cardiac surgery in solid organ transplant recipients with functioning allografts.
Methods: Sixty four transplant recipients (40 kidney, 16 liver, 5 heart, 2 lung, and 1 liver/kidney) underwent 66 cardiac procedures that included: 30 CABG, 24 single or combined valve replacement/repair, 3 combined CABG/valve, 4 aortic repairs, 3 pericardiectomy, 1 transmyocardial laser revascularization, and 1 native cardiectomy. The mean interval from transplant to cardiac surgery was 53 months (range 1 day to 220 months) (range 19 to 77 years); 50% (32/64) were diabetic, and 97% (62/64) were hypertensive. The surgical and medical management was similar in all patients.
Results: There were 2 (3%) peri-operative deaths, one of which was an arrhythmia induced cardiac arrest, and 7 (11%) late deaths of non-cardiac causes. Sixteen of 64 (25%) transplant recipients had chronic renal failure (serum creatinine levels > 3 mg/dl), including 13 of 40 (33%) kidney tranplant patients. Seven (54%) of these 13 patients developed acute renal failure post-operatively, of which three (23%) grafts failed permanently. No liver or thoracic organ transplant recipient experienced graft failure. Three patients (5%), 2 kidney and 1 lung transplant recipient, experienced transient acute rejection. Major complications included 12 infections (19%), 10 mediastinal re-explorations for bleeding (16%), and 9 others (15%). Fifty of 55 surviving patients, at a mean follow-up of 22 months, are in NYHA Class I or II without recurrent cardiac disease.
Conclusion: Although short term morbidity was significant, the low incidence of mortality and permanent graft dysfunction indicates that solid organ transplant recipients can safely and effectively undergo subsequent cardiac surgical procedures.

References

1. Beauchamp GD, Sharma JN, Crouch T, et al. (1976) Coronary bypass surgery after renal transplantation. Am J Cardiol 37: 1107–1110
2. Bolman RM, Anderson RW, Molina JE, et al. (1984) Cardiac operations in patients with functioning renal allografts. J Thorac Cardiovasc Surg 88: 537–543
3. Chawla R, Gailiunas P, Lazarus JM, et al. (1977) Cardiopulmonary bypass surgery in chronic hemodialysis and transplant patients. Trans Am Soc Artif Intern Organs 23: 694–697
4. Copeland JG, Rosado LJ, Sethi G, Huston C, Lee RW (1991) Mitral valve replacement 6 years after cardiac transplantation. Ann Thorac Surg 51 (6): 1014–1016
5. Crawford FA, Selby JH, Bowers JD, et al. (1977) Coronary revascularization in patients maintained on chronic hemodialysis. Circulation 56: 684–687
6. David CA, Horowitz MD, Burke GW (1992) Aortic valve endocarditis in a liver transplant recipient – successful management by aortic valve replacement. Transplantation 1992; 53(6): 1366–1377

7. Dillow JR, Larrieu AJ, Fine RH (1995) Emergency coronary revascularization in a liver transplant recipient. Chest 108(6): 1763–1764
8. Dunton RF, Karlson KJ, Leonardi HK, Jenkins RL, Berger RL (1994) Coronary artery bypass grafting in patients with transplanted livers. Ann Thorac Surg 58: 1054–1058
9. Frazier OH, Vega JD, Duncan JM, et al. (1991) Coronary artery bypass two years after orthotopic heart transplantation : a case report. Jrnl Hrt Lung Transplant 10(6): 1036–1040
10. Lamberti JJ, Cohn LH, Collins JJ, et al. (1975) Cardiac surgery in patients undergoing renal dialysis or transplantation. Ann Thorac Surg 19: 135–141
11. Laws KH, Merrill WH, Hammon JW, Prager RL, Bender HW (1986) Cardiac surgery in patients with chronic renal disease. Ann Thorac Surg 42: 152–157
12. Lindner A, Charra B, Sherrard D, Scribner BH (1974) Accelerated atherogenesis in prolonged maintenance hemodialysis. N Engl J Med 290: 647–650
13. Menzoian JO, Davis RC, Idelson BA, Mannick JA, Berger RL (1974) Coronary artery bypass surgery and renal transplantation : a case report. Ann Surg 179: 63–66
14. Monson BK, Wickstrom PH, Haglin JJ, et al. (1980) Cardiac operation and end-stage renal disease. Ann Thorac surg 30: 267–272
15. Najarian JS, Sutherland DER, Simmons RL, et al. (1979) Ten year experience with renal transplantation in juvenile onset diabetes. Ann Surg 190: 487–500
16. Nakhjavan FK, Kahn D, Rosenbaum J, Ablaza S, Goldberg H (1975) Aortocoronary vein graft surgery in a cadaver kidney transplant recipient. Arch Intern Med 135: 1511–1513
17. Shafei H, Briggs JD, Bain WH (1989) Follow-up after coronary revascularization in patients with renal transplants. Eur Jrnl Cardiothoracic Surg 3: 262–266
18. STS Cardiac Surgery National Database : an update. Ann Thorac Surg 1995; 59(6): 1376–1381
19. Swift C, Steinmuller DR, Novick AC, et al. (1989) Open heart surgery in patients undergoing renal transplantation : Comparison of surgery pre- vs. post- transplant. Transplant Proc 21(1): 2137–2138
20. Votapka TV, Appleton RS, Pennington DG (1994) Tricuspid valve replacement after orthotopic heart transplantation. Ann Thorac Surg 57(3): 752–754

Author's address
Si M. Pham, MD
Assistant Professor of Surgery
Division of Cardiothoracic Surgery
University of Pittsburgh School of Medicine
Suite C-700 PUH
200 Lothrop Street
Pittsburgh, PA 15213, USA

Patients with severe concomitant disease and advanced coronary artery disease: The role of supporting devices

W. Konertz, L. Pietsch, H. Laube, H. Hotz, W. Rutsch[1], G. Baumann[1]

Dept. of Cardiac Surgery and Dept. of Cardiology[1], Charité, Humboldt-University Berlin, Germany

Introduction

Today cardiac surgery is performed in patients becoming older and sicker, in patients with previous often multiple cardiac interventions and/or operations, and in patients with disorders that may increase the risk of an open heart procedure. It has been known for a long time that extracorporeal circulation damages cellular components of the blood, impairs the coagulation system, and endorgan failure may occur in patients after an uneventful operation.

In 1983 Kirklin (8) described the damaging effect of complement activation by means of extracorporeal circulation and subsequent work in this field showed a whole array of disorders induced by the heart lung machine, most strikingly neurological and mental abnormalities occur.

Because of the well known damaging effects of cardiopulmonary bypass and cardioplegic arrest, methods were sought to minimize the risk of extracorporeal circulation or to avoid it at all. Supporting devices were developed to enhance beating heart surgery by technicals means, i.e., stabilizers or devices to improve exposure of remote coronary territories for off pump beating heart revascularization. On the other hand hemodynamic support other than open heart surgery with

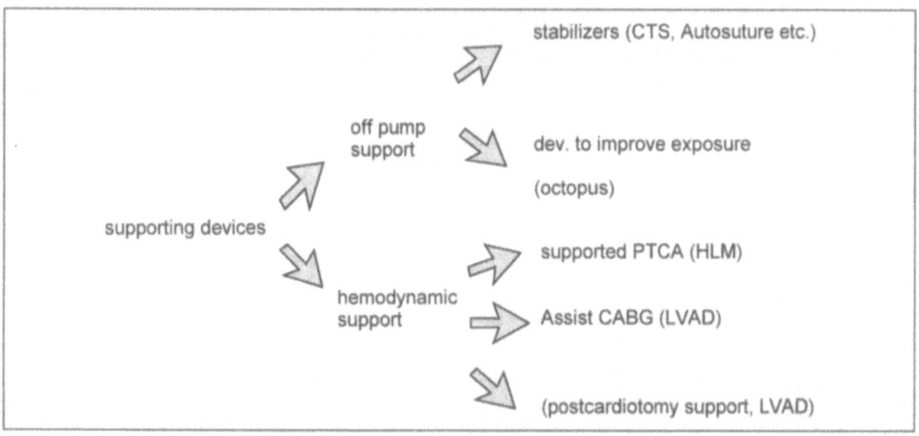

Fig. 1. The role of supporting devices in coronary patients with severe concomitant disease

cardiopulmonary bypass in the form of supported PTCA or revascularization under support with a pump emerged (Fig. 1). The purpose of this work is to summarize our experience with all of the above mentioned methods to improve treatment of severely sick patients.

Off pump coronary heart surgery

After pioneering work of Benetti (2) and Buffolo (6) with large series of patients operated upon for coronary heart disease without cardiopulmonary bypass, it become evident that revascularization of the heart can be performed effectively this way. Progress in this field brought up innovative stabilizing devices which made surgery on the anterior part of the heart possible with only a small anterior thoracotomy (7).

MIDCAB

Minimally Invasive Direct Coronary Bypass is performed on a increasing number of patients (3), and soon it became evident that the patients did very well after the procedure, could be extubated on the table, and leave the ICU environment sooner and stay in hospital shorter (1). The definition of minimally invasive cardiac surgery (MICS) became subject of dispute. For coronary procedures there exists unanimosity that avoidance of cardiopulmonary bypass is the main contributing factor for MICS, regardless of the operative access. Valvular procedures require extracorporeal circulation anyway, and in this group of patients MICS may be defined as limited access and/or endoscopic cardiac surgery (12).

MICS has been performed at our institution since February 1996 in a growing number of patients (Table 1). Coronary, calvular, and congenital MICS procedures make up 10–15% of today's total case load. Especially minimally invasive coronary

Table 1. Distribution of 412 MICS patients operated between February 1996 and September 1997: A/M/DVR: Aortic/mitral/double valve replacement/repair, ASD: atrial septal defect; VSD ventricular septal defect, BDG: bidirectional Glenn

Coronary	
MIDCAB	107
OCTOPUS	19
ASSIST-CABG	119
Valvular	
AVR	87
MVR	15
DVR	2
Congenital	
ASD	25
VSD	6
BDG	6
Miscellaneous	26

Table 2. Patient characteristics of MIDCAB patients. 1-2-3 VD: 1-2-2 vessel disease; LVEF: left ventricular ejection fraction; Redo: reoperative patient; (A)MI: (acute) myocardial infarction

Total	107
1 VD	64
2 VD	25
3 VD	30
LVEF < 35%	37
Redo	16
Re-redo	4
AMI	6
old MI	32

Table 3. Noncardiac comorbity in a cohort 107 MIDCAB patients. COLD: chronic obstructive lung disease; DM: diabetes mellitus; PVD: peripheral vascular disease

COLD	18
DM	4
pVD	17
renal failure	10
Malignancy	8

Table 4. Results of 107 Consecutive MIDCAB procedures. Redo: reoperative patient; Hybrid: MIDCAB plus PTCA; LVEF: Left ventricular ejection fraction

	n	deaths
Redo	20	1
Hybrid	32	0
LVEF < 35%	37	0
Other	18	1
Total	107	2

heart surgery expanded rapidly. What showed to be an advantage for otherwise healthy people suffering from one – vessel-disease involving the LAD only, might be also beneficial for patients with comorbidity that may be prohibitive to the application of cardiopulmonary bypass.

After establishment of the procedure MIDCAB was used in a group of severely ill patients with significant cardiac (Table 2) and noncardiac (Table 3) comorbidity. All patients received the LIMA to the LAD; one patient received an additional graft to the right coronary artery. Most of the patients with multivessel disease underwent a so-called hybrid procedure. Coronary intervention by means of PTCA and/or stenting preceeded the MIDCAB procedure in 6 patients and was performed after the operation in 26 patients. Results of the MIDCAB procedure are shown in Table 4. Two Patients died, making a total mortality of 1.8%. In the patients with increased operative and/or cardiac risk 1 of 80 patients died after his third revascularization procedure from multiorgan failure. No patient from the hybrid procedures died and in 37 patients with impaired LV function also no fatality occurred. In the patients with noncardiac comorbidity (n=56), a 79 years old patient died 12 days after the procedure from pneumonia and sepsis. From this experience it became obvious that MIDCAB may be a reliable and beneficial adjunct to cardiac surgery. Complications after the operation were rare and no neurologic, psychiatric or neurocognitive disorders occurred after the procedure.

Though MIDCAB is not applicable to all patients, involves a learning curve, and may be associated with incomplete revascularization as PTCA is, it is a valuable tool in the armamentarium for revascularization of the heart especially under conditions of increased operative risk with conventional surgery.

Octopus

Borst and Jansen from the University of Utrecht, the Netherlands, developed an innovative instrument that improves exposure and stabilization of remote coronary arteries for revascularization with the heart beating by means of a suction device called Octopus. So multivessel revascularization became feasible under conditions of beating heart surgery. Fig. 2 shows the exposure of the LAD with this device. Since July 1997, we performed revascularization in 19 patients with multivesel disease with the Octopus. Table 5 shows cardiac and noncardiac concomitant disease in these patients. All patients received the LIMA to the LAD, and 16 patients received 1 or 2 additional grafts either as saphenous vein grafts or the RIMA. No patient died, and in only two patients complications occurred. One obese patient with severe COLD required long-term ventilation and tracheostomy. Another patient required postoperatively PTCA and stenting of the RCA due to malinsertion

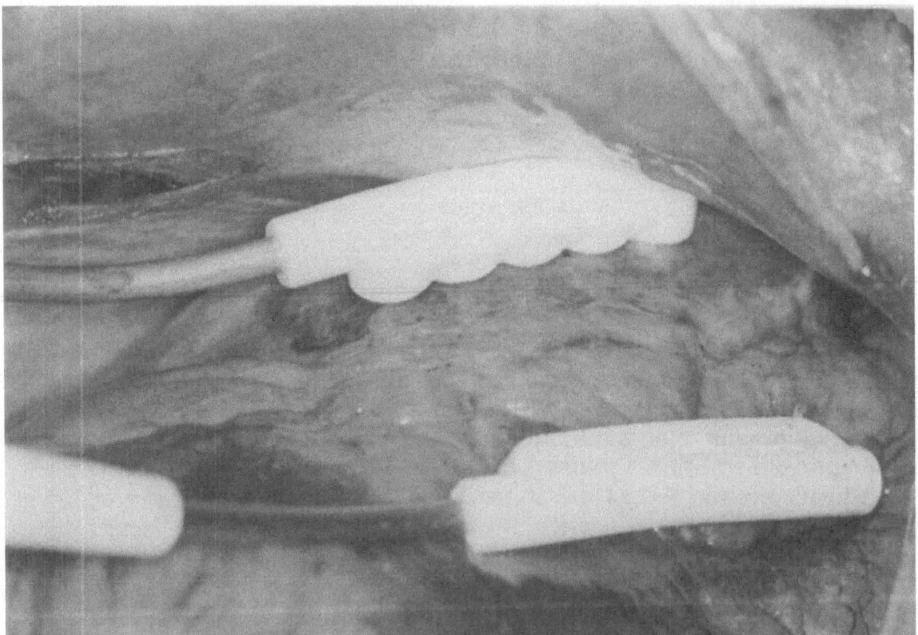

Fig. 2. Intraoperative exposure of the left anterior descending coronary artery with the Octopus® device

Table 5. Comorbidity in 19 patients operated on the beating heart with aid of Octopus®. LVEF: left ventricular ejection fraction; COLD: chronic obstructive lung disease; PVD: peripheral vascular disease; DM: diabetes mellits

LVEF < 35%	3
COLD	4
PVD	4
DM	5
porcellaine aorta	1

of the RCA bypass, which was anastomosed only to a posterolateral branch of the RCA. The Octopus seems to become a valuable adjunct for revascularization of patients with multivessel disease. The technical and methodological limits are expanded cautiously with ongoing experience.

Revascularization under Circulatory support

Circulatory support is thought to stabilize a patient in hemodynamic compromize or to prevent deterioration of cardiac performance during complex and risky revascularization procedures through either PTCA or CABG.

Supported PCA

PTCA always implies temporary blockade of flow in the target vessel. The increasing ability of cardiologists to do intervention also in complex anatomy and multivessel disease led to the concept of high-risk PTCA, under support of the IABP. To go even one step further supported PTCA either by intercardiac axial flow pump (9) or by means of femoro – femoral bypass with a heart lung machine (4) became feasible. From Aug. 1, 1994 to Aug. 31, 1997 28 patients 44 to 76 years old (mean 62.5 years) were treated with this modality. The indications for the procedure were either prohibitive surgical risk due to recent MI, multiple previous cardiac operations in combination with poor left ventricular function and vessels suitable for PTCA (Personett score > 20). From the cardiologist's standpoint the target vessels should support more than 50% of the viable myocardium.

For the procedure both groins are draped and in the only lightly sedated patient the left femoral vessels are exposed and cannulated under local anaesthesia. The patient is connected to the heart lung machine and arterial access for the cardiologist is gained at the contralateral femoral artery. The extracorporeal circulation is started in the nonintubated, awake patient and coronary intervention proceeded.

60 vessels, 2.5 per patient were treated. Table 6 shows the distribution of these vessels and the main interventional technique used to receive patency of the target vessel. The primary success rate was 88%. Fig. 3 a–c shows treatment of a severe, left main stenosis by means of the Rotablator. In this series 2 early deaths occurred due to myocardial infarction in one and cardiac failure in another patient. 30 day mortality is 6.5%, which is considerably less than for patients with such high Parsonett scores undergoing conventional surgery. Late mortality occurred in two

Table 6. Vessel treated and interventional technique used in 28 patients undergoing supported PTCA: LM: left main; LAD: left anterior descending; $D_{1/2}$: first/second diagonal branch; RCA: right coronary artery; RCX: circumflex coronary artery; $M_{1/2}$: obtuse marginal branch; SVG: saphenous vein graft; PTCA: percutaneous translumina coronary angioplasty; DCA: directional coronary atherectomy

LM:	5	RCX:	13
LAD:	18	M1/M2:	6
D1/D2:	4	SVG:	2
RCA:	12		
PTCA:	44	Rotablator:	1
DCA:	9	Stents:	6

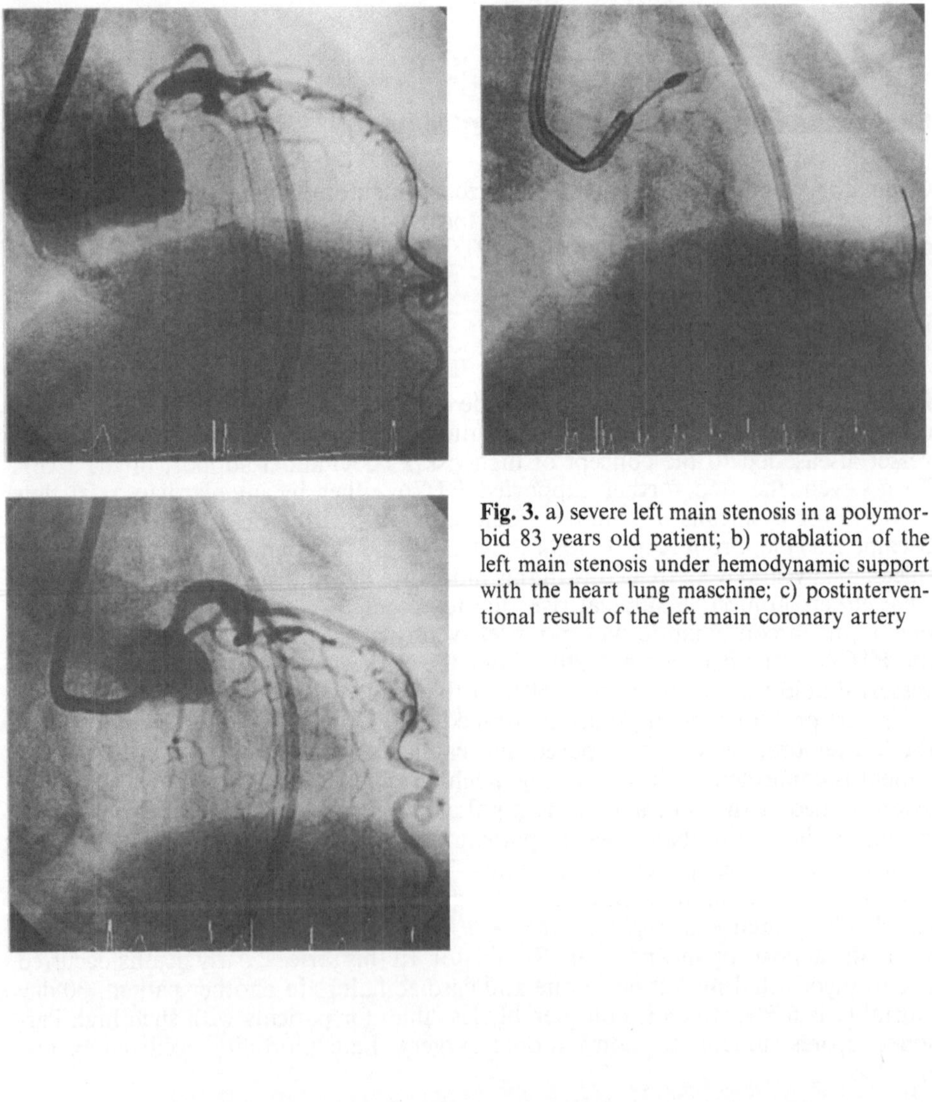

Fig. 3. a) severe left main stenosis in a polymorbid 83 years old patient; b) rotablation of the left main stenosis under hemodynamic support with the heart lung maschine; c) postinterventional result of the left main coronary artery

other patients 3 and 27 months after the procedure. One fatality occurred due to stroke and the late course of death in the other patient is unknown. Cardiac and local groin complications were rare and periprocedural transfusion requirements low. One unit of packed red cells was used in 1 patient, two units in 3, and three units in another patient. During follow up, 3 reinterventions, 1 of them again with support of cardiopulmonary bypass became necessary. One patient received uneventful CABG three months after his supported PTCA. In this patient LVEF had improved markedly during the interval, thus, making surgery successful. The heart lung machine supported coronary intervention has been shown to be feasible with a low procedural risk, enhanced patient survival and is considered useful in a select subgroup of coronary patients.

Assist-CABG

1992 Sweeney and Frazier published a landmark paper on revascularization on the beating heart and circulatory support with one or two centrifugal pumps (13). The technique was taken over by Lönn; instead of centrifugal pumps this group used axial flow pumps (10). The advantage of this approach lies as with all sort of beating heart surgery in the avoidance of cardioplegic arrest and excess hemodilution, and continuous perfusion and ventilation of the lung.

From Oct. 1, 1994 to Aug. 31, 1997, 119 patients underwent coronary artery bypass grafting under circulatory support with the centrifugal pump. Patients suffered from substantial cardiac impairment and comorbidity (Table 7). Patients included in this study had to have an increased risk for standard cardiopulmonary bypass and a favorable coronary anatomy. Technical details of the operation are described elsewhere (14). The operation is performed with cannulation of the aorta and the left atrium. Access to the left atrium is gained through the right superior pulmonary vein or through the atrial dome. After establishing circulatory support the heart is slowed with generous amounts (8–10 μg/kg) of the short acting β-blocker Esmolol (Breviblock). After completion of all anastomoses, the patient is weaned from assist and the chest closed as usual. Should hemodynamic instability occur at the termination of perfusion, the assist is left in place, the chest closed with a Goretex-Membrane, and the patient transferred to the ICU for prolonged support and gradual weaning. This was the case in 5 patients in this series, all of

Table 7. Cardiac and noncardiac comorbidity in a cohort of 105 patients udnergoing LVAD-assisted coronary artery bypass surgery. AMI: acute myocardial infarction; LVEF: left ventricular ejection fraciton; Redo: reoperative patients, COLD: chronic obstructive lung disease; PVD peripheral vascular disease; CLD: cerebrovascular disease; DVM: diabetes mellitus

ASSIST-CABG

AMI	17	PVD	19
LVEF < 35%	25	CVD	10
Redo	8	DM	24
COLD	23	Malignancy	3
renal failure	14		

them had fresh myocardial infarction and were brought to the OR hemodynamically compromised or under cardiopulmonary resucitation.

A single graft, most often LIMA to LAD was performed in 57 patients; 38 patients received double and 4 triple grafting. Coronary reconstruction became necessary in 5 patients, in whom an endarterectomy of the LAD with patch angioplasty and LIMA insertion became necessary, a technique, which has been described earlier by Johnson (5) and Reul (11). An average of 1.4 distal anastomes was performed in all coronary territories. Revascularization of the second marginal branch and the distal circumflex artery, however, proved to be difficult and was later in the study no longer considered. 5 patients died, three of them in the group of 15 patients with fresh or ongoing myocardial infarction who had brought to the OR in extremis. No patient out of the group of 25 patients with poor left ventricular function (LVEF < 35%) died and two from the remaining patients died due to noncardiac comorbidity and complications. No perioperative infarction could be detected by means of ECG (new Q waves) and biochemistry (CKMB). Complications in survivors were rare. Four patients required temporary dialysis postoperatively; other complications were ileus or gastrointestinal hemorrhage in 3 patients and prolonged respiratory treatment in four. No neurologic complications could be found, and in no patient laboratory evidence of inflammatory response to extracorporeal circulation could be detected.

Through the recent advent of stabilizing devices as the Octopus device, this technique faded in our routine use; however there seem to be still indications in certain subsets of patients as in patients with hemodynamic compromise, patients requiring extensive coronary reconstruction, and patients who tolerate coronary occlusion only poorly.

Conclusions

From this experience we conclude that innovative devices deliver intraoperative technical and circulatory support and these devices bear a high potential for making surgery for sick patients easier and saver. A dedicated team approach covering the whole spectrum of interventional cardiology and cardiac surgery is necessary.

References

1. Arom KV, Emery RW, Nocoloff DM, Flavin TF, Emery A (1997) Minimally invasive direct coronary artery bypass grafting: experimental and clinical experiences. Ann Thorac Surg 63 (Suppl): 48–52
2. Benneti FJ, Noselli G, Wood M, Geffner L (1991) Direct myocardial revascularization without extracorporeal circulation: experience in 700 patients. Chest 100: 312–316
3. Benetti F, Mariani MA, Sani G, Boonstra PW, Grandjean JG, Giomarelly P, Toscano M (1996) Video-assisted minimally invasive coronary operations without cardiopulmonary bypass: A multicenter study. J Thorac Cardiovasc Surg 112: 1478–1484
4. Borges AC, Waldenberger FR, Wolf C, Reindl I, Habedank D, Haisjackl M, Kox WJ, Konertz W, Baumann G, Kleber FX (1996) Die perkutane „Hochrisiko"-Angioplastie unter prophylaktischen kardiopulmonalen Support. Z Kardial 85: Suppl 4: 21–28
5. Brenowitz JB, Kayer KL, Johnson WD (1988) Triple vessel coronary artery endarterectomy and reconstruction: Results in 144 patients. J Am Coll Cardiol 11: 706–711

6. Buffolo E, Antrade JCS, Branco JNR, Aguiar LF, Ribeiro EE, Jatene AD (1990) Myocardial revascularization without extracorporeal circulation: 7 years experience in 593 cases. Eur J Cardiothorac Surg 4: 504–508
7. Calafiore A, Angelin GD, Bergsland JB, Salerno TA (1996) Minimally invasive coronary artery bypass grafting. Ann Thorac Surg 62: 1545–1548
8. Kirklin JK, Westaby S, Blackstone EH, Kirklin JW, Chenowith DE, Pacifico AD (1983) Complement and the damaging effects of cardiopulmonary bypass. J Thorac Cardiovasc Surg 86: 845–852
9. Loisance D, Dubois-Rande JI, Deleuz Ph, Okude J, Rosenval O, Geschwind H (1990) Prophylactic intraventricular pumping in high risk coronary angioplasty. Lancet 335: 438–440
10. Lönn U, Peterzen B, Granfeld H, Casimir-Ahn H (1994) Coronary artery operation with support of the Hemopump cardiac assist system. Ann Thorac Surg 58: 519–523
11. Reul G (1985) Present status of the internal mammary artery as a coronary artery bypass conduit of the Texas Heart Institute. Texas Heart Inst Gown 12: 211–219
12. Schwartz DS, Ribakove GH, Grossi EA, Stevens JH, Siegel LC, St Goar FG, Peters WS, McLoughlin D, Baumann FG, Colvin SB, Galloway AC (1996) Minimally invasive cardiopulmonary bypass with cardioplegic arrest: A closed chest technique with equivalent myocardial protection. J Thorac Cardiovasc Surg 111: 556–566
13. Sweeney MS, Frazier OA (1992) Device supported myocardial revascularisation: Safe help for sick hearts. Ann Thorac Surg 54: 1065–1070
14. Waldenberger FR, Hotz H, Haisjackl M, Konertz W (1996) Chirurgische Koronarrevaskularisation am schlagenden Herzen. Z Kardiol 85: Suppl 4: 35–41

Author's address:
Prof. Dr. W. Konertz
Dept. Cardiac Surgery
Charité
Schumannstraße 20/21
10098 Berlin
Germany

Cardiac Echinococcosis – Acute cardiac tamponade and emergency excision under cardiopulmonary bypass

G. Rupp, C. Vicol, E. Struck

Herzchirurgische Klinik, Zentralklinikum Augsburg, Germany

Introduction

Primary echinococcosis of the heart is a very rare event (0.2–2% of all cases of human hydatosis). Echinococcosis prevails in regions with extensive cattle or sheep raising, e.g., Northern Africa or the Near East region. Diagnosis is often difficult because of long latency between infection and manifestation. In only 8% of reported cases the right vetricular myocardium is involved.

Clinic

The 56 year old male patient, a Turkish resident, is admitted because of sharp thoracic pain of sudden onset rediating to the back between the shoulders. Auscultatory findings were a 2/6 systolic bruit over the aorta, the lungs were clear. Blood pressure, pulse, and temperature were in the normal range. Electrocardiographically there were no signs of myocardial infarction; the myocardial enzymes were not elevated. Aortic dissection was ruled out by echocardiography. Magnetic resonance imaging and echocardiography showed a round-shaped cyst at the anterior-inferior right-ventricular myocardial wall. Blood eosinophilic rate was 6.4%, the echinococcus antibody titer 1 : 6.400. Cardiac catheterization was done and elective surgical removal of the cyst was planned. An oral anthelminthic therapy with Albendazol (R) was started. Sudden signs of acute pericardial tamponade necessitated emergency surgery for cardiac relief and cyst removal.

Operation

After median sternotomy and pericardial incision 500 ml of serous pericardial fluid were collected. The cyst of about 7 cm in diameter and of elastic consistency showed intact and partially buried in the right anterior-inferior ventricular wall. The cyst contents were sterilized by 10% formalin solution in a closed circuit system with simultaneous infusion of the formalin and removal of the cyst contents. Contact of formalin with mediastinal structures was strictly avoided. The cyst was removed in part during cardiopulmonary bypass with the heart beating. Remnants of the cyst were "marsupialized" to control bleeding.

Outcome

The clinical course was uneventful. Follow-up after three months showed no cyst recurrence or new cyst formation in other organs. The patient was well and orally administered anthelminthic therapy was continued.

Conclusion

Surgical removal of hydatid cysts of the myocardium is the sole therapeutic approach because of the possibly lethal complications of this infectious disease. Cardiopulmonary bypass with the heart beating or under cardioplegic arrest depending on the localization of the cyst is the method of choice. Concomittant anthelminthic therapy is mandatory as well as regular follow-up to rule out new cyst formation.

Author's address:
Gerald Rupp, M.D.
Herzchirurgische Klinik am Zentralklinikum Augsburg
Stenglinstr. 5
86156 Augsburg, Germany

Effects of coronary bypass grafting on the prevalence of ventricular late potentials

C. Hanefeld, K. Weber, J. Böckenforde, C. Israel, D. Ricken

Department of Cardiology, Ruhr-Universität Bochum, St. Josef-Hospital, Bochum, Germany

Introduction

Ventricular late potentials (LP) in the signal-averaged electrocardiogram represent the electrophysiological substrate of morphological changes in the myocardial tissue that may constitute a reentry tachycardia. They indicate electrophysiological vulnerability of the myocard and may the prognostic value to identify patients with a high risk for ventricular tachycardia.

The purpose of this study was to evaluate the influence of revascularization on the prevalence of late potentials. It may be suggested that coronary revascularization reduces ischemia and, thus, may alter the conditions for reentry. On the other hand, if surviving fibers rather than ischemia within scarred tissue represent the anatomic basis for reentry, coronary artery bypass grafting will not change the prevalence of LP.

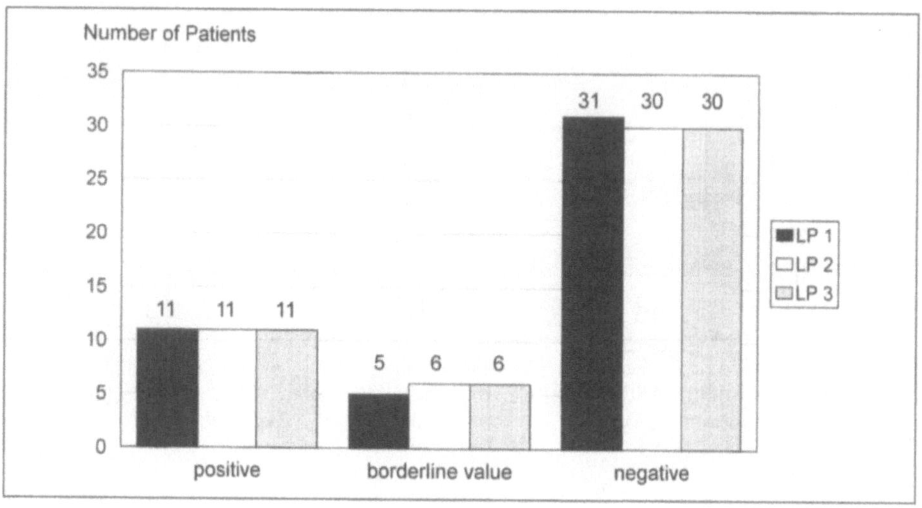

Fig. 1. Late potentials of the study cohort at baseline (LPI) an all follow-up visits (LP2, LP3)

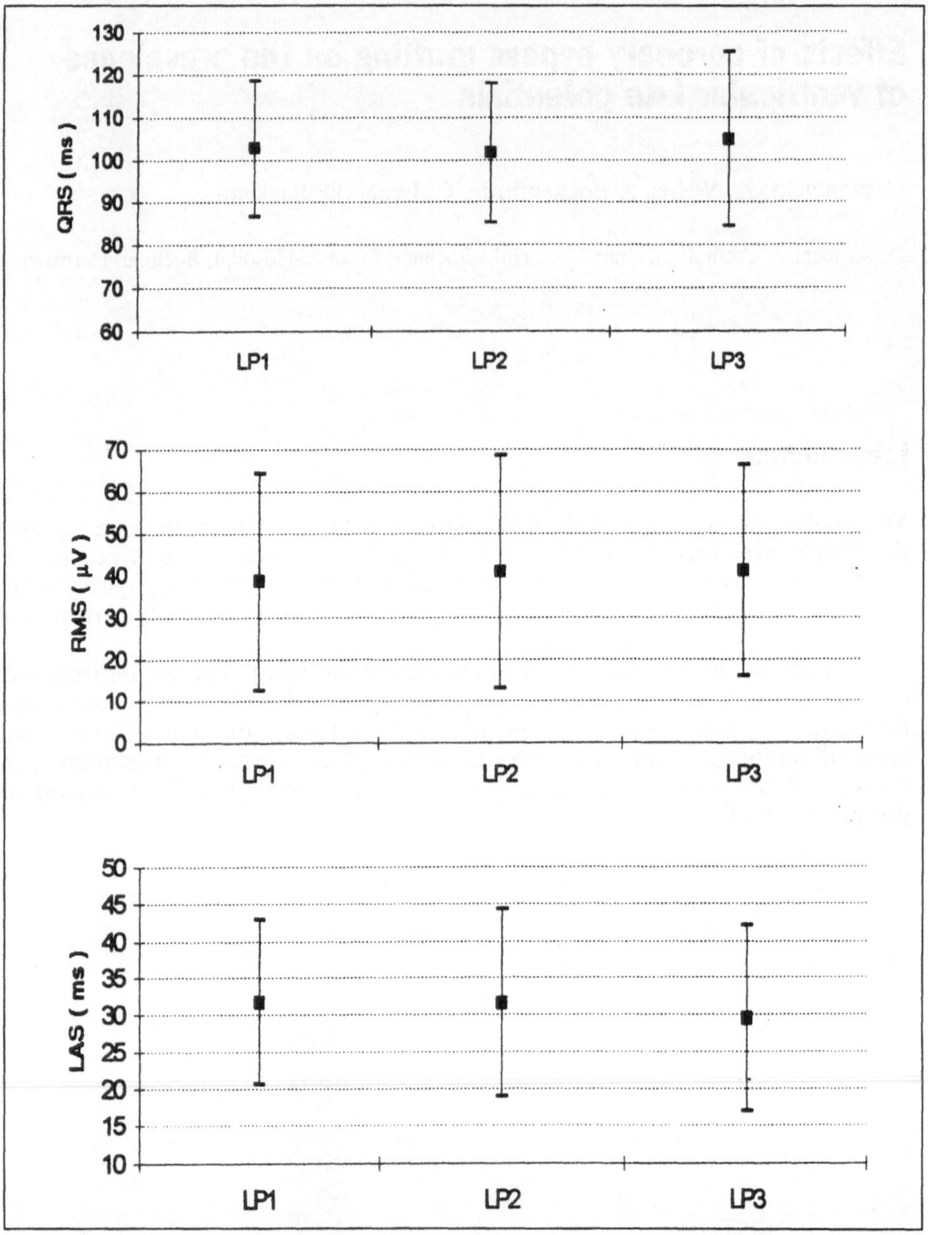

Fig. 2. QRS, RMS and LAS in the whole study group at baseline (LP1) and all follow-up visits (LP2, LP3)

Patients and methods

In a prospective study we evaluated the prevalence of ventricular late potentials using electrocardiographic signal averaging in 53 patients (female = 7, male = 46; mean age 60.8 years), who underwent coronary bypass surgery. Three measurements were performed on an average of 84 days before (LP1) as well as 15 days (LP2) and 100 days (LP3) after surgery.

The signal-averaged electrocardiogram was recorded with a Fidelity Medical 3000 recorder, using the method of Simson for time domain analysis. The signals of the three surface ECG leads were amplified (200 heart beats), averaged, and filtered with cutoff-frequencies at 40 to 250 Hz.

Late potentials were defined by the presence of two of the three following parameters:

- QRS: total duration of the filtered QRS > 115 mS
- RMS: amplitude of signals in the last 40 mS of the QRS < 25 μV
- LAS: duration of the terminal high-frequency, low amplitude signals of less than 40 μV > 38 mS

Results

There was no change in late potentials neither in the whole study cohort nor in specific subgroups (preoperative infarct, no infarct preoperatively, ejection fraction below or above 40 %).

Using the arithmetical means the separate comparison of the three measured parameters (QRS, RMS, LAS) exhibited no significant differences in LP1, LP2 and LP3.

Conclusions

The results indicate that the underlying mechanisms of late potentials are not affected by revascularization following coronary bypass surgery. Thus, myocardial ischemia may not be a significant contributor to changes in late potentials but it might rather be affected by irreversible changes in myocardial anatomy. The reversal of arrhythmic events following coronary bypass surgery is potentially induced by the protective effect of reduced myocardial ischemia while late potentials remain unchanged.

References

1. Borbola J, Serry C, Goldin et al. (1988) Short-term effect of coronary artery bypass grafting on the signal averaged electrocardiogram. Am J Cardiol 61: 1001–1005
2. Breithardt G, Cain ME, El-Sherif et al. (1991) Standards for analysis of ventricular late potentials using high resolution or signal-averaged electrocardiography. Eur Heart J 12: 473–480

3. Every NR, Fahrenbruch CE, Hallstrom AP et al. (1992) Influence of coronary artery bypass surgery on subsequent outcome of patients resuscitated from out of hospital cardiac arrest. J Am Coll Cardiol 19: 1435–1439
4. El-Sherif N (1993) Electrophysiologic basis of ventricular late potentials. Prog in Cardiovasc Dis 6: 417–427
5. Hammermeister KE, De Rouen TA, Murrey JA et al. (1977) Effect of aortocoronary saphenous vein bypass grafting on death and sudden death. Am J Cardiol 39: 925–934
6. Holmes DR, Davis K, Gersh BJ et al. (1989) Risk factor profiles of patients with sudden cardiac death from other cardiac causes: a report from the coronary artery surgery study (CASS). J Am Coll Cardiol 13: 524–530
7. Simson, MB (1981) Use of signals in the terminal QRS complex to identify patients with ventricular tachycardia after myocardial infarction. Circulation 64: 235–242
8. Weber K, Bergbauer M (1991) Nicht-invasive Registrierung von Spätpotentialen zur Feststellung einer erhöhten ventrikulären Vulnerabilität. DMW 116: 665–669

Author's address:
C. Hanefeld, MD
Department of Cardiology
St. Josef-Hospital
Ruhr-Universität Bochum
Gudrunstr. 56
44791 Bochum